Single Best Answers in
SURGERY

Second edition

Single Best
Answers in

SURGERY

Second edition

Darren K Patten BSc(Hons) MBBS MRCS(Eng) Wellcome Trust Clinical Research
Fellow and Specialist Trainee in General Surgery (London Deanery), Department of
Surgery and Cancer, The Imperial Centre for Translational and Experimental Medicine,
Imperial College, London, UK

David M Layfield BSc(Hons) MBBS MRCS(Eng) CRUK Clinical Research Fellow
and Specialist Trainee in General Surgery (Yorkshire and Humber Deanery),
University of Southampton, UK

Shobhit Arya BSc(Hons) MBBS MRCS(Eng) Clinical Research Fellow, Department
of Biosurgery and Surgical technology, QEQM , St Mary's Hospital, Imperial College,
London, UK

Daniel R Leff MBBS PhD FRCS(Gen Surg) Clinical Lecturer in Surgery, Hamlyn
Centre for Robotic Surgery, Imperial College, London, UK

Paraskeva A Paraskevas MBBS(Hons) PhD FRCS(Gen Surg) Reader in Surgery and
Consultant Colorectal Surgeon, St Mary's Hospital, Imperial College Healthcare NHS
Trust, London, UK

Editorial Advisor
Professor the Lord Darzi of Denham KBE HonFREng FMedSci Professor of Surgery
and Head of Department, Paul Hamlyn Chair of Surgery, Department of Biosurgery
and Surgical Technology, Division of Surgery, Oncology, Reproductive Biology and
Anaesthetics, Faculty of Medicine, Imperial College, London, UK

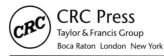

CRC Press
Taylor & Francis Group
Boca Raton London New York

CRC Press is an imprint of the
Taylor & Francis Group, an **informa** business

CRC Press
Taylor & Francis Group
6000 Broken Sound Parkway NW, Suite 300
Boca Raton, FL 33487-2742

© 2015 by Taylor & Francis Group, LLC
CRC Press is an imprint of Taylor & Francis Group, an Informa business

No claim to original U.S. Government works

Printed on acid-free paper
Version Date: 20140911

International Standard Book Number-13: 978-1-4441-7597-4 (Paperback)

This book contains information obtained from authentic and highly regarded sources. While all reasonable efforts have been made to publish reliable data and information, neither the author[s] nor the publisher can accept any legal responsibility or liability for any errors or omissions that may be made. The publishers wish to make clear that any views or opinions expressed in this book by individual editors, authors or contributors are personal to them and do not necessarily reflect the views/opinions of the publishers. The information or guidance contained in this book is intended for use by medical, scientific or health-care professionals and is provided strictly as a supplement to the medical or other professional's own judgement, their knowledge of the patient's medical history, relevant manufacturer's instructions and the appropriate best practice guidelines. Because of the rapid advances in medical science, any information or advice on dosages, procedures or diagnoses should be independently verified. The reader is strongly urged to consult the relevant national drug formulary and the drug companies' printed instructions, and their websites, before administering any of the drugs recommended in this book. This book does not indicate whether a particular treatment is appropriate or suitable for a particular individual. Ultimately it is the sole responsibility of the medical professional to make his or her own professional judgements, so as to advise and treat patients appropriately. The authors and publishers have also attempted to trace the copyright holders of all material reproduced in this publication and apologize to copyright holders if permission to publish in this form has not been obtained. If any copyright material has not been acknowledged please write and let us know so we may rectify in any future reprint.

Visit the Taylor & Francis Web site at
http://www.taylorandfrancis.com

and the CRC Press Web site at
http://www.crcpress.com

To my Mother, Father (June 1948–February 1994) and
Brother for their everlasting support.

Darren K Patten

Contents

Contributors   ix
Foreword   xi
Preface   xiii
Acknowledgements   xv
How to approach an SBA exam   xvii
Abbreviations   xix
Common reference intervals   xxi

SECTION 1: APPLIED ANATOMY 25   1
Questions   2
Answers   9

SECTION 2: PRE- AND POSTOPERATIVE MANAGEMENT 25   19
Questions   20
Answers   29

SECTION 3: FLUID BALANCE AND NUTRITION 20   39
Questions   40
Answers   47

SECTION 4: ANAESTHETICS AND SURGICAL CRITICAL CARE 25 55
Questions   56
Answers   64

SECTION 5: TRAUMA 30   75
Questions   77
Answers   86

**SECTION 6: ABDOMEN: UPPER GASTROINTESTINAL AND
HEPATOBILIARY SURGERY** 35   101
Questions   103
Answers   112

SECTION 7: ABDOMEN: LOWER GASTROINTESTINAL SURGERY   131
Questions   30   133
Answers   141

SECTION 8: ABDOMEN: THE ACUTE ABDOMEN 30   157
Questions   159
Answers   168

SECTION 9: BREAST SURGERY AND ENDOCRINE DISEASE 25   183
Questions   184
Answers   192

SECTION 10: VASCULAR SURGERY 25   203
Questions   204
Answers   212

SECTION 11: UROLOGY 30   227
Questions   229
Answers   238

SECTION 12: ORTHOPAEDICS 30   257
Questions   259
Answers   267

SECTION 13: NEUROSURGERY 20   281
Questions   282
Answers   289

SECTION 14: ENT SURGERY 20   303
Questions   304
Answers   311

SECTION 15: OPHTHALMIC SURGERY 20   317
Questions   318
Answers   325

SECTION 16: LUMPS, BUMPS, SKIN AND HERNIAS 20   333
Questions   334
Answers   340

SECTION 17: PRACTICE EXAM 100   351
Questions   354
Answers   384

Index   290   510   431

Contributors

Authors

Mr Darren K Patten BSc(Hons) MBBS MRCS(Eng), Wellcome Trust Clinical Research Fellow and Specialist Trainee in General Surgery (London Deanery), Department of Surgery and Cancer, The Imperial Centre for Translational and Experimental Medicine, Imperial College London, UK

Mr David M Layfield BSc(Hons) MBBS MRCS(Eng), CRUK Clinical Research Fellow and Specialist Trainee in General Surgery (Yorkshire and Humber Deanery), University of Southampton, UK

Mr Shobit Arya BSc(Hons) MBBS MRCS(Eng), Clinical Research Fellow, Department of Biosurgery and Surgical Technology, QEQM, St Mary's Hospital, Imperial College, London, UK

Mr Daniel R Leff MBBS PhD FRCS(Gen Surg), Clinical Lecturer in Surgery, Hamlyn Centre for Robotic Surgery, Imperial College, London, UK

Mr Paraskevas A Paraskeva MBBS(Hons) PhD FRCS(Gen Surg), Reader in Surgery and Consultant Colorectal Surgeon, St Mary's Hospital, Imperial College Healthcare NHS Trust, London, UK

Editorial Advisor

Professor the Lord Darzi of Denham KBE HonFREng FMedSci, Professor of Surgery and Head of Department, Paul Hamlyn Chair of Surgery, Department of Biosurgery and Surgical Technology, Division of Surgery, Oncology, Reproductive Biology and Anaesthetics, Faculty of Medicine, Imperial College, London, UK

Foreword

Preparation and practice are vital for undergraduate clinical trainees as they journey the long series of examinations and assessments towards qualification as a junior doctor. With a significant proportion of testing now conducted in the *single best answer* format, it is vital for students to have access to high-quality practice questions to aid learning and feedback to improve their clinical acumen and decision-making. The second edition of *Single Best Answers in Surgery* contains a revised question bank and the addition of two new chapters: 'Applied Anatomy' and 'Surgical Critical Care'. With a mix of both junior and senior authors, it strives to address the modern needs of medical students while at the same time providing expertly described examples and advice. *Single Best Answers in Surgery, Second Edition* provides a much-needed framework to facilitate surgical education and will undoubtedly prepare students for optimised exam performance.

Professor the Lord Ara Darzi of Denham
PC KBE HonFREng FMedSci FRS

Preface

The single best answer (SBA) question format is gradually being implemented across a vast number of medical schools in the UK, for the written component of the undergraduate medicine and surgery curricula. Single best answers have been shown to be a better modality, not only for testing knowledge but also for testing judgment in clinical practice.

The second edition of *Single Best Answers in Surgery* contains 510 SBAs and includes a 100-question practice exam and the addition of two new chapters ('Applied Anatomy' and 'Surgical Critical Care'). In addition, the question bank has undergone revision to accommodate changes in clinical practice.

The questions are arranged in a topic by topic format, and test core and advanced knowledge across the undergraduate surgical curriculum and also cater to final-year medical students sitting the written papers in surgery. Detailed explanations for each question are provided at the end of each topic section, describing how the correct answer is reached over the other possible options to the question.

Not only will this book act as a question bank, it will also act as a useful revision aid, providing the reader with the fundamental knowledge to sit the undergraduate surgical written exam with confidence!

Darren K Patten
David M Layfield
Shobhit Arya
Daniel R Leff
Paraskevas A Paraskeva

Acknowledgements

We would like to express our gratitude to the following for contributing their invaluable advice and expertise during the review stages of this book:

Miss Stella Vig BSc(Hons) MB BCh MCh FRCS(Eng) FRCS(Ed) FRCS(Gen Surg)
Consultant Vascular and General Surgeon
Croydon University Hospital
Croydon Health Services NHS Trust
Croydon, UK

Mr Dimitri J Hadjiminas MD MPhil FRCS(Ed) FRCS(Eng)
Consultant Breast and Endocrine Surgeon
Imperial College NHS Health Care Trust
Charing Cross and St Mary's Hospitals
London, UK

Mr Kasim A Behranwala MS DNB FRCS(Glas) FRCS(Ed) FRCS(Gen Surg) EBSQ(Surg Oncol)
Consultant Oncoplastic Breast and Emergency General Surgery
North Middlesex University Hospital NHS Trust
London, UK

Dr Alex EJ Trevatt BSc MB ChB
Foundation Year One Doctor
Department of General Surgery
North Middlesex University Hospital NHS Trust
London, UK

Miss Upekha Karunarathna BSc(Hons) MRes PhD Student
Department of Surgery and Cancer
Imperial College School of Medicine
London, UK

We would also like to thank Dr Joanna Koster, Rachael Russell and the rest of the Taylor & Francis team for their invaluable support and advice during the writing and publication of the second edition of *Single Best Answers in Surgery*.

How to approach an SBA exam

The first step in perfecting your exam technique is to follow the format set by your medical school and practise answering many of these questions well in advance of the exam. For example, little benefit is drawn from using true/false questions as a revision tool when the exam format is based on a bank of single best answer (SBA) questions.

In the context of SBA questions, you will usually be awarded one mark for every question that is answered correctly. Some medical schools implement negative marking, where one mark is deducted per wrong answer. This makes guesswork highly unfavourable and may result in you obtaining significantly low marks. However, in the majority of UK medical schools there is no negative marking so you should aim to answer all of the questions.

The SBA question consists of an introductory theme, a question stem (which in most cases consists of a clinical vignette but may occasionally be a theory-based fact), followed by five possible responses (A–E), of which one of them is the most likely suited answer to the question.

How to answer SBAs

First, we recommend that you attempt to answer an SBA question in just under a minute. This can be hard at first but, through practice, it is achievable and will leave you with some spare time to re-check your responses or go over questions that you are unsure about.

A method of answering an SBA is to cover up (with a piece of paper or your hand) the five possible options and carefully read just the theme and stem. By doing this, you may be able to think of the answer which will usually be one of the five options given for that question. In some cases where questions tend to be less straightforward, the method of delineating the wrong options first is usually very helpful as this will leave you with fewer possible options and with a higher chance of opting for the correct answer.

Some students tend to lose marks by blindly answering SBAs and extended matching questions (EMQs) by using pattern recognition of the words used in the stems. In some cases this may prove to be successful, but distracters may be placed in the stem which may change the entire meaning of the question, which would in turn demand an alternative response to the one initially thought. The best way to avoid this is to read the question carefully and understand fully what the SBA question is asking of you. In an SBA, all of the options available may not be ideal, but you still have to select the best of those available.

SBA terminology

It is vitally important to understand the terminology used in questions; for example:

- **Always** means 100 per cent of the time and is unlikely to be true.
- **Never** is another absolute term and may often be wrong.
- **Occasionally** can make many options potentially viable as correct answers and confuse you.
- **Commonly** means more than 75 per cent or even more of the time.
- **Rarely** is equivalent to something which occurs less than 1 per cent of the time.
- **Associated with** means that there is a definable link between the theme and this option.
- **Pathognomonic** means that if this particular item is not present in the stem it would cause the diagnosis to be in doubt.

How are SBA examinations set?

In the past, questions were selected for examinations in a random manner by the academics setting the paper. In modern exams, the question paper should be representative of the curriculum that the medical school has provided for the student and hence examine knowledge within these limits. To aid this, many papers are now 'mapped' against the curriculum to ensure that most topics are represented, and that different areas of a topic are covered. When the composition of the paper is being decided the questions are selected to give a spread of difficulty. It is important that the exam tests core knowledge, but at the same time has enough challenging questions to spread and stratify to allow ranking. This therefore means some questions will deliberately be very easy and some will be almost impossible to allow the stratification process. Multiple-choice questions of all varieties are now graded for difficulty which helps to calculate the pass mark for the paper. One such system is the Ebel system where six or more separate assessors score each question on its relevance and difficulty, hence a less relevant or more fringe topic that is difficult will be given a low score, indicating that the examiners expect only a minor percentage of candidates to get this right. Conversely very relevant core knowledge will be given a high score as examiners expect most candidates to get this correct. From the average scores of all the questions from all the assessors the pass mark is calculated.

Reading the explanations to the SBAs in this book will not only reinforce your clinical and theoretical knowledge, but will also teach you an assertive exam technique for answering SBAs. By applying the recommended methodologies explained above, we hope that you will be able to use this book to its maximum potential and we wish you the very best of luck in your exams.

Darren K Patten and Paraskevas Paraskeva

Abbreviations

5-HT	5-hydroxytryptamine	CHRPE	congenital hypertrophy of retinal pigment epithelium
A&E	accident and emergency	CNS	central nervous system
AAA	abdominal aortic aneurysm	COPD	chronic obstructive pulmonary disease
ABG	arterial blood gas		
ABPI	ankle–brachial pressure index	CREST	calcinosis, Raynaud's, oesophageal and gut dysmotility, sclerodactyly, telangiectasia
ACE	angiotensin converting enzyme		
ACTH	adenocorticotrophin hormone	CRP	C-reactive protein
ADH	antidiuretic hormone	CSF	cerebrospinal fluid
ADP	adenosine diphosphate	CT	computed tomography
AF	atrial fibrillation	CVA	cerebrovascular accident
AFP	a-feta protein	CVP	central venous pressure
AIDS	acquired immune deficiency syndrome	DCIS	ductal carcinoma *in situ*
		DCSS	diffuse cutaneous systemic sclerosis
ALI	acute lung injury		
ANCA	anti neutrophil cytoplasmic antibody	DEXA	dual X-ray energy absorptiometry
APKD	adult polycystic kidney disease	DIPJ	distal interphalangeal joint
		DMSA	dimercaptosuccinic acid
APTT	activated partial thromboplastin time	DPL	diagnostic peritoneal lavage
		DRE	digital rectal examination
APUD	amine precursor uptake and decarboxylation	DSA	digital subtraction angiography
ARDS	acute respiratory distress syndrome	DTPA	diethylene triamine pentaacetic acid
ASIS	anterior superior iliac spine	DVT	deep vein thrombosis
AST	aspartate aminotransferase	ECG	electrocardiogram
ATLS	advanced trauma and life support	EEG	electroencephalogram
		ERCP	endoscopic retrograde cholangiopancreatography
ATP	adenosine triphosphate		
BCC	basal cell carcinoma	ESR	erythrocyte sedimentation rate
BCG	Bacillus Calmette–Guérin		
BMD	bone mineral density	ESWL	extracorporeal shock wave lithotripsy
BMI	body mass index		
BPH	benign prostatic hypertrophy	EVAR	endovascular aneurysm repair
BPPV	benign paroxysmal positional vertigo	FAST	focused assessment with sonography for trauma
CA	carbohydrate antigen	FBC	full blood count
CBD	common bile duct	FSH	follicle stimulating hormone
CCP	combined contraceptive pill		
CEA	carcinoembryonic antigen	GCS	Glasgow Coma Scale

GORD	gastro-oesophageal reflux disease	NSAID	non-steroidal anti-inflammatory drug
GTN	glyceryl trinitrate	NSGCT	non-seminomatous germ cell tumours
HCC	hepatocellular carcinoma		
hCG	human chorionic gonadotrophin	OGD	oesophageal gastroduodenoscopy
HDU	high-dependency unit	PBC	primary biliary cirrhosis
HIV	human immunodeficiency virus	PCA	patient controlled analgesia
		PCOS	polycystic ovary syndrome
HNPCC	hereditary non-polyposis colon cancer	PCR	polymerase chain reaction
		PE	pulmonary embolus
HPV	human papilloma virus	PIPJ	proximal inter-phalangeal joint
IBD	inflammatory bowel disease		
		PPI	proton pump inhibitor
ICP	intracranial pressure	PSA	prostate specific antigen
IM	intramuscular	PSC	primary sclerosing cholangitis
INR	international normalized ratio		
		PTFE	polyfluorotetraethylene
ITU	intensive care unit	PVD	peripheral vascular disease
IV	intravenous	RA	rheumatoid arthritis
IVP	intravenous pyelogram	RBC	red blood cell
IVU	intravenous urogram	SAH	subarachnoid haemorrhage
KUB	kidneys, ureters, bladder	SCC	squamous cell carcinoma
LDH	lactate dehydrogenase	SCM	sternocleidomastoid
LH	luteinizing hormone	SFA	superficial femoral artery
LMN	lower motor neuron	SFJ	saphenofemoral junction
LMWH	low molecular weight heparin	SIJ	sacroiliac junction
		SIRS	systemic inflammatory response syndrome
LOS	lower oesophageal sphincter		
LRTI	lower respiratory tract infection	SLE	systemic lupus erythematous
		TB	tuberculosis
LUTS	lower urinary tract symptoms	TIA	transient ischaemic attack
		TIPSS	transjugular intrahepatic portosystemic stent shunt
MCPJ	metacarpophalangeal joint		
MEN	multiple endocrine neoplasia	TNM	tumour, node, metastases
		TPN	total parenteral nutrition
MRCP	magnetic resonance cholangiopancreatogram	TURP	transurethral resection of prostate
MRCS	Membership of the Royal College of Surgeons		
		UMN	upper motor neurone
MRI	magnetic resonance imaging	UTI	urinary tract infection
		VAC	vacuum-assisted closure
NG	nasogastric	VIP	vasoactive intestinal peptide
NICE	National Institute for Health and Clinical Excellence	VTE	venous thromboembolism
		WHO	World Health Organization
		WLE	wide local excision

Common reference intervals

Haematology
Haemoglobin
    Men   13–18 g/dL
    Women   11.5–16 g/dL
Mean cell volume (MCV)   76–96 fL
Platelets $150–400 \times 10^9/L$
White cells (total) $4–11 \times 10^9/L$
Neutrophils   40–75%
Lymphocytes   20–45%
Eosinophils   1–6%

Blood gases	kPa	mmHg
pH		7.35–7.45
paO_2	>10.6	75–100
$paCO_2$	4.7–6	35–45
Base excess		± 2 mmol/L

Urea and electrolytes
Sodium   135–145 mmol/L
Potassium   3.5–5 mmol/L
Creatinine   70–150 mmol/L
Urea   2.5–6.7 mmol/L
Calcium (total)   2.12–2.65 mmol/L
Albumin   35–50 g/L
Proteins   60–80 g/L

Liver function tests
Bilirubin   3–17 mmol/L
Alanine aminotransferase (ALT)   3–35 IU/L
Aspartate transaminase (AST)   3–35 IU/L
Alkaline phosphatase   30–35 IU/L

Cardiac enzymes
Troponin T   <0.1µg/L
Creatine kinase   25–195 IU/L
Lactate dehydrogenase (LDH)   70–250 IU/L

Lipids and other biochemical values

Cholesterol	<5 mmol/L (desired)
Triglycerides	0.5–1.9 mmol/L
Amylase	0–180 IU/L
C-reactive protein (CRP)	<10 mg/L
Glucose (fasting)	3.5–5.5 mmol/L
Prostate-specific antigen (PSA)	0–4 ng/mL
T4 (total thyroxine)	70–140 mmol/L
Thyroid-stimulating hormone (TSH)	0.5–5 mU/L

SECTION 1:
APPLIED ANATOMY

Questions

1. Anatomy of the inguinal canal 2
2. Anatomy of the spermatic cord 2
3. Midline laparotomy 2
4. The diaphragm 3
5. Anatomy of the thyroid gland (1) 3
6. Anatomy of the thyroid gland (2) 3
7. Axillary lymph node clearance 3
8. The parotid gland 4
9. Organs of the abdomen 4
10. Vascular anatomy of the lower limb 4
11. Insertion of a chest drain 5
12. Transpyloric plane of Addison 5
13. The marginal artery of Drummond 5
14. Liver laceration 5
15. The mediastinum 6
16. The thoracic aorta 6
17. Duodenum 6
18. Portosystemic anastomoses 7
19. The skull foramina 7
20. Inserting a tracheostomy 7
21. Lower limb fracture 7
22. Carpal tunnel decompression 8
23. The blood supply to the rectum 8
24. The manubriosternal junction 8
25. Scrotal exploration 8

Answers 9

QUESTIONS

1. Anatomy of the inguinal canal

You are assisting with a primary open right inguinal hernia repair in a 27-year-old male. During the operation, the lead surgeon asks you to define the boundaries of the inguinal canal. Which of the following does not form part of the boundaries of the inguinal canal?

A.   Transversalis fascia and the conjoint tendon
B.   Inguinal ligament
C.   Pectineal ligament
D.   Aponeuroses of the external and internal oblique fibres
E.   Arching fibres of the internal oblique and transversus abdominis muscles

2. Anatomy of the spermatic cord

During a repair of a primary inguinal hernia, you are asked to name the nerve that is located within the spermatic cord. Which of the following is the nerve that is found within the spermatic cord?

A.   Ilioinguinal nerve
B.   Genitofemoral nerve
C.   Genital branch of the genitofemoral nerve
D.   Iliohypogastric nerve
E.   Lateral femoral cutaneous nerve

3. Midline laparotomy

You are asked to assist the lead surgeon with a midline laparotomy in theatre. The patient has small bowel obstruction confirmed by CT imaging. Before the start of the operation, you are asked what layers, from superficial to deep, would be cut through during a midline laparotomy incision. Which of the following is the most likely answer?

A.   Skin, subcutaneous fat, Scarpa's fascia, external oblique, internal oblique, transversalis fascia, extraperitoneal fat and peritoneum
B.   Scarpa's fascia, skin, linea alba, transversalis fascia, extraperitoneal fat, subcutaneous fat and peritoneum
C.   Skin, Scarpa's fascia, linea alba, transversalis fascia, extraperitoneal fat, subcutaneous fat and peritoneum
D.   Linea alba, Scarpa's fascia, skin, external oblique, internal oblique, transversalis fascia, extraperitoneal fat, subcutaneous fat and peritoneum
E.   Skin, subcutaneous fat, Scarpa's fascia, linea alba, transversalis fascia, extraperitoneal fat and peritoneum

4. The diaphragm

During an open repair of an abdominal aortic aneurysm, the consultant asks you to discuss the openings in the diaphragm. You discuss the structures that pass through the three main openings as well as the several smaller ones. Which of the following structures does not pass through one of the three main diaphragmatic openings?

    A. Aorta
    B. Left gastric artery
    C. Left phrenic nerve
    D. Inferior vena cava
    E. Oesophagus

5. Anatomy of the thyroid gland (1)

You are assisting with a total thyroidectomy for a patient who has a goitre and is experiencing compressive symptoms. The Surgical Registrar asks you to name the artery supplying the thyroid gland, which originates from the external carotid artery. From the list below, choose the most likely answer.

    A. Inferior thyroid artery
    B. Thyroid ima artery
    C. Superior thyroid artery
    D. Ascending pharyngeal artery
    E. Lingual artery

6. Anatomy of the thyroid gland (2)

During a total thyroidectomy, the lead surgeon tells you that he must first identify and then preserve a nerve that is situated near the thyroid gland. He also tells you that this nerve is at risk of injury during thyroidectomy procedures. Which of the following nerves is he referring to?

    A. External laryngeal nerve
    B. Vagus nerve
    C. Phrenic nerve
    D. Recurrent laryngeal nerve
    E. None of the above

7. Axillary lymph node clearance

You are shadowing the Breast Surgery Consultant during a clinical consultation. He begins to explain that he has a patient who is due for a right-sided axillary lymph node clearance the following day. He tells you that he will perform a Level 3 axillary lymph node clearance. From the list below, please select the answer that best describes the location of Level 3 axillary lymph nodes.

    A. Lateral to pectoralis minor
    B. Posterior to pectoralis minor

C. Posterior to pectoralis major
D. Anterior to pectoralis major
E. Superomedial to pectoralis minor

8. The parotid gland

You examine a 35-year-old female patient who presents with a right parotid swelling. Which of the following structures does not lie within the parotid gland?

A. Mandibular nerve
B. External carotid artery
C. Facial nerve
D. Marginal mandibular nerve
E. Retromandibular vein

9. Organs of the abdomen

A patient is admitted following a road traffic accident. He has a suspected liver laceration and is taken to theatre for a laparotomy. The surgeon performing the procedure asks you to name the other intraperitoneal organs within the abdomen. Which of the following abdominal organs is not classified as intraperitoneal?

A. Ureters
B. Transverse colon
C. Stomach
D. Gallbladder
E. Caecum

10. Vascular anatomy of the lower limb

You are assisting a bypass grafting procedure in theatre. Your senior colleague asks you to show him from where the common femoral artery arises. From the list below, choose the statement that best describes the anatomical landmark and course of the common femoral artery.

A. As the external iliac artery passes over the inguinal ligament, it becomes the common femoral artery, and gives off the superficial femoral artery before continuing down to the thigh, medial to the femur, as the profunda femoris artery
B. As the internal iliac artery passes under the inguinal ligament, it becomes the common femoral artery, and gives off the profunda femoris artery before continuing down to the thigh, medial to the femur, as the superficial femoral artery
C. As the external iliac artery passes under the inguinal ligament, it becomes the common femoral artery, and gives off the profunda femoris artery before continuing down to the thigh, medial to the femur, as the superficial femoral artery
D. As the internal iliac artery passes over the inguinal ligament, it becomes the common femoral artery and gives off the profunda

femoris artery before continuing down to the thigh, medial to the
femur, as the superficial femoral artery

E. As the external iliac artery passes under the inguinal ligament, it
becomes the common femoral artery and gives off the superficial
femoral artery before continuing down to the thigh, medial to the
femur, as the profunda femoris artery

11. Insertion of a chest drain

A 35-year-old female has suffered a road traffic accident while coming off her
motorbike at 25 mph during a head-on collision with a car. On arrival to the
emergency department, she is found to have a pneumothorax following review
of her trauma series imaging. You assist the Surgical Registrar in siting a chest
drain. Which of the following structures does not form part of the layers encountered when inserting a chest drain?

A. Serratus anterior
B. External intercostal muscle
C. Scarpa's fascia
D. Innermost intercostal muscle
E. Endothoracic fascia

12. Transpyloric plane of Addison

During a radiological meeting at your local hospital, the Consultant Radiologist is
commenting on the intra-abdominal structures found at the level of the transpyloric
plane of Addison on a CT scan. At what vertebral level does this plane pass through?

A. At the level of the first lumbar vertebra (L1)
B. At the level of the fourth lumbar vertebra (L4)
C. At the level of the third lumbar vertebra (L3)
D. At the level of the second lumbar vertebra (L2)
E. None of the above

13. The marginal artery of Drummond

A patient undergoes a laparotomy for large-bowel obstruction secondary to an
obstructing sigmoid colonic lesion confirmed on a CT scan. The Surgical Registrar
asks you about the formation of the marginal artery of Drummond. Which two
vessels from the list below anastomose to form the marginal artery of Drummond?

A. Inferior mesenteric artery and the splenic artery
B. Superior mesenteric artery and the splenic artery
C. Inferior mesenteric artery and middle rectal artery
D. Superior mesenteric artery and inferior mesenteric artery
E. Inferior mesenteric artery with superior rectal artery

14. Liver laceration

A 45-year-old man undergoes emergency laparotomy for suspected intra-
abdominal trauma. A large liver laceration is detected during laparotomy and the

bleeding is difficult to control. The Consultant locates the free edge of the lesser omentum and performs Pringle's manoeuvre to control the haemorrhage. From the list below, which structures are found within the free edge of the lesser omentum?

A. Common hepatic artery, cystic duct and hepatic vein
B. Hepatic artery and inferior vena cava
C. Hepatic artery and common bile duct
D. Hepatic portal vein, cystic duct and hepatic artery
E. Hepatic portal vein, hepatic artery and common bile duct

15. The mediastinum

During a ward round, you are asked to review a chest radiograph of a 45-year-old female who experienced difficulty breathing 1 day post laparoscopic cholecystectomy. You are quizzed about the contents of the mediastinum. From the list below, which structure does not form part of the contents of the mediastinum?

A. Thymus
B. Trachea
C. Great vessels
D. Thoracic duct
E. None of the above

16. The thoracic aorta

You are reviewing a contrast CT of the thoracic aorta of a 65-year-old patient who has suspected aortic dissection. The radiologist asks you to name the branches of the thoracic aorta. Which of the following is not a branch of the thoracic aorta?

A. Subcostal artery
B. Bronchial artery
C. Coeliac trunk
D. Oesophageal artery
E. Pericardial artery

17. Duodenum

You are in the endoscopy unit observing an endoscopic retrograde cholangio pancreatogram for a patient with deranged liver function tests also presenting with jaundice. The Consultant explains to you that he must get to the part of the duodenum where the duodenal papilla is located. From the list of answers below, which part of the duodenum is the Consultant referring to?

A. First part (D1)   at L1
B. Second part (D2)   at L2
C. Third party (D3)   at L3
D. Fourth part (D4)   at L2
E. Fifth part (D5)

18. Portosystemic anastomoses

You see a 60-year-old female presenting with haematemesis. An upper gastro-intestinal endoscopy reveals bleeding oesophageal varices. From the list below, select the answer that corresponds to the correct number of areas of portosystemic anastomoses present in the abdomen.

    A. 1
    B. 2
    C. 3
    D. 4
    E. 5

19. The skull foramina

A 16-year-old male suffers a head injury and subsequent loss of consciousness while playing rugby. The site of impact was the right temporoparietal region and a CT scan of the head reveals a right-sided extradural haematoma with minimal midline shift. The Radiologist suspects that a branch of the middle meningeal artery is the cause of the extradural haematoma. The patient is taken urgently to theatre to evacuate the haemorrhage. From the list below, select the skull foramina through which the middle meningeal artery passes.

    A. Foramen ovale
    B. Foramen spinosum
    C. Foramen lacerum
    D. Jugular foramen
    E. Carotid canal

20. Inserting a tracheostomy

You are observing a tracheostomy being sited in theatre for a patient who has suffered extensive facial trauma. Which of the following structures is not encountered and traversed during insertion of a tracheostomy?

    A. Platysma muscle
    B. Thyroid isthmus
    C. Strap muscles
    D. Sternocleidomastoid muscle
    E. Investing layer of deep cervical fascia

21. Lower limb fracture

A 25-year-old male sustains a right tibia and fibula fracture. He is unable to dorsiflex his right foot and has lost sensation to the dorsum of his right foot. From the list below, select the nerve that is likely to have been damaged.

    A. Medial plantar nerve
    B. Lateral plantar nerve
    C. Sciatic nerve

D. Tibial nerve
E. None of the above

22. Carpal tunnel decompression

You are observing an open carpal tunnel decompression in theatre. Which of the following structures is not at risk during this procedure?

A. Posterior interosseous nerve
B. Palmar cutaneous branch of the median nerve
C. Median nerve
D. Superficial palmar arch
E. Recurrent branch of the median nerve

23. The blood supply to the rectum

A 49-year-old male is undergoing an elective low anterior resection for a rectal adenocarcinoma. Having studied the blood supply to the large bowel, you are asked about the arterial supply to the rectum. From the list below, choose the artery that contributes to the vascular supply to the rectum.

A. Superior mesenteric artery
B. Left gastric artery
C. Gastroduodenal artery
D. Splenic artery
E. Internal pudendal artery

24. The manubriosternal junction

You are examining a patient and looking for the second intercostal place by finding the manubriosternal junction (also known as the 'angle of Louis'). From the list below, choose the vertebral level that corresponds to the manubriosternal junction.

A. T1
B. T2
C. T3
D. T4
E. T5

25. Scrotal exploration

A 12-year-old boy is suspected to have a right-sided testicular torsion and is taken urgently to theatre for a scrotal exploration. Which of the following structures is not encountered during a scrotal exploration?

A. Dartos muscle
B. Tunica vaginalis
C. External oblique muscle
D. Cremaster fascia and muscle
E. External spermatic fascia

ANSWERS

Anatomy of the inguinal canal

1 C Pectineal ligament
The boundaries of the inguinal canal are as follows:

Anteriorly: The aponeuroses of the external and internal oblique

Posteriorly: The transversalis fascia, and medially, the conjoint tendon that is made up of the merging pubic attachments of the internal oblique and transversus abdominis aponeurosis

Superiorly (the roof): Arching fibres of the internal oblique and transversus abdominis

Inferiorly (the floor): The inguinal ligament which is the folded lower margin of the aponeurosis of the external oblique muscle

Answer C is the correct option due to the fact that the pectineal ligament, also known as the ligament of Sir Astley Cooper, forms the inferior border of the femoral canal. Please refer to Chapter 16 for more information regarding the boundaries of the femoral canal.

Anatomy of the spermatic cord

2 C Genital branch of the genitofemoral nerve
The genital branch of the genitofemoral nerve forms part of the structures found within the spermatic cord and supplies the cremasteric muscle (motor) and anterior scrotal skin (sensory). Other structures include the vas deferens, the testicular artery, cremasteric and vas deferens, the pampiniform plexus, sympathetic nerve fibres and lymphatic vessels. The ilioinguinal nerve, which supplies sensation to the scrotum and medial aspect of the thigh, runs anteriorly to the spermatic cord. The iliohypogastric nerve and lateral femoral cutaneous nerve are not found within the spermatic cord. In addition to the genitofemoral nerve, ilioinguinal nerve, femoral nerve and obturator nerve, these nerves originate from the lumbar plexus (L1–L3 ventral primary rami and the superior branch of spinal nerve L4).

Midline laparotomy

3 E Skin, subcutaneous fat, Scarpa's fascia, linea alba, transversalis fascia, extraperitoneal fat and peritoneum
The layers encountered during a midline laparotomy are skin, subcutaneous fat, Scarpa's fascia, linea alba, transversalis fascia, extraperitoneal fat and peritoneum. In the midline, the external and internal oblique muscles are absent. The linea alba is a fibrous aponeurotic

structure that runs from the xiphoid process to the pubic symphysis. It divides the right and left rectus abdominis muscles.

The diaphragm

4 C Left phrenic nerve

The diaphragm has three main openings as well as several smaller openings that transmit many structures. All structures mentioned in Answers A, B, D and E pass through the main openings of the diaphragm.

The three main openings are the following:

1   The vena caval opening (at the level of T8 vertebra), which transmits the inferior vena cava and the right phrenic nerve
2   The oesophageal opening (at the level of T10 vertebra), which transmits the oesophagus, the left gastric artery and vein, and the vagus nerve
3   The aortic opening (at the level of the T12 vertebra), which transmits the aorta, the azygous vein and the thoracic duct

The other smaller openings transmit the splanchnic nerves, sympathetic trunk, subcostal nerve and vessels, left phrenic nerve, superior epigastric vessels and extraperitoneal lymph vessels.

Anatomy of the thyroid gland (1)

5 C Superior thyroid artery

The superior thyroid artery is the first branch of the external carotid artery and enters the upper pole of each lateral lobe of the thyroid gland. The main arterial supply of the lower pole of the thyroid gland is the inferior thyroid artery originating from the thyrocervical trunk, which is a branch of the first part of the subclavian artery. The thyroid ima artery, which is not always present, originates from either the aortic arch or the brachiocephalic trunk and enters the lower aspect of the thyroid isthmus. The ascending pharyngeal and lingual artery are branches of the external carotid that do not supply the thyroid gland.

Anatomy of the thyroid gland (2)

6 D Recurrent laryngeal nerve

The recurrent laryngeal nerve is most at risk of damage during thyroid operations. This nerve must be visualized and protected before the removal of thyroid gland. In the case of thyroid lobectomies, the ipsilateral recurrent laryngeal nerve to the thyroid lobe being resected must be visualized and protected. Damage to this nerve will cause temporary or permanent hoarseness of voice, dependent on the extent of the nerve injury.

The recurrent laryngeal nerve passes upwards in the trachea-oesophageal groove to lie immediately behind the cricothyroid joint. The recurrent laryngeal nerve then enters the larynx deep to the inferior constrictor of the pharynx. The nerve tends to divide into two branches at the level of the thyroid isthmus. The recurrent laryngeal nerve is closely related to the inferior thyroid artery, but this may vary. On the left side, the nerve lies behind the inferior thyroid artery while on the right it can be situated behind or between the branches of the inferior thyroid artery.

The external laryngeal nerve (Answer A) is situated posterior to the superior thyroid artery and is unlikely to be injured providing that the superior thyroid artery is ligated close to the upper pole.

In addition, the phrenic and vagus nerves are also not usually at risk of injury during thyroid procedures.

Axillary lymph node clearance

7 E   Superomedial to pectoralis minor
Axillary lymph nodes can be described anatomically with regard to their positional relationship with the pectoralis minor muscle. Level 1 nodes are positioned below the inferior edge of the pectoralis minor muscle, Level 2 nodes are found behind the pectoralis minor and Level 3 nodes are superomedial to the pectoralis minor muscle. There are interpectoral nodes (Rotter's nodes) situated between the pectoralis major muscle and pectoralis minor muscle.

The parotid gland

8 A   Mandibular nerve
From superficial to deep, the following structures all lie within the parotid gland:

- Facial nerve
- Retromandibular vein
- External carotid artery

The marginal mandibular nerve is a branch of the facial nerve. The facial nerve enters the parotid gland as it emerges from the stylomastoid foramen, giving rise to five branches (temporal branch, zygomatic branch, buccal branch, marginal mandibular nerve and cervical branch) within the parotid gland.

Answer A is correct as the mandibular nerve (V_3) is the third main branch of the trigeminal nerve (cranial nerve 5) and does not lie within the parotid gland. The other two main branches of the trigeminal nerve are the ophthalmic (V_1) and the maxillary (V_2) nerves.

Organs of the abdomen

9 A Ureters

Intraperitoneal organs are found between the parietal peritoneum and the abdominal wall and are suspended by mesentery. Retroperitoneal organs lie behind the peritoneum in the abdominal cavity.

The ureters are retroperitoneal structures along with the following:

- Kidneys
- Adrenal glands
- Ascending and descending colon
- Splenic and hepatic flexures
- Most of the pancreas except the tail
- Second to fourth parts of the duodenum
- Inferior vena cava
- Aorta (including surrounding lymph nodes)
- Urinary bladder
- Vagina

Intraperitoneal organs include the following:

- Stomach
- First part of the duodenum
- Jejunum
- Ileum
- Transverse colon
- Tail of the pancreas
- Appendix
- Caecum
- Gallbladder
- Uterus
- Ovaries

Vascular anatomy of the lower limb

10 C As the external iliac artery passes under the inguinal ligament, it becomes the common femoral artery and gives off the profunda femoris artery before continuing down to the thigh, medial to the femur, as the superficial femoral artery

Bypass grafting is usually performed on patients with critical ischaemia and when percutaneous transluminal angioplasty (with or without stenting) has failed or is not suitable. The procedure involves diverting blood from the proximal artery, above the site of occlusion, distally. Reversed autologous vein (e.g. long saphenous vein) grafts or synthetic polytetrafluoroethylene or Dacron grafts can be used. Vein grafts are more effective and remain patent longer compared with synthetic grafts. Vein grafts are indicated for occlusions below the inguinal ligament, whereas synthetic

grafts are indicated for occlusions above the inguinal ligament. Bypass
procedures can be classified as anatomical (e.g. femoropopliteal bypass)
and extra-anatomical (e.g. axillofemoral or axillobifemoral bypass).

Insertion of a chest drain

11 C   Scarpa's fascia
On insertion of the chest drain, the following structures are encountered from superficial to deep:

- Skin
- Subcutaneous fat
- Superficial fascia
- Serratus anterior muscle
- External intercostal muscle
- Internal intercostal muscle
- Innermost intercostal muscle
- Endothoracic fascia
- Parietal pleura

Scarpa's fascia is the deep layer of superficial fascia found in the layers of the anterior abdominal wall. It is deep to Camper's fascia and
lies superficial to the external oblique muscle. In the midline, it lies
between the subcutaneous fat and the linea alba. As Scarpa's fascia is
found in the abdominal wall, it does not form part of the layers encountered during insertion of a chest drain.

Transpyloric plane of Addison

12 A   At the level of the first lumbar vertebra (L1)
The transpyloric plane of Addison passes through the body of the first
lumbar vertebra. This plane is a point midway between the suprasternal
notch of the manubrium and the upper border of the symphysis pubis.
This plane marks the level at which many important structures are
seen, which include the hilum of the kidneys and their corresponding
vascular supply, termination of the spinal cord, junction of the superior
mesenteric and splenic vein to form the origin of the hepatic portal
vein, pylorus, the first (see Question 17) part of the duodenum, hilum
of the spleen, duodenojejunal junction, attachment of the transverse
mesocolon, the origin of the superior mesenteric artery at the aorta, the
neck of the pancreas and the fundus of the gallbladder.

The marginal artery of Drummond

13 D   Superior mesenteric artery and inferior mesenteric artery
The superior mesenteric artery and the inferior mesenteric artery form
an important anastomosis that runs along the whole length of the
large bowel forming a continuous vascular arcade. This is known as

the marginal artery of Drummond. There is a watershed area, formed between these two vascular territories at the splenic flexure of colon.

Liver laceration

14 E   **Hepatic portal vein, hepatic artery and the common bile duct**
The free edge of the lesser omentum, which also forms the anterior border of the foramen of Winslow, contains the portal triad of the hepatic portal vein (posteriorly), the common bile duct on the right and the hepatic artery on the left (anteriorly).

Pringle's manoeuvre is performed by compressing the portal triad with the finger and thumb. This manoeuvre is performed to temporarily arrest the inflow of blood to the liver to control haemorrhage from the liver.

The mediastinum

15 E   **None of the above**
The mediastinum is the central compartment of the thorax situated between the two pleural sacs. The mediastinum can be divided into two parts:

1   The superior mediastinum that extends from the thoracic inlet to a plane at the level of the sternal angle and the T4/5 intervertebral disc
2   The inferior mediastinum that extends from the sternal angle and T4/5 intervertebral disc to the diaphragm

The contents of the superior mediastinum include the superior vena cava, arch of the aorta, trachea, phrenic nerves, thoracic duct, oesophagus, vagus nerves, left recurrent laryngeal nerve and thymus gland.

The inferior mediastinum can be further divided into the following:

1   Anterior (containing fat and remnants of the thymus gland)
2   Middle (containing the heart, surrounding pericardium and the roots of the great vessels; ascending aorta, superior vena cava and pulmonary trunk)
3   Posterior (containing the lower part of the oesophagus, descending aorta, thoracic duct, tracheobronchial lymph nodes, azygous and hemiazygous veins, thoracic sympathetic trunks and thoracic splanchnic nerves)

Answer E is correct as Answers A–D are all found within the mediastinum.

The thoracic aorta

16 C   Coeliac trunk
The thoracic aorta commences at the lower border of T4 and ends at T12 where the aorta leaves the thorax, by passing through the diaphragm between the crura, and continues as the abdominal aorta. The branches of the thoracic aorta include nine pairs of posterior intercostal arteries,

subcostal arteries, bronchial arteries, oesophageal arteries, pericardial arteries and a branch of the phrenic artery.

The abdominal aorta continues as it leaves the thorax through the diaphragm and ends at the level of L4 where it bifurcates into the common iliac arteries. The branches of the abdominal aorta include the inferior phrenic arteries, coeliac trunk, superior mesenteric artery, inferior mesenteric artery, suprarenal arteries, renal arteries, testicular/ovarian arteries and four pairs of lumbar branches.

Duodenum

17 B   Second part (D2)

The duodenum is anatomically divided into four parts. The first part (D1) lies at the level of L1, the second part (D2) lies at the level of L2, the third part (D3) lies at the level of L3 and the fourth part (D4) at the level of L2.

Within the second part (D2), the major duodenal papilla is situated where the ampulla of Vater, made up of the common bile duct and major pancreatic duct, opens into the duodenum.

Portosystemic anastomoses

18 E   (5)

Portosystemic anastomoses do not become clinically significant until there is evidence of portal hypertension that prevents normal portal venous drainage. This results in the development of a collateral circulation leading to clinical conditions such as bleeding oesophageal varices.

There are five areas of portosystemic anastomoses: (1) lower oesophagus, (2) rectal, (3) bare area of the liver, (4) peri-umbilical area and (5) retroperitoneum.

The skull foramina

19 B   Foramen spinosum

The middle meningeal vessels run through the foramen spinosum to supply the dura mater. The middle meningeal artery is the largest of the three arteries that supply the meninges. The other two arteries are the anterior and posterior meningeal arteries. The anterior branch of the middle meningeal artery courses underneath the pterion where it is at risk of injury.

The mandibular division of the trigeminal nerve passes through the foramen ovale. The carotid canal transmits the internal carotid artery and sympathetic plexus. The jugular foramen transmits the internal jugular vein, glossopharyngeal nerve, vagus and accessory nerve. The internal carotid artery passes into the foramen lacerum from the carotid canal.

Inserting a tracheostomy

20 D Sternocleidomastoid

The following structures are encountered and divided to allow for passage of the tracheostomy tube, from superficial to deep: skin, subcutaneous fat, platysma muscle, investing layer of deep cervical fascia, strap muscles (sternohyoid and sternothyroid muscles that are retracted as opposed to being cut), pre-tracheal fascia, thyroid isthmus (which is ligated and divided) and the trachea.

Lower limb fracture

21 E None of the above

This patient is suffering from a common peroneal (fibular) nerve injury. The sciatic nerve runs down to the posterior aspect of the mid-thigh in the region of the apex of the popliteal fossa where it divides into its terminal branches: the tibial nerve and the common peroneal nerve (or common fibular nerve). The tibial nerve innervates both superficial and deep muscles of the posterior compartment of the leg and provides sensory innervation to the posterior aspect of the leg and the sole of the foot. The tibial nerve terminates by bifurcating into the medial and lateral plantar nerves in the sole of the foot.

The common peroneal nerve travels around the neck of the fibula in the superficial position where it is vulnerable to injury. Near the neck of the fibula, the common peroneal nerve divides into superficial (motor to the lateral compartment of the leg and sensory to the anterolateral aspect of the leg and the dorsum of the foot) and deep branches (motor to the anterior compartment of the leg, which involves muscles that dorsiflex the foot and extend the toes, and sensory to the webspace between the hallux and the second digit).

Carpal tunnel decompression

22 A Posterior interosseous nerve

In an open carpal tunnel decompression, the structures that are at risk of damage are the flexor tendons passing through the carpal tunnel, the superficial palmar arch, the median nerve, the ulnar nerve as it passes through the flexor retinaculum, the recurrent branch of the median nerve that provides motor innervation to the thenar muscles and the palmar cutaneous branch of the median nerve.

The posterior interosseous nerve is a continuation of the deep branch of the radial nerve. This nerve does not pass through the carpal tunnel but courses down the arm to the dorsal surface of the forearm supplying all the muscles on the radial side and dorsal surface of the forearm (excluding anconeus, brachioradialis and extensor carpi radialis longus that are supplied by the radial nerve).

The blood supply to the rectum

23 E Internal pudendal artery

The rectum is supplied by the superior, middle and inferior rectal arteries. The superior rectal artery is a continuation of the inferior mesenteric artery. The middle rectal artery is a branch of the internal iliac artery and the inferior rectal artery is a branch of the internal pudendal artery.

The superior mesenteric artery supplies the bowel (midgut) from the second part of the duodenum through two-thirds of the transverse colon. It also supplies the pancreas via the inferior pancreatoduodenal artery.

The left gastric, splenic and gastroduodenal arteries are branches of the coeliac axis that supplies structures of the foregut (oesophagus, stomach, spleen, liver and superior parts of the duodenum and pancreas).

The manubriosternal junction

24 D (T4)

The manubriosternal junction, also known as the sternal angle or 'angle of Louis', is at the level of the second costal cartilage towards the lower border of the T4 vertebra.

Scrotal exploration

25 C External oblique muscle

The external oblique muscle is not encountered during a scrotal exploration; however, the external spermatic fascia, derived from the aponeurosis of the external oblique muscle, covers the testis during embryological descent and is encountered during scrotal exploration.

From superficial to deep, the structures that must be traversed are the skin, subcutaneous tissue containing the dartos fascia and muscle (which is a continuation of Camper's fascia) instead of fat, external spermatic fascia, cremaster muscle and fascia (derived from the internal oblique muscle), internal spermatic fascia (from the transversalis fascia) and the tunica vaginalis derived from the abdominal peritoneum.

SECTION 2:
PRE- AND POSTOPERATIVE MANAGEMENT

Questions

1.	Postoperative analgesia	20
2.	Postoperative urine output decline	20
3.	Right upper quadrant pain	20
4.	Postoperative breathlessness	21
5.	Abdominal distension	21
6.	Perioperative steroid therapy	21
7.	Health and safety in the surgical environment	22
8.	Postoperative pyrexia (1)	22
9.	Postoperative pyrexia (2)	22
10.	Acid–base balance	23
11.	Postoperative wound dehiscence	23
12.	Informed surgical consent	23
13.	Venous thromboembolism prophylaxis	24
14.	Preoperative blood transfusion	24
15.	Postoperative confusion	24
16.	Postoperative pyrexia (3)	25
17.	Preoperative coagulation assessment	25
18.	Emergency preoperative management	25
19.	Perioperative glycaemic control (1)	26
20.	Perioperative glycaemic control (2)	26
21.	Investigating postoperative pyrexia	27
22.	Postoperative pain and pyrexia	27
23.	Presurgical optimization for laparoscopic cholecystectomy	27
24.	Presurgical assessment	28
25.	Confusion	28
Answers		29

QUESTIONS

1. Postoperative analgesia

You are asked to review a 45-year-old man on the surgical ward by the nursing staff. Checking through the notes, you observe that he is 1 day following an open anterior resection for rectal carcinoma. He describes severe central abdominal pain associated with dyspnoea. The abdomen is soft but generally tender throughout. His symptoms have occurred despite an epidural that was inserted prior to surgery. What is the most effective form of analgesia in this setting?

epidural is usually first choice

A. Four-hourly intramuscular morphine
B. Patient-controlled opiate analgesia (PCA)
C. Intravenous paracetamol
D. Per rectum diclofenac
E. Intravenous oxycodeine hydrochloride

2. Postoperative urine output decline

A 64-year-old man undergoes a laparoscopic gastric bypass for obesity. His baseline blood pressure is 150/80 mmHg. Intraoperatively, there was a small serosal tear which was sutured laparoscopically. The patient had some bleeding during the dissection of the lesser omentum, which was controlled with diathermy. The patient did not require intraoperative transfusion. Postoperatively on return to the high dependency unit, the patient is mechanically ventilated and his blood pressure is 80/40 mmHg. His urine output is 15 mL/h. Which of the following is the best means of improving his urine output?

not in hypovol patient

A. Commence an infusion of furosemide
B. A trial of dobutamine
C. O-negative blood transfusion
D. Insert a Swan–Ganz catheter
E. Give a fluid challenge and monitor the clinical response

3. Right upper quadrant pain

A 46-year-old woman re-presents to the emergency department 48 hours following an 'uncomplicated' laparoscopic cholecystectomy and on-table cholangiogram. She describes a history of progressive, constant, right upper quadrant pain radiating to the shoulder tip since the surgery. The pain is worse on coughing and moving. On direct questioning, she describes a 24-hour history of nausea and vomiting. The abdomen is rigid. Her liver function tests are abnormal as follows: bilirubin 60 μmol/L, alkaline phosphatase 550 IU/L and alanine aminotransferase 220 IU/L. Her international normalized ratio is <1.5. Which single investigation is more likely to be diagnostic?

- (A) Endoscopic retrograde cholangiopancreatography
- B. Computed tomography scan of the abdomen and pelvis
- C. Erect chest radiograph
- D. Amylase or lipase levels
- E. Urine Ketostix to detect ketonuria

handwritten note: → slipped stone?
✗ First investigation?
CT / US : to see the leak

✗ 4. Postoperative breathlessness

You are called urgently to see a 67-year-old man who is 24 hours following uncom-✱ plicated laparoscopic cholecystectomy. The patient is human immunodeficiency virus-positive and has a past history of thrombocytopenia and at pre-assessment his platelet count was 60 × 10⁹/L. He is complaining of chest pain and breathless-ness and his abdomen is noticeably more distended than in the initial postoperative ✗ period with significant peri-umbilical tenderness. His postoperative electrocardio-gram shows lateral ischaemia and his current haemoglobin level is 7.5 g/dL. He is tachycardic and his blood pressure is 115/75 mmHg. The next appropriate step is

- A. Bleep the on-call cardiologist
- B. Start treatment dose heparin
- C. Start an infusion of glyceryl trinitrate
- (D) Start blood transfusion
- E. Return the patient to operating theatre for re-look laparoscopy

handwritten note: • periumbilical hematoma (complication of laparoscopic surgery)

5. Abdominal distension

The nursing staff asks you to review an erect chest radiograph of a 60-year-old ✱ woman who has undergone open colonic surgery for a pelvic mass 3 days ago. She is comfortable at rest. Her abdomen is distended, with absent bowel sounds. Free air under the hemi-diaphragms is likely to be due to

- A. Perforated peptic ulcer
- B. Anastomotic leakage (will result in peritonitis)
- C. Perforated sigmoid diverticulum
- (D) A normal finding 4 days post laparotomy
- E. A diaphragmatic injury

6. Perioperative steroid therapy

A 22-year-old woman with known Crohn's disease is about to undergo an emer-gency subtotal colectomy with ileostomy. Prior to surgery the patient has been on 30 mg of prednisolone daily for more than 3 months. The best management to prevent an addisonian crisis would be

- A. Additional steroid cover is not required
- B. Usual preoperative dose only (30 mg oral prednisolone)

major operation
↓

C. 50 mg of hydrocortisone intravenously preoperatively, followed by 50 mg of hydrocortisone intravenously 8-hourly for 72 hours

D. 25 mg of hydrocortisone intravenously preoperatively, then resume the normal steroid dose postoperatively

Minor op

E. 25 mg of hydrocortisone intravenously preoperatively, followed by 25 mg of hydrocortisone intravenously for 24 hours
↓
Moderate op.

7. Health and safety in the surgical environment

You are asked to assist your consultant who is operating on a 43-year-old human immunodeficiency virus-positive man involved in a road traffic accident. The following precautions have been shown to decrease risk of HIV transmission, with the exception of

A. Gowns

B. Double glove with indicator system

C. Protective eye wear

D. Laminar flow ventilation

E. Surgical masks

8. Postoperative pyrexia (1)

You are called to the ward to review a 72-year-old man who is pyrexial at 38.0°C, 8 hours following an anterior resection for rectal adenocarcinoma without defunctioning stoma. He is asymptomatic and pain-free with an epidural. A urinary catheter inserted in theatre is draining concentrated urine. He has a history of chronic airways disease controlled with inhalers. He has no respiratory distress, but both lung bases sound quiet. The most likely explanation for the patient's pyrexia is

asymptomatic AT aft OT

A. Epidural abscess

B. Systemic response to surgical trauma

C. Basal atelectasis *24-48 h postoperatively*

D. Infective exacerbation of chronic airways disease *3-7 d as a typical complication of atelectasis*

E. Urinary sepsis

9. Postoperative pyrexia (2)

You are called to see the same patient 7 days postoperatively as he has become unwell and pyrexial with a temperature of 39.0°C. The patient has generalized abdominal discomfort. The abdomen is tender with generalized guarding and rebound. The chest is clear to auscultation. The patient's catheter and epidural were removed 2 days ago. The most likely explanation for the patient's pyrexia is

A. Deep vein thrombosis

B. Infective exacerbation of chronic airways disease

C. Pulmonary embolus

D. Anastomotic leakage
E. Pre-existing chest infection

10. Acid–base balance

A 62-year-old man is admitted to the emergency department with abdominal pain. The patient has a past history of ischaemic heart disease and atrial fibrillation. Computed tomography scan features are highly suggestive of ischaemic bowel. The patient's blood gases are as follows:

- pH = 7.25 ↓   *acidosis*
- paO_2 = 10
- $paCO_2$ = 2.8 ↓   *compensated*
- HCO_3 = 18 ↓   *acidosis metabolic*
- Base excess = −8   *acidosis*

* if fully compensated
  → pH should be close to normal

* If uncompensated
  → paO2 should be normal.

Which of the following best describes the patient's acid–base status?

A. Metabolic acidosis
B. Metabolic acidosis with respiratory compensation
C. Respiratory acidosis with metabolic compensation
D. Metabolic acidosis with inadequate respiratory compensation
E. Cannot be sure without a serum lactate level

11. Postoperative wound dehiscence

You are called urgently to see an 80-year-old man who is 6 days following open anterior resection for rectal carcinoma with defunctioning stoma. The patient reported seeing a gush of pink fluid from the central laparotomy wound. You notice that the small bowel is eviscerating from the wound. Following initial resuscitation, the next best step is to

① A. Cover the small bowel with a sterile saline-soaked gauze
② B. Call for senior help   — *cover then call.*
③ C. Administer intravenous cefuroxime 1.5 g
④ D. Return the patient to theatre for deep-tension abdominal wall closure   → *not first step.*
E. Apply vacuum-assisted closure therapy   → *If no evisceration*

12. Informed surgical consent

The surgical registrar is about to obtain informed consent from a 16-year-old boy for an open appendicectomy. Which of the following statements regarding consent in minors is most correct?   *Legal age for consent in UK = 18 years.*

A. Parental consent must be sought prior to obtaining patient consent
B. If the child refuses treatment, the parent's consent is required
C. The registrar must determine if the child is competent to obtain informed consent

D. A court order is required
E. None of the above

13. Venous thromboembolism prophylaxis

A 72-year-old woman is about to undergo an elective total hip replacement for osteoarthritis. She has a history of hypertension and type 2 diabetes mellitus but no ischaemic heart disease or peripheral vascular disease. Which of the following is the most appropriate thromboembolic prophylaxis?

A. Intermittent pneumatic calf compression
B. Calf-length thromboembolic deterrent elastic stockings and early ambulation
C. Full-dose unfractionated heparin to increase the activated partial thromboplastin time to two time control
D. Insertion of an inferior vena cava filter → if anticoagulation is C/I
E. Subcutaneous low-molecular-weight heparin

14. Preoperative blood transfusion

A 22-year-old man (O blood group) sustained a splenic injury in a road traffic accident. He is undergoing a transfusion of 4 units prior to surgery. You are asked to review the patient 10 minutes into the transfusion as he has become unwell and agitated. He has pyrexia (39.5°C) with associated tachycardia (120 beats/min) and hypotension (80/50 mmHg). Which of the following is the most likely cause?

A. Non-haemolytic febrile transfusion reaction — patient is well   >30 min of starting trans
B. Transfusion-related acute lung injury? not likely
C. Bacterial contamination
D. Air embolus
E. Haemolytic transfusion reaction (ABO incompatibility) within minutes usually.

15. Postoperative confusion

You are called to the ward to see an agitated 68-year-old man who is 3 days following radical prostatectomy. He is wandering aimlessly around the ward convinced that he is the Duke of Wellington. His Mini-Mental Test score is 4/10. His latest observations reveal pyrexia of 37.6°C, pulse 100 beats/min, blood pressure 146/88 mmHg and respiratory rate 20 breaths/min. You note that the urinary catheter bag contents are cloudy. Which is the most likely explanation for the patient's confusion?

→ not acute development
A. Preoperative dementia
B. Delirium secondary to chest infection
C. Delirium secondary to reactionary haemorrhage → occurs sooner
D. Delirium secondary to urinary tract sepsis
E. Stroke   What?!?

16. Postoperative pyrexia (3)

A 49-year-old woman weighing 65kg is 5 days following gastrectomy for gastric carcinoma. Her observations are as follows:

- ↑Temperature = 39.0°C
- ↑Pulse = 110 beats/min   *tachycardia*
- ↓Blood pressure = 90/50 mmHg   *hypotension*
- ↓Urine output = 10mL/h
- ↑Respiratory rate = 30 breaths/min   *tachypnea*

Which of the following best describes this patient's pathophysiological status?

A. Sepsis   *? need source of infection*
B. Septic shock
C. Systemic inflammatory response syndrome
D. Multiple organ dysfunction syndrome → *involves 2 or more systems*
E. None of the above

Indication = atrial fib; so can stop warfarin
if DVT/PE ⇒ need to convert to IV heparin

17. Preoperative coagulation assessment

A 62-year-old man is about to undergo an elective abdominoperineal resection for a low rectal carcinoma. He usually takes 5 mg warfarin per day for atrial fibrillation. His most recent international normalized ratio (INR) is 2.9. Which of the following is the best preoperative strategy?

A. Admit the patient 1 day prior to surgery to stop warfarin and check the INR
B. Admit the patient 3–5 days prior to surgery to stop the warfarin and check the INR <1.5
C. Admit the patient 3–5 days prior to surgery to stop the warfarin, check the INR <1.5 and start aspirin → *no*
D. Admit the patient 3–5 days prior to surgery to stop the warfarin, check the INR <1.5 and start heparin infusion → *no. will ↑ risk of bleeding.*
E. Admit the patient 1 day prior to surgery to stop warfarin, check the INR <1.5 and start low-molecular-weight heparin

18. Emergency preoperative management

DVT
A patient on warfarin for multiple deep vein thrombosis is about to undergo an emergency laparotomy for a perforated sigmoid colon. Which of the following is the best preoperative strategy?

A. Discontinue warfarin therapy, administer vitamin K (2–3 mg) and check the international normalized ratio (INR) every 6–8 hours preoperatively
B. Discontinue warfarin therapy and check the INR every 6–8 hours preoperatively
C. Continue warfarin therapy as prescribed

D. Discontinue warfarin therapy, administer vitamin K (2–3 mg), check the INR every 6–8 hours preoperatively, request fresh frozen plasma to cover the procedure

E. None of the above as the surgery should be postponed

19. Perioperative glycaemic control (1)

A 34-year-old man is about to undergo a left hemicolectomy for colorectal carcinoma. He is an insulin-dependent diabetic. The most appropriate perioperative management is

A. Preoperatively commence 0.9% normal saline (3 L in 3 hours), along with 20 units of intramuscular Actrapid insulin to 6 units per hour thereafter along with potassium supplementation

B. Preoperatively start 50 units of insulin in 500 mL of normal saline and continue through to postoperative period, then restart normal subcutaneous insulin when the patient is eating and drinking normally

C. Start an intravenous infusion of 5% or 10% dextrose (500 mL bags) over 4–6 hours and add insulin and potassium chloride to each bag, titrated to blood glucose and potassium levels

D. Continue usual subcutaneous insulin until and including the day of surgery. Place first on the list and monitor blood glucose preoperatively, intraoperatively and in recovery

E. None of the above

20. Perioperative glycaemic control (2)

A 55-year-old man is about to undergo a diagnostic knee arthroscopy as a day case. He has type 2 diabetes mellitus for which he takes metformin 850 mg/day. The most appropriate perioperative management is

A. Start an intravenous infusion of 5% or 10% dextrose (500 mL bags) over 4–6 hours and add insulin and potassium chloride to each bag, titrated to blood glucose and potassium levels

B. Continue oral hypoglycaemic agents until and including the day of surgery

C. Provided that blood glucose <10mmol/L, continue oral hypoglycaemic agents until the day of surgery, then omit morning dose, restart oral hypoglycaemic with first meal

D. Provided that blood glucose <10mmol/L, preoperatively start 50 units of insulin in 50mL of normal saline and continue through to postoperative period, then restart oral hypoglycaemics with first meal

E. None of the above as management depends on HbA1c levels

21. Investigating postoperative pyrexia

A 17-year-old Caucasian woman who underwent a laparotomy 2 weeks ago for a perforated appendix develops a swinging fever, dry cough, and pain in the tip of her right shoulder. Her latest observations are as follows:

*Sub diaphragmatic Collection. *

- ↑ Temperature = 38.9°C
- Blood pressure = 120/76 mmHg
- ↑ Pulse rate = 110 beats/min
- Respiratory rate = 20 breaths/min

Examination shows tenderness over the lower lateral ribcage. Abdominal and rectal examinations are normal. The white blood cell count is 18000 × 10⁹/L. Which one of the following is the *best* diagnostic test for this patient?

- A. Erect chest radiograph → non specific findings (hemidiaphragm)
- B. Abdominal radiograph
- C. Abdominal ultrasound
- Ⓓ Abdominal CT scan
- E. Gastrografin follow-through

22. Postoperative pain and pyrexia

A 45-year-old African Caribbean man is approximately 5 days following right femoropopliteal bypass for superficial femoral artery atherosclerosis. The nursing staff has asked you to see the patient, who is complaining of increasing pain over the right groin wound. The patient has a low-grade pyrexia of 37.6°C. On examination the wound is erythematous, hot and tender on palpation. There is no obvious collection, abscess or crepitation. The right leg is mildly swollen and the calf is soft. All peripheral pulses are palpable. The most likely diagnosis is

- A. Cellulitis secondary to *Staphylococcus epidermidis* infection → in HIV patient
- B. Deep vein thrombosis → needs to be excluded
- Ⓒ Cellulitis secondary to *Streptococcus pyogenes* infection → In immunocompetent patient
- D. Lymphoedema secondary to filariasis → tropical Infection
- E. Occlusion secondary to graft thrombosis — unlikely 5 d after operation — also pulses are palpable

23. Presurgical optimization for laparoscopic cholecystectomy

A 74-year-old Caucasian man with obstructive jaundice secondary to gallstones is about to undergo urgent laparoscopic cholecystectomy and bile duct exploration following failed endoscopic retrograde cholangiopancreatography. His latest blood tests are as follows:

- Bilirubin = 180
- ↑ Alkaline phosphatase = 700 IU/L
- ↑ Alanine aminotransferase = 250 IU/L
- ↑ White cell count = 18 × 10⁹/L
- ↑ Urea = 9.0 mmol/L
- Creatinine = 180 μmol/L

Which one of the following is the best statement regarding perioperative management considerations?

→ need generous fluids

A. Rehydration should be approached with caution to prevent the risk of hepatorenal syndrome

B. The patient is at increased risk of bleeding to reduced absorption of clotting factors II, VII, IX and X

C. There is a lower risk of infection so prophylactic antibiotics are not necessary *↳ no higher*

D. Analgesics are less effective so doses of opiates should be increased

E. Surgery should not be performed in a jaundiced patient

↳ can be if optimized first
↳ But preferable if jaundice relieved first.

24. Presurgical assessment

A 62-year-old man is awaiting an elective femoropopliteal bypass for peripheral vascular disease. He is a smoker of 60 pack years and is being treated for hypertension and hypercholesterolaemia with ramipril 5 mg each morning and simvastatin 10 mg orally at night. Three weeks ago he was admitted following an ST elevation myocardial infarction. His current blood pressure is 170/110 mmHg. Which of the following best describes the preoperative strategy?

A. Preoperative control of blood pressure with nifedipine is mandatory

B. Preoperative unfractionated heparin should be started, with 4-hourly monitoring of the patient's activated partial thromboplastin time

C. Intensive chest physiotherapy three times a day is vital postoperatively

D. A preoperative echocardiogram is required

E. None of the above, as the surgery should be deferred for 6 months

25. Confusion

A 37-year-old man is admitted with abdominal pain and treated for pancreatitis; 48 hours following his admission you are asked to assess the patient as he has become increasingly confused and aggressive. Observations are not possible, but you note he appears to be breathing hard, he is tremulous and has pruritus. Choose an appropriate management strategy:

A. Septic screen; urine dip, chest radiograph and blood cultures

B. Chlordiazepoxide 20 mg intravenously, four times daily for 1 week

C. Haloperidol 2 mg intramuscularly and confine to side room

D. Lorazepam infusion

E. Oral chlordiazepoxide-reducing regimen with 48 hours intravenous thiamine (B1)

✱ alcohol withdrawal ✱

ANSWERS

Postoperative analgesia

1 B   Patient-controlled opiate analgesia (PCA)

This patient is 1 day following a major bowel resection. The best form of analgesia in this setting is an epidural; however, this appears not to be functioning. Hence, a PCA system is indicated. This mode of delivery has been shown to be effective for control of postoperative pain. In addition, it reduces the risk of development of basal atelectasis and other respiratory complications. The drawback with PCA is that it requires a level of patient cooperation and understanding, and the patient has to be able to use the device.

Best is an epidural

if not → PCA

Intravenous oxycodeine hydrochloride and intramuscular morphine are strong and effective analgesics. The rationale for preferring PCA is that it has been shown to provide a superior background of analgesia, with fewer episodes of breakthrough pain. The parental opioid administration is preferred in patients who are less suitable for PCA, that is those unable to understand instructions, those under sedation and those with vision impairment or mobility/coordination issues. Paracetamol and diclofenac are simple analgesics, which you are told have not relieved the patient's pain. These drugs may be appropriate to use in conjunction with a PCA system or other morphine analgesia, although candidates must be aware that PR drugs should be strictly avoided in patients with a recent low rectal resection.   *PR ⇒ per rectum*

Postoperative urine output decline

2 E   Give a fluid challenge and monitor the clinical response

In a surgical patient, it is typically safe to assume that the cause of postoperative hypotension is hypovolaemia until proved otherwise. This patient may be suffering from a reactionary haemorrhage from a vessel within the lesser omentum. The most appropriate management plan would be to give a fluid challenge and monitor the clinical response while simultaneously checking the full blood count and clotting.

post op hypotn = hypovolaemia until proven otherwise

Inotropic support with drugs such as noradrenaline and dobutamine is the reserve of patients who are fluid replete but who still struggle to maintain their urinary output. Use of these drugs might be indicated once there is confirmation that the patient is adequately filled. There is little value to be gained from inserting a Swan–Ganz catheter, unless there is a clear cardiac cause for shock. Insertion of pulmonary artery catheters is controversial and some studies even suggest their use is associated with increased mortality. Furosemide may play a role in the management of a patient with low urine output and fluid overload but not in cases of hypovolaemia.

[handwritten: Furosemide →]

Right upper quadrant pain

3 A Endoscopic retrograde cholangiopancreatography

This question requires careful consideration because of its wording: 'Which *single* investigation is more likely to be *diagnostic*'. An urgent CT scan of the abdomen and pelvis will reveal a small amount of free air secondary to the recent laparoscopy and free fluid; however, it would not be able to determine the source of the fluid. In this setting, ERCP would be required to determine the site of a leak and a CT would help in the assessment. If the question had asked which investigation is likely to be performed first, the correct answer might be a CT or ultrasound scan. Optimal care would be for a scan to confirm a collection followed by an operation to identify a cause.

[handwritten margin: post cholecystectomy; first Inv. → CT scan; diagnostic → ERCP → Can determine source of leak]

The most likely diagnosis in this case is of a biliary leak (commonly secondary to either slipped Ligaclip, a high pressure ductal system, or a duct of Luschka). An erect chest plain film radiograph is an appropriate investigation in the work-up of a patient with an acute abdomen, but in this setting it is likely to reveal a small amount of free air secondary to the recent laparoscopic cholecystectomy. Urgent amylase or lipase levels should be performed as a matter of routine to exclude pancreatitis secondary to the on-table cholangiogram. However, pancreatitis is unlikely to be the cause of this patient's peritonism or subphrenic irritation. Urine Ketostix to detect ketonuria should be performed as part of the assessment. It is likely to show dehydration-associated ketonuria, but this will not aid the diagnosis.

Postoperative breathlessness

4 D Start blood transfusion

It is likely that this patient has had an umbilical port-site bleed/ haematoma (not uncommon following laparoscopic procedures). Subsequent blood loss and anaemia are the likely precipitant of the angina-like chest pain and dyspnoea. Note that atherosclerosis is more common in retroviral-positive individuals, and they are therefore at increased risk of underlying undiagnosed cardiovascular disease. Treating the cause of the anaemia is likely to be the most important step. It may be appropriate to call a cardiologist and ultimately commence a GTN infusion, although GTN should be avoided in haemodynamic compromise as it can cause profound hypotension. Heparin should be used cautiously in patients with thrombocytopenia and the advice of a haematologist should be sought.

[handwritten margin: Chest pain due to anemia and blood loss.]

Abdominal distension

5 D A normal finding 4 days post laparotomy

The presence of free air under the diaphragm is not uncommon following open and laparoscopic surgery and is the most likely explanation for this finding. This represents a normal finding 3 days post laparotomy. Other less likely causes of free intraperitoneal air in this setting include anastomotic leakage, perforated sigmoid diverticulum and perforated peptic ulcer; however, these are extremely unlikely in a patient who is otherwise well.

Perioperative steroid therapy

6 C 50 mg of hydrocortisone intravenously preoperatively, followed by 50 mg of hydrocortisone intravenously 8-hourly for 72 hours

The amount of steroid cover required perioperatively relates to the duration of preoperative steroid use, the amount used and the nature of the surgery. The following table shows a guide to pre- and postoperative steroid regimens for different types of surgery.

Preoperative steroid use	Nature of surgery	Suggested steroid regimen
<10 mg daily	Minor	No cover required
>10 mg daily	Minor	25 mg intravenous hydrocortisone preoperatively. Resume normal steroid use postoperatively
>10 mg daily	Intermediate	25 mg intravenous hydrocortisone preoperatively. 25 mg intravenous hydrocortisone every 8 hours for 24 hours then resume normal steroid dose
>10 mg daily	Major	50 mg intravenous hydrocortisone preoperatively. 50 mg intravenous hydrocortisone every 8 hours for 72 hours then resume normal steroid dose

Health and safety in the surgical environment

7 D. Laminar flow ventilation

The US Centers for Disease Control and Prevention recommends wearing gloves and surgical masks for all invasive procedures. Protective eyewear or face shields should be worn for procedures that commonly result in the generation of droplets, splashing of blood or other body fluids, or the generation of bone chips. Gowns or aprons made of materials that provide an effective barrier should be worn during invasive procedures that are likely to result in the splashing of blood or other body fluids. There is no evidence that laminar flow ventilation reduces the risk of contraction of HIV.

Postoperative pyrexia (1)

8 B   Systemic response to surgical trauma
This patient is only 8 hours following major abdominal surgery. The pyrexia is likely to be due to the systemic response to surgical trauma. *atelectasis 24-48h*The patient is at risk of pulmonary atelectasis, but this would be a more likely answer 24–48 hours postoperatively. An infective exacerbation *Inf exacer. 3-7d* of chronic airways disease is less likely in the absence of respiratory symptoms or signs and more commonly occurs as a consequence of pulmonary atelectasis between 3 and 7 days postoperatively. The urinary catheter was inserted in theatre, making urinary catheter sepsis less likely. While an epidural abscess is a recognized cause of postoperative pyrexia, it is unlikely to be responsible for early postoperative pyrexia.

Postoperative pyrexia (2)

9 D   Anastomotic leakage
The patient is 7 days following an anterior resection without a defunctioning stoma. The patient has generalized peritonitis. The most likely answer is an anastomotic leakage. Pulmonary embolus and deep vein thrombosis are recognized causes of postoperative pyrexia and should be excluded but are less likely. Pre-existing chest infection and infective exacerbations are common in patients with COPD but are less likely to be responsible for increasing abdominal pain and peritonitis.

Acid–base balance

10 D   Metabolic acidosis with inadequate respiratory compensation
This patient probably has ischaemic bowel. This is a common cause of metabolic acidosis. However, the patient's $paCO_2$ level is low, suggesting that there is an element of respiratory compensation, but the continued low pH suggests that the respiratory compensation is inadequate. The most likely answer therefore is metabolic acidosis with inadequate respiratory compensation. A serum lactate level may help determine the underlying cause of the metabolic acidosis, but is not a consideration when determining the nature of the acid–base derangement.

Postoperative wound dehiscence

11 A   Cover the small bowel with a sterile saline-soaked gauze
The most appropriate next step following resuscitation is to protect the bowel from the atmosphere with a saline-soaked gauze. This should precede the subsequent management, which would include calling a senior colleague, administering intravenous antibiotics and returning the patient to theatre for immediate closure of the abdomen using deep tension sutures. Vacuum-assisted closure therapy can be used in cases of wound dehiscence, but not where the bowel is eviscerated. (Note that

the use of VAC dressings in full abdominal dehiscence, evisceration and fistula formation has been described, but involves the use of a protective layer of the bowel; trials are ongoing to determine efficacy.)

Informed surgical consent

12 C **The registrar must determine if the child is competent to obtain informed consent**
The law regarding consent of a minor is complex and often confusing. Remembering a few basic rules, however, will aid understanding. First, the legal age of consent is 18 in the UK. Second, no person may consent to or refuse treatment for another person, not even the parents of the child concerned. Children aged 16–18 may consent to treatment if it is thought that they comprehend the decision they are being asked to make; the medical professional seeking consent is responsible for deciding whether this is the case. Children aged less that 18 cannot refuse treatment, although this area of law is muddied and a court order is often necessary to force treatment, with the burden of proof being on the medical professional to argue that the management is beneficial and life-saving.

Although not legally required, it is good medical practice to seek the consent of the parents of the child concerned. In the event of parents refusing consent for a child to have life-saving treatment, such as an appendicectomy, medical professionals can overrule the decision of the parents if they consider treatment is undoubtedly in the child's best interest.

Venous thromboembolism prophylaxis

13 E **Subcutaneous low-molecular-weight heparin**
Venous thromboembolism is an important cause of hospital morbidity and mortality. It is estimated that between 5% and 10% of all hospital deaths are directly caused by thromboembolic complications. Postmortem studies show up to 70% of all patients who die in hospital have some venous thrombus formation. Effective prophylaxis is therefore paramount. A systematic review published in the *New England Journal of Medicine* in 1988 demonstrated that LMWH administration alone reduced risk of all venous thrombus formation by 67%, with a reduction in the incidence of pulmonary embolism by 47% and fatal pulmonary embolism by 64%.

This question may seem confusing to candidates as most will recognize that optimal management in a patient of this age and co-morbidities undergoing hip surgery would be a combination of different prophylactic measures; a combination of LMWH and intermittent calf compression stockings would give the optimum protection. Correct answering of this question, therefore, requires knowledge of the relative efficacy of the different prophylaxis methods. According to published data, following hip surgery elasticised stockings alone reduce risk of VTE by 23%, intermittent compression stockings reduce the incidence by 63% and LMWH alone reduces the risk by 70%. Unfractionated heparin is no better at preventing VTE than LMWH, it is more difficult to administer and is associated with a greater incidence of bleeding complications. The correct answer is therefore option E.

Preoperative blood transfusion

14 E   Haemolytic transfusion reaction (ABO incompatibility)
Patients becoming unwell within minutes of starting a blood transfusion should arouse the suspicion of a haemolytic transfusion reaction (ABO incompatibility) especially in a patient with O group status. In this scenario we are not told whether the blood was cross-matched or type specific. Non-haemolytic febrile transfusion reactions are more likely to occur >30 minutes following transfusion, and generally, the patient remains well. Bacterial contamination is a possibility and should be excluded, but is less likely than ABO incompatibility. Air embolus and transfusion-related acute lung injury are recognized complications of blood transfusions, but are less likely given the patient's symptoms.

Postoperative confusion

15 D   Delirium secondary to urinary tract sepsis
Acute confusion is common in elderly patients in the early postoperative period. A history of dementia should be sought, but is unlikely to be responsible for the acute confusion in this patient. The most common causes include dehydration and sepsis. This patient has had a urological procedure and was noted to have cloudy urine. Therefore the most likely explanation is delirium secondary to urinary tract sepsis. Confusion may occur following reactionary haemorrhage, but this is less likely in a patient 3 days following their operation.

Postoperative pyrexia (3)

16 C   Systemic inflammatory response syndrome
This patient is displaying features of SIRS, which is defined as two or more of the following:

- Temperature >38°C or <36°C
- Heart rate >90 beats/min
- Tachypnoea (respiratory rate >20 breaths/min) or hyperventilation ($paCO_2$ <4.25 kPa)
- White blood cell count >12 × 10^9/L or <4 × 10^9/L or the presence of more than 10% immature neutrophils

Sepsis and septic shock by definition require a confirmed source of infection, which is not supported by the information supplied in the clinical scenario. The multiple organ dysfunction syndrome is the presence of altered organ function in acutely ill patients such that homeostasis cannot be maintained without intervention. It usually involves two systems and there are specific scoring systems required to make the diagnosis.

Preoperative coagulation assessment

17 B Admit the patient 3–5 days prior to surgery to stop the warfarin and check the INR <1.5
The patient is about to undergo a major colonic resection with risk of haemorrhage. As the indication for the warfarin therapy is atrial fibrillation, the best strategy is to admit the patient 3–5 days prior to surgery to stop the warfarin and check the INR is <1.5 the day prior to the procedure. No intervening aspirin or heparin is necessary, and indeed these may exacerbate haemorrhage at the time of surgery.

Greater consideration needs to be given if the indication for warfarin is recurrent DVT/PE or metallic heart valves. These patients may require admission for conversion of warfarin to heparin injections/infusions. Guidance regarding specific circumstances varies between centres and opinion varies among surgeons. Not all surgery requires cessation of warfarin; for very minor procedures such as examinations under anaesthesia where the risk of serious bleeding is very low, there is no need to stop warfarin.

Emergency preoperative management

18 D Discontinue warfarin therapy, administer vitamin K (2–3 mg), check the INR every 6–8 hours preoperatively, request fresh frozen plasma to cover the procedure
This patient has a serious intra-abdominal pathology that requires urgent surgery. Delay in operative management in such a patient increases morbidity and mortality. Therefore, rapid correction of established anticoagulation is necessary in this case. The current recommendation for urgent surgery (i.e. <24 hours) in patients taking oral anticoagulants is to discontinue warfarin therapy, administer vitamin K (2–3 mg), check the INR every 6–8 hours preoperatively and request fresh frozen plasma and cryoprecipitate to cover the procedure.

In addition, because of the real risk of major haemorrhage, additional blood and platelets should be requested. It is advisable to liaise with a haematologist in all complex cases such as this.

Perioperative glycaemic control (1)

19 C   Start an intravenous infusion of 5% or 10% dextrose (500 mL bags) over 4–6 hours and add insulin and potassium chloride to each bag, titrated to blood glucose and potassium levels

Insulin-dependent diabetic patients undergoing major elective surgery should continue their normal subcutaneous insulin until nil by mouth the night before surgery. Two preoperative regimens are commonly used: PIG (= potassium, insulin and glucose) as per option C or 50 units of insulin in 50 mL normal saline (i.e. 1:1 regimen) administered according to a sliding scale, run with fluids supplemented with KCl. Option B cannot be considered as the correct answer as it does not take into consideration the need to supplement potassium when infusing insulin.

Option A is the appropriate therapy for diabetic ketoacidosis. Note that insulin-dependent diabetic patients undergoing minor surgery may not require additional insulin, and only require close monitoring of blood glucose in the perioperative period.

Perioperative glycaemic control (2)

20 C   Provided that blood glucose <10 mmol/L, continue oral hypoglycaemic agents until the day of surgery, then omit morning dose, restart oral hypoglycaemics with first meal

The management of type 2 diabetic patients undergoing (minor to intermediate surgery is to continue oral hypoglycaemic agents until the day of surgery, then omit the morning dose, restarting oral hypoglycaemics with the first meal. If the patient's blood glucose is >10 mmol/L or they are undergoing major surgery, one of the two commonly used regimens for insulin-dependent diabetic patients should be followed, i.e. either PIG (potassium, insulin and glucose) or an insulin sliding scale. Perioperative management does not depend on HbA1c levels, but this is a reasonably good marker of long-term diabetic control.

Investigating postoperative pyrexia

21 D   Abdominal CT scan

This patient probably has a subphrenic collection/abscess which is not uncommon 15–20 days following laparotomy for a perforated intra-abdominal viscus. The swinging pyrexia and shoulder tip pain are pointers to the diagnosis. An abdominal CT scan is the most accurate at delineating intra-abdominal fluid collection and may be required to guide radiological aspiration or drainage. The chest radiograph may show non-specific signs (pulmonary atelectasis, elevated hemidiaphragm and pleural effusion) that are not diagnostic. Abdominal radiographs and Gastrografin follow-through are unlikely to be helpful in

[handwritten margin notes:] minor surgery → no need insulin during surgery. major → as for IDDM 50:50 sliding scale or as above cf

making the diagnosis of a subphrenic abscess, but are useful postoperative tests if there is suspicion of postoperative ileus or obstruction.

Postoperative pain and pyrexia

22 C   Cellulitis secondary to *Streptococcus pyogenes* infection
In an immunocompetent patient, the most likely cause of postoperative
pain and erythema surrounding an operative wound is cellulitis secondary to *Streptococcus pyogenes* or *Staphylococcus aureus* (*S. epidermidis*
is more likely in an immunocompromised patient). Low-grade pyrexia
and leg swelling should give rise to a suspicion of deep vein thrombosis,
which must be excluded. It is a less likely diagnosis in the present question, given the set of symptoms and signs. Filariasis is a tropical para-
sitic infection that can give rise to lymphoedema. Occlusion secondary
to graft thrombosis is unlikely 5 days following primary reconstruction, especially in the presence of palpable distal pulses.

Presurgical optimization for laparoscopic cholecystectomy

23 B.   The patient is at increased risk of bleeding to reduced absorption of
clotting factors II, VII, IX and X
Patients suffering from jaundice are at increased risk of bleeding owing
to reduced absorption of clotting factors II, VII, IX and X. Perioperative
rehydration should be generous to prevent the risk of dehydration and
hepatorenal syndrome. Jaundiced patients are at increased risk of infection and therefore prophylactic antibiotics should not be withheld. The
effects of opiate analgesics may be prolonged due to abnormalities with
drug metabolism and first pass elimination. Surgery can be safely performed in a jaundiced patient provided the necessary steps are taken
toward optimization. It is preferable to relieve jaundice where possible
prior to surgery, but in this instance ERCP has failed.

Presurgical assessment

24 E   None of the above, as the surgery should be deferred for 6 months
The best strategy would be to postpone the surgery for 6 months. The
risk of postoperative reinfarction after a previous myocardial infarction is

- 0–3 months = 35%
- 3–6 months = 15%
- >6 months = 4%

The decision is more straightforward in benign disease (vascular
disease) versus carcinoma. Unfractionated heparin may be beneficial as an initial therapy in critical ischaemia. Preoperative control of
blood pressure is important, but deferring surgery to obtain control is
more advantageous than acute control with calcium channel blockers.

Routine chest physiotherapy postoperatively should be adequate management of this patient.

Confusion

25 E **Oral chlordiazepoxide-reducing regimen with 48 hours intravenous thiamine**

alcohol withdrawal

This patient is withdrawing from alcohol; he has been admitted with a condition commonly caused by alcohol excess and the timing (24–72 hours post-cessation of drinking) is classic. The symptoms and signs of acute alcohol withdrawal should be familiar with candidates – tachycardia with hypotension followed by tremor, confusion, seizure, coma and death. Patients commonly have acute psychosis, typically extremely unpleasant and vivid tactile and visual hallucinations.

tachycardia
hypotension
Confusion
Seizures
coma
tremor
acute psychosis

Patients suffering withdrawal should be commenced immediately on a reducing regimen of benzodiazepines to wean or 'detox' from alcohol. The single best drug to use is chlordiazepoxide, which is given orally. Regimens differ between centres. If oral medication is impossible, IM diazepam or lorazepam is the next drug of choice. IV infusion is inappropriate, as is prolonged administration of a set dose since the patient will simply become dependent on the benzodiazepine and require weaning from this. A septic screen is probably also indicated, but failure to treat the withdrawal will lead to further morbidity and possible mortality.

1) first choic oral
2) then IV/IM
} benzodiazepines
↳ oral prefered → IV → may lead to dependance
first Rx withdrawal → then septic screen

SECTION 3:
FLUID BALANCE AND NUTRITION

Questions

1. Postoperative fluid therapy (1)   40
2. Intravenous access in the trauma patient   40
3. Intravenous fluid management in the trauma patient   40
4. Fluid and nutrition management   40
5. Postoperative fluid therapy (2)   41
6. Fluid balance management   41
7. Fluid resuscitation in the critically ill   41
8. Complications of blood transfusion   42
9. Colloid replacement in a postsurgical patient   42
10. Hartmann's solution   42
11. Hyponatraemia   43
12. Nutritional management (1)   43
13. Complications of enteral nutrition   43
14. Nutritional management (2)   44
15. Total parenteral nutrition (1)   44
16. Total parenteral nutrition (2)   44
17. Postoperative pyrexia   44
18. Management of breathlessness   45
19. Nutritional management (3)   45
20. Complications of enteral feeding   46

Answers   47

QUESTIONS

1. Postoperative fluid therapy (1)

A 70 kg patient is 1 day following total hip replacement. He has not started eating and drinking. He is being rehydrated with dextrose/saline (4% dextrose and 0.18% saline). Which one of the following best describes this type of fluid therapy?

    A. It is an inappropriate fluid therapy for a postoperative patient
    B. It contains 120 mmol of Na$^+$ ions
    C. Potassium supplementation is not required
    D. Its osmolality is almost isotonic with plasma (286 mOsm/kg)
    E. It has a pH of 7.35   *only for Post-op*

2. Intravenous access in the trauma patient

A 22-year-old man is admitted following a stab injury to the right groin. He is bleeding profusely from the wound. His blood pressure is 80/40 mmHg and his pulse is 140 beats/min. He is agitated and mildly confused. His skin is cool and mottled. In this scenario, which is the best mode of fluid delivery? *hypotensive shock II*

    A. Left subclavian central line
    B. Long saphenous vein cut down
    C. Right internal jugular approach central line
    D. Left femoral long line
    E. Two wide-bore cannulae inserted bilaterally to the antecubital fossae *: wide vessels*

3. Intravenous fluid management in the trauma patient

For the patient described in Question 2, which one of the following statements regarding fluid resuscitation is most correct?

    A. Hartmann's solution should not be used
    B. The best fluid replacement is cross-matched blood
    C. It is mandatory to use colloid over crystalloid
    D. Colloids are preferable to expand the intracellular volume
    E. Crystalloids should be avoided as they may cause anaphylaxis

4. Fluid and nutrition management

A 40-year-old man weighing approximately 70 kg is being kept nil by mouth due to small bowel obstruction. He is afebrile at 36.7 °C. Which of the following regimens best describe the patient's requirements over the first 24 hours?

    A. 1–2 mmol/kg of sodium is required *: normal*
    B. 0.5–1 mmol/kg of potassium is required *: normal*

C. At least 100–1000 kcal/kg/day are required   30–40

D. 2700 mL of water is required   1– 2 L

E. None of the above

5. Postoperative fluid therapy (2)

A 68-year-old man is 6 days following open anterior resection with defunctioning ileostomy. The patient is afebrile at 36.7 °C. He is eating and drinking normally. The nursing staff informs you the stoma output is 3 L/day. His mucous membranes are dry and the patient feels thirsty. Which one of the following statements regarding fluid therapy is most correct? ✗

A. Continue to push oral fluids   he is dehydrated

B. 5% dextrose is most appropriate given nutritional content   doesn't have   Na

C. 0.9% normal saline with potassium supplementation is most appropriate

D. Potassium supplementation is not required

E. None of the above

6. Fluid balance management

A 59-year-old woman is admitted with central abdominal pain. Serum amylase is 1800 IU/L. Her initial Glasgow Coma Scale score is 4. You are asked to review her the next day as the nurses have noticed that her urine output has been just 15 mL in the past 3 hours. The rest of her observations are as follows:

Complicated
Pancreatitis

- Blood pressure = 105/45 mmHg   ↓
- Pulse = 113 beats/min   ↑
- Respiratory rate = 28 breaths/min
- Saturation 93% on 8 L of oxygen

On auscultation of her chest you hear widespread crepitations. What is the most appropriate next course of action?

A. Fluid restriction   : initial mgt

B. Colloid bolus

C. Furosemide   : toxic to   kidny

D. Transthoracic echocardiogram

E. Central line insertion   : to monitor ? ARDS
guide fluid mgt

7. Fluid resuscitation in the critically ill

The patient in Question 6 had a central line inserted and was transferred to the high-dependency unit. Her observations remained the same and in the last hour only 5 mL of urine is passed. Her saturations remain poor. Her central venous pressure initially is 11 cmH$_2$0. You attempt a fluid bolus of 250 mL of colloid, following which her central venous pressure increases and remains

normal
↳ (0 −5)

RUF

at 15 cmH$_2$O. Her urine output over the next hour is 10 mL. Which one of the following statements is the most correct?

- A. This patient is septic
- B. Noradrenaline is the next most appropriate step
- C. A further fluid bolus is warranted
- Ⓓ This patient has left ventricular failure
- E. This patient will require dialysis

8. Complications of blood transfusion

A 22-year-old patient is brought to the emergency department in class III shock following multiple penetrating stab injuries to the torso, chest and abdomen. He undergoes an emergency thoracotomy and laparotomy. In theatre, he requires a total of 30 units of blood. Which of the following is the best statement regarding complications of massive blood transfusion?

- A. Thrombocytosis is inevitable   ✓ Platelet
- B. Depletion of factor XI and X is a common problem   5,8
- Ⓒ Hypocalcaemia may ensue   citrate
- D. Hyperkalaemia is uncommon   ↑k common
- E. Hypothermia is rare   common

9. Colloid replacement in a postsurgical patient

A 70 kg, 56-year-old patient is 12 hours following a difficult colectomy for colorectal carcinoma. During the procedure, the patient experienced bleeding, which needed to be controlled with diathermy coagulation. You are asked to review the patient who has become increasingly unwell and is complaining of abdominal pain. Physical examination reveals marked left-sided tenderness. His pulse is 130/min and blood pressure is 80/40 mmHg. He is pale and clammy and the urine output is 15 mL for the last hour. His haemoglobin is 6.0 g/dL having been 13 g/dL preoperatively. You decide to start rehydration using Gelofusine colloid. Which one of the following is the most appropriate statement regarding fluid resuscitation in this patient?

- A. Colloid is a useful fluid therapy as it rapidly enters the intercellular compartment
- B. Colloid decreases the plasma oncotic pressure
- C. Colloid is less likely than crystalloid to induce allergic reactions
- D. Colloids are better than crystalloids as they are of low molecular weight
- Ⓔ Colloid should be changed for blood as soon as is possible

10. Hartmann's solution

You are called to review a 70 kg, 60-year-old man who is 2 days following an emergency laparotomy for adhesion-related small bowel obstruction (adhesiolysis).

Close to physiological

He is currently being infused with Hartmann's solution (Ringer's lactate). Which one of the following statements regarding this type of fluid therapy is most appropriate?

    A. It contains more sodium than normal 0.9% saline solution
    B. It does not contain bicarbonate
    C. 3 L contains sufficient K+ ions for this patient
    D. It has a composition that is closer to plasma than dextrose saline
    E. None of the above

11. Hyponatraemia

You have been asked to see a 72-year-old Caucasian woman who is 52 hours following uncomplicated laparoscopic cholecystectomy for gallstone disease. She was found unconscious on the ward with generalized tonic-clonic seizures, requiring 20 mg diazepam. Her sodium level is 112 mmol/L. During surgery she received 3 L of 5% dextrose with 20 mmol/L potassium chloride. Her potassium and urea and creatinine are within normal limits. There are no signs of heart failure. Her plasma osmolality is 265 mOsm/kg and her urinary osmolality is 566 mOsm/kg. Which of the following is the most likely cause for her low sodium?

Plasma Osm ↓
• Urine ,, ↑ ? / so the problem is not due to ↑ fluid given
• serum Na ↑

    A. Excess 5% dextrose
    B. Addison's disease → *K+ is increased*
    C. Syndrome of inappropriate antidiuretic hormone secretion
    D. Nephrotic syndrome ⎫ *edema*
    E. Congestive cardiac failure ⎭

12. Nutritional management (1)

A 45-year-old patient is 1 week following an attack of severe acute pancreatitis. He has been unable to start eating as this precipitates severe pain. Physical examination reveals a soft abdomen with epigastric tenderness. Bowel sounds are scanty. He is afebrile. His amylase in normal and C-reactive protein is 200 mg/L. Which of the following statements regarding management of nutrition is correct?

    A. No supplementary nutrition is required
    B. Total parenteral nutrition should be commenced *if enteral fails, cause sepsis*
    C. Nasogastric feeding should be commenced *→ results in high aspirates*
    D. Nasojejunal feeding should be commenced *→ delivers nutrition beyond the point*
    E. None of the above   *of small bowel ileus*

13. Complications of enteral nutrition

After a multidisciplinary review, a 55-year-old patient is commenced on enteral feeding. After 24 hours, he complained of severe diarrhoea. What is the most appropriate step in managing this patient?

Diarrhea – most common complication of enteral feeding.

A. Speed up enteral feed
B. Stop the enteral feed
C. Slow down the enteral feed
D. Continue the enteral feeding at current rate and exclude other causes
E. None of the above

14. Nutritional management (2)

Ileus

A 75-year-old Caucasian man is on the intensive care unit following an emergency Hartmann's procedure for an obstructing sigmoid carcinoma. He is currently 6 days post-procedure. His past history includes chronic obstructive pulmonary disease. The nursing staff report high nasogastric aspirates despite slow enteral feeding at 10 mL/hour. On examination, his abdomen is mildly distended, and generally tender with no peritonism. His stoma looks healthy, but has not started to work yet. His bowel sounds are absent. What is the best way to manage this patient's nutrition?

A. Continue nasogastric feeding
B. Site nasojejunal tube and start feeding
C. Commence total parenteral nutrition
D. Site a percutaneous gastrostomy tube → need functioning GI tract
E. None of the above

15. Total parenteral nutrition (1) → mostly lipids

A patient is commenced on total parenteral nutrition. You are asked by the nutrition team to ensure that adequate monitoring takes place. Which one of the following statements regarding monitoring of total parenteral nutrition is most correct?

A. Daily liver function tests – 2x a week
B. Weekly blood capillary glucose → should be daily
C. Monthly full blood count → daily due to ↑ risk of sepsis
D. There is no need to monitor phosphate → daily. Electrolyte disturbances common in TPN.
   → hypophosphatemia common.
E. None of the above

16. Total parenteral nutrition (2)

Which one of the following is the best statement regarding total parenteral nutrition?

A. The nutritional content should be specifically tailored to the patient rarely
B. Feed usually hypo-osmolar → hyper osmolar.
C. Contains 14 g of nitrogen as D-amino acids L– amino acids
D. Should be higher in glucose content versus lipid content lipids more
E. None of the above

17. Postoperative pyrexia

You are called to see a 50-year-old Asian man who has been receiving total parenteral nutrition for 6 days via his central line. He is 15 days following sub-total colectomy and ileostomy. The nursing staff is concerned as he appeared to have a rigor. He is febrile at 38.0 °C. His pulse rate is 100 beats/min, and his blood pressure is 130/70 mmHg. His lung bases sound quiet and his notes document that a urinary catheter was removed day 6 postoperatively. His abdomen is mildly tender with no signs of peritonism. Which of the following is the most likely source of sepsis?

A. Peritoneal collection → no s/s of peritonism
B. Central line sepsis
C. Respiratory tract infection — less likely 15d post op.
D. Urinary sepsis — usually 24-72h after removal of catheter
E. Contaminated total parenteral nutrition

18. Management of breathlessness

You are asked to see a 45-year-old African Caribbean female patient on the ward. She is approximately 30 minutes following the insertion of a left internal jugular vein catheter sited for total parenteral nutrition. A plain film chest radiograph has not yet been performed following the procedure. The nursing staff is concerned as the patient is breathless. On arrival, the patient's airway is patent, but she is breathless at rest. Her respiratory rate is 30 breaths/min. The trachea is central. Her pulse is 110 beats/min and blood pressure is 160/90 mmHg. There are reduced breath sounds on the left and the left chest is hyper-resonant to percussion. Select the most appropriate diagnosis and management strategy.

A. Tension pneumothorax; tube thoracostomy 5th intercostal space, anterior to mid-axillary line → tracheal deviation not present
B. Simple pneumothorax; tube thoracostomy 5th intercostal space, anterior to mid-axillary line
C. Chylothorax; immediate insertion of large-bore cannula, 2nd intercostal space, mid-clavicular line — not definitive Mx.
D. Tension pneumothorax; immediate needle thoracocentesis → no tracheal deviation
E. Haemothorax; tube thoracostomy 5th intercostal space, anterior to mid-axillary line

percussion will be dull.

19. Nutritional management (3)

A 30-year-old man is on the surgical ward following an assault resulting in severe head injury. The speech and language therapist is unhappy with the patient's swallow as he regurgitates fluid and is at risk of aspiration. Which of the following is the best long-term strategy for addressing this patient's nutritional requirements? → long term Nutrition

A. Nasogastric feeding
B. Nasojejunal feeding — not suitable for long term nutrition.
C. Percutaneous gastrostomy tube
D. Total parenteral nutrition
E. None of the above

→ GI tract functioning well, but oral intake not possible

20. Complications of enteral feeding

You are called to the ward to review a patient who is now 1 week into percutaneous endoscopic gastrostomy (PEG) feeding. The nursing staff is concerned because he grimaces when the feed is running, and has now developed a tachycardia. On examination, he is febrile at 38 °C, pulse is 110 beats/min, and blood pressure is 110/80 mmHg. The PEG site is clean and healthy. Physical examination reveals marked upper abdominal tenderness with guarding and rebound tenderness. Which of the following complications is most likely?

- A. Peritonitis from tube malplacement
- B. Perforation at time of insertion
- C. PEG tube infection
- D. Tube-related fistulation
- E. None of the above

ANSWERS

only for post op.

Postoperative fluid therapy (1)

1 D Its osmolality is almost isotonic with plasma (286 mOsm/kg)

Isotonic
Alkaline
30 mmol

Dextrose/saline is a useful fluid therapy in the early postoperative period because it does not cause salt and water overload and provides some energy to the patient. Dextrose/saline solution, otherwise known as one-fifth normal saline, has an osmolality that is nearly isotonic with plasma because of the 4% content of dextrose. It has a slightly alkaline pH and contains approximately 30 mmol of sodium and chloride ions. It does not contain K^+ ions and so potassium supplementation is important if the patient is not yet established on oral intake. It predominantly replaces pure water losses that are common following surgery. It is less useful in hypovolaemic resuscitation as it is a less effective plasma expander than colloid or normal saline and in patients who are losing excess salts.

Intravenous access in the trauma patient

2 E Two wide-bore cannulae inserted bilaterally to the antecubital fossae

Optimal fluid volume delivery is through large-bore access achieved with cannulae inserted into the antecubital fossae. Central lines (answers A and C) are generally long conduits with narrow lumens and are therefore less effective at delivering large volumes to hypotensive trauma patients. The same is true of long lines inserted through a femoral approach. It may be necessary to perform a long saphenous venous cut-down, but this approach should be reserved for patients where attempts to obtain standard peripheral venous access have failed.

Intravenous fluid management in the trauma patient

3 B The best fluid replacement is cross-matched blood

This patient has sustained a significant vascular injury and is in class III shock. During resuscitation, the guiding principle is that the best form of fluid therapy is to replace 'like with like'. Since he is continuing to lose blood, cross-matched blood would be the best form of fluid replacement. The transfusion should be started while arrangements are made for emergency exploration and repair of the injury.

Two litres of warmed Hartmann's is the ATLS standard initial resuscitation fluid given as first line therapy for trauma patients. Colloids are useful fluid therapy in hypotensive trauma patients when blood is not immediately available as they expand the intravascular compartment, but they are used following initial crystalloid therapy. Crystalloids rarely induce allergic reactions, although colloids have been known to.

Fluid and nutrition management

4 E   None of the above

Despite the question stating that the patient has no overt fluid losses, this patient is likely to have significant covert losses. Patients with small bowel obstruction sequester huge volumes of fluid within their bowel (so called 'third space losses'). In addition, the fluid lost into the bowel will be salt rich.

Typical daily requirements for a normal, healthy adult are approximately 1–2.5 L of water, with 1–2 mmol/kg of sodium and 0.5–1 mmol/kg of potassium. The requirements of this patient are far likely to exceed this. In terms of energy requirements in this patient, in the absence of sepsis 30–40 kcal/kg/day should be sufficient. Therefore, none of the options are correct.

In patients such as this, the best fluid regimen would be 0.9% normal saline (150 mmol/L Na) with 20–40 mmol potassium chloride added to each litre bag. The rate of fluid therapy should be titrated to vital signs and findings on serial examinations. Additional electrolyte supplementation is often necessary, and this should be guided by serial blood tests.

Postoperative fluid therapy (2)

5 C   0.9% normal saline with potassium supplementation is most appropriate

This patient is losing salt-rich fluid. Ileal fluid contains approximately 130 mmol/L Na$^+$, 110 mmol/L Cl$^-$ and 10 mmol/L K$^+$. The most appropriate therapy would be 0.9% normal saline with potassium supplementation. Continuing to push oral fluids is likely to exacerbate losses from a high output ileostomy, worsening dehydration. Five per cent dextrose does not contain the required composition of sodium and chloride ions, and is not preferred in this setting.

Fluid balance management

6 E   Central line insertion

This scenario describes a presentation of severe pancreatitis. Pancreatitis is a systemic inflammatory insult; this patient has a Glasgow Coma Scale score of 4 indicating her disease is severe. These patients often present appearing surprisingly well; however, this patient should be expected to deteriorate quickly in the subsequent 24–72 hours. The initial priority in managing acute pancreatitis is fluid resuscitation; losses in pancreatitis are considerable and can be divided into external (vomiting, reduced intake, sweating) and internal. Internal loss is often far greater, comprising pooling within the gastrointestinal tract following ileus and intercellular loss; the 'cytokine storm' which results from pancreatitis increases the permeability of tissues, particularly in the retroperitoneum and lung parenchyma. This is problematic as these insensible losses cannot be measured or reliably estimated.

This patient has evidence of ALI, a complication of systemic inflammation broadly similar to acute respiratory distress syndrome. The injured lung is increasingly susceptible to fluid overload. In addition, without invasive monitoring, it is impossible to reliably differentiate between the effects of ALI and cardiac failure. This patient requires a central line to guide fluid management as a matter of urgency. A further bolus at this time may further compromise respiratory function and fluid restriction would exacerbate the acute renal injury. There is no evidence that furosemide in these circumstances improves outcome of renal failure; furosemide itself is toxic to the renal system and its administration would only deplete intravascular volume further. This patient needs an echocardiogram, but central monitoring and guided fluid resuscitation takes priority.

Acute lung injury [handwritten margin note]

Fluid resuscitation in the critically ill

7 D This patient has left ventricular failure

The placement of a central line was well conceived; a sustained rise in CVP following fluid bolus is indicative of a fluid overloaded system. This patient almost certainly has left ventricular failure and a cause of this should be sought. This scenario is unusual, however; the majority of low blood pressure and oliguria encountered in acute pancreatitis will be due to hypovolaemia; this question is purely designed to assess a candidate's understanding of CVP monitoring.

if CVP ↑
→ Fluid overload
or Cardiac failure [handwritten margin notes]

The CVP depends on the venous return to the great veins and the efficiency of the cardiac pump. Increased CVP indicates either an expanded circulating volume or cardiac failure. Causes of non-cardiac pulmonary oedema would not increase the CVP. There is no defined 'normal range' for CVP and therefore a one-off reading is not useful. A reading before and after a fluid challenge is of more use; if the CVP remains unchanged, then the patient is hypovolaemic. A rise of 2–4 cmH$_2$O which reverses after around 30 minutes indicates the patient is approximately euvolaemic. A sustained rise of >5 cmH$_2$O is indicative of overload or cardiac failure.

Complications of blood transfusion

8 C Hypocalcaemia may ensue

Massive blood transfusion is defined as the replacement of an individual's entire circulating volume (>10 units) within 24 hours. Such large transfusions are associated with specific complications, which occur in addition to standard transfusion reactions. These complications occur due to inherent differences between stored blood and blood in circulation.

Stored blood is deficient in platelets and clotting factors (V and VII), the function of which declines rapidly while the blood is in storage. Patients receiving large transfusions should therefore receive additional platelets and cryoprecipitate in order to avoid disseminated intravascular coagulation and transfusion-related haemorrhage. Most centres have their own established massive transfusion protocol. In addition, blood is stored below body temperature, and therefore people receiving large transfusions have commonly become hypothermic.

Electrolyte disturbance is also common; stored blood has a high potassium content. Post-transfusion potassium overload is a common problem. Transfusion in dialysis dependant renal failure is particularly hazardous. Hypocalcaemia results from the use of the anticoagulant citrate in stored blood. Citrate binds calcium ions and in doing so prevents coagulation. Its anticoagulant effects are reversed when stored blood enters the circulation and the clotting factors are exposed to serum calcium. However, in massive transfusion the citrate load may overwhelm the body's circulating calcium, causing hypocalcaemia.

Colloid replacement in a postsurgical patient

9 E Colloid should be changed for blood as soon as is possible
This patient is most likely experiencing reactionary haemorrhage. Therefore, colloid should be changed for blood as soon as is possible. Inevitably, there will be some delay obtaining cross-matched blood so O-negative blood should be obtained if possible. Colloids are often used as a bridge to transfusion while cross-matched blood is prepared. Cross-matched samples should be obtained prior to starting colloids since colloids can interfere with the cross-matching process.

Colloids have high molecular weights and do not readily diffuse across semipermeable membranes. Colloids are therefore thought to be more efficient at expanding the intravascular compartment when compared with crystalloid solutions. One disadvantage is that colloids are more likely to cause allergic/anaphylactic reactions.

Hartmann's solution

10 D It has a composition that is closer to the plasma than dextrose saline
Hartmann's solution contains:

- $Na^+ = 131$ mmol/L
- $Cl^- = 111$ mmol/L
- $HCO_3^- = 29$ mmol/L

- $K^+ = 5$ mmol/L
- $Ca^{2+} = 2$ mmol/L
- Lactate $= 29$ mmol/L

Hartmann's solution is designed to more closely resemble the electrolyte composition of plasma than normal saline or dextrose/saline fluids. It is extremely useful in the replacement of pure plasma losses in trauma and acute haemorrhage and is the first-choice resuscitation fluid according to current ATLS guidance. It contains a lower level of sodium ions than 0.9% normal saline (150 mmol/L) and also a lower level of chloride ions. Its pH is close to that of plasma due to the lactate and bicarbonate ion content.

Hartmann's solution is less useful in the provision of maintenance fluids and electrolytes, particularly when the patient is experiencing excessive salt losses. Unlike normal saline, it is not possible to increase the potassium content of the fluids. Three litres of Hartmann's would only provide 15 mmol/L of potassium; the daily requirement of potassium for an average adult is 0.5–1 mmol/L/kg and therefore 15 mmol/L would not be an adequate maintenance dose for this patient, especially in the presence of small bowel obstruction.

Hyponatraemia

11 C Syndrome of inappropriate antidiuretic hormone secretion
The SIADH consists of hyponatraemia, inappropriately elevated urine osmolality (>200 mOsm/kg), excessive urine sodium excretion (urinary Na >30 mEq/L), and decreased serum osmolality. These findings occur in a euvolaemic patient without signs of oedema. The hyponatraemia is a result of excess water and not a sodium deficiency. Therefore, treatment is fluid restriction. Excess 5% dextrose can cause hyponatraemia, but will not result in inappropriately concentrated urine. The electrolyte changes that accompany Addison's disease include an elevated plasma K^+ level. Nephrotic syndrome and congestive cardiac failure usually give rise to oedema.

Nutritional management (1)

12 D Nasojejunal feeding should be commenced
Published studies have shown that over 30% of all hospital inpatients are malnourished and that a poor nutritional state protracts recovery, increases the incidence of complications and prolongs admission. As a general rule, enteral feeding is preferable to TPN in all patients; IV nutrition should be the reserve of patients in whom enteral feeding is impossible or has failed. This is because of the risk of sepsis, thrombus,

metabolic imbalance and lipid overload (over 50% of calories in TPN are provided by lipids) as well as the negative effects of prolonged disuse of the alimentary tract.

Nasojejunal feeding has the greatest chance of successfully supplementing nutritional requirements as enteral feeding is delivered beyond the upper small bowel ileus. Nasogastric feeding is likely to result in high aspirate volumes. Total parenteral nutrition may be required if enteral feeding fails.

Complications of enteral nutrition

13 C Slow down the enteral feed
Diarrhoea is the commonest complication of enteral feeding, occurring in 2%–63% of patients depending on the definition. Diarrhoea may respond to slowing down the rate of enteral feeding. Concurrently concomitant causes (e.g. antibiotic therapy) should be identified and modified. Other strategies include switching to nutritional regimens that contain higher fibre content.

Nutritional management (2)

14 C Commence total parenteral nutrition
Prolonged ileus is not uncommon following major abdominal surgery for obstruction. Continuing nasogastric feeding is unlikely to be successful. Nasojejunal feeding is a useful route for ensuring enteral nutrition in patients with upper small bowel ileus in conditions such as acute pancreatitis. However, this patient is an ideal candidate for short-term total parenteral nutrition, which should continue until the ileus resolves, whereupon the patient should be re-established on oral intake. Percutaneous endoscopic gastrostomy tubes are useful in patients who have a functioning gastrointestinal tract, but where oral feeding is considered unsafe or not possible (e.g. patients with swallowing insufficiency following cerebrovascular accident).

Total parenteral nutrition (1)

15 E None of the above
Blood glucose should be monitored daily as hyper/hypoglycaemia is common on total parenteral nutrition regimens. Electrolyte disturbance is also common and therefore urea, creatinine, potassium, sodium, magnesium and phosphate levels must also be checked daily. Hypophosphataemia is a particular problem with TPN and additional supplementation is almost always required. There is significant risk of sepsis, therefore daily FBC is also required.

Daily weights should be taken, along with meticulous fluid balance charting. Liver function tests should be performed twice weekly to monitor any sign of cholestatic jaundice and fatty infiltration.

Total parenteral nutrition (2)

16 E   None of the above

Total parenteral nutrition is rarely tailored to the specific individual. The feed is usually hyper-osmolar, which means that a dedicated large central feeding line is required. Usually, the feed contains 14 g of nitrogen as L-amino acids. The lipid content is usually higher than the glucose content, as the latter is converted to CO_2 resulting in more respiratory work for an acutely ill surgical patient.

Postoperative pyrexia

17 B   Central line sepsis

This patient is at high risk of central line sepsis. This should be considered as a source in any patient who develops a sepsis with a central venous catheter *in situ*, especially if there are local signs and symptoms. This risk is far greater in individuals who are receiving TPN through their central line; TPN is the perfect media for bacterial growth. Ideally central lines should be changed every 5 days. If a line is being used for TPN, a dedicated port should be allocated solely for this purpose to minimize risk of colonization. In this case, blood cultures should be sent from both the line and a peripheral site, the line should be removed and the tip sent for microbiological culture.

Anastomotic leakage should always be considered and excluded, but is less likely in patients who have a stoma and in the absence of peritonism. Basal atelectasis and lower respiratory tract infection commonly complicate major abdominal surgery, especially if abdominal pain limits tidal volume and expectoration, but are decreasingly likely 15 days postoperatively. Urinary tract infection should be excluded, but is unlikely to be the cause in this patient; catheter associated UTIs typically occur within 24–72 hours following removal.

Management of breathlessness

18 B   Simple pneumothorax; tube thoracostomy 5th intercostal space, anterior to mid-axillary line

This patient has the features of a simple pneumothorax secondary to CVP line insertion. The appropriate management is to insert a tube thoracostomy in the 5th intercostal space, just anterior to the mid-axillary line. Tension pneumothorax should be suspected in the presence of trachea deviation and signs of impaired venous return, but these do not feature in this scenario. Haemothorax and chylothorax can also complicate CVP access, but are unlikely in the absence of a dull percussion note.

Nutritional management (3)

19 C Percutaneous gastrostomy tube
This patient's gastrointestinal tract is functioning normally, but the oral route is not an option. This is an ideal patient for a percutaneous gastrostomy tube. Nasogastric and nasojejunal feeding and total parenteral nutrition are not suitable long-term strategies.

Complications of enteral feeding

20 A Peritonitis from tube malplacement
This patient has signs of peritonitis secondary to misplacement of the feeding tube. The tachycardia, pyrexia and abdominal guarding with rebound tenderness are all suggestive of an infective peritonitis. In addition, marked abdominal tenderness while the feed is running indicates that the abdominal cavity is being irritated by the feed content which makes option (A) more likely than option (B).

SECTION 4:
ANAESTHETICS AND
SURGICAL CRITICAL CARE

Questions

1.	Stages of anaesthesia	56
2.	Uses of a central venous cannula	56
3.	Difficulty breathing	56
4.	Postoperative acute confusion	57
5.	Abdominal aortic aneurysm repair	57
6.	Shortness of breath	57
7.	Tension pneumothorax	58
8.	ASA grading	58
9.	Head injury	58
10.	Preoperative starvation	59
11.	Thyroid storm	59
12.	Hypokalaemia	59
13.	Disseminated intravascular coagulation	60
14.	The oxygen dissociation curve	60
15.	Cardiac tamponade	60
16.	Acute respiratory distress syndrome	60
17.	Acute hypocalcaemia	61
18.	Nutrition	61
19.	Gram negative bacteria	61
20.	Sepsis	62
21.	Lactic acidosis	62
22.	Respiratory failure	62
23.	Local anaesthetic	62
24.	Aortic dissection	63
25.	Intraoperative complication	63

Answers | 64

QUESTIONS

1. Stages of anaesthesia

You are observing a 45-year-old female being prepared for induction of anaesthesia for a laparoscopic cholecystectomy. You discuss the stages of anaesthesia with the Consultant anaesthetist. From the list below, select the answer corresponding to the correct number of stages of anaesthesia.

     A.   1   *Induction → slowly lose conscioumess*
     B.   2   *Excitation phase → full loss but involuntary movement present*
     C.   3   *'Surgical anethesia phase → skeletal muscles relax, pt ready for surgery*
     D.   4   *Overdose phase: received too much.*
     E.   5

2. Uses of a central venous cannula

You see a patient on the Intensive Care Unit who has been admitted with severe pancreatitis. He is having a central venous catheter inserted for intravenous fluid monitoring. Other than using a central venous cannula to measure central venous pressure during fluid resuscitation, from the list below choose the answer which correctly describes a long-term use of a central venous cannula.

     A.   Haemodialysis
     B.   Total parenteral nutrition   *Longterm*
     C.   Pulmonary artery catheterisation
     D.   Drug administration
     E.   Transvenous cardiac pacing

short term

3. Difficulty breathing

A 57-year-old lady is post total thyroidectomy for thyromegaly with retrosternal extension. During the transfer of the patient from theatre to recovery, she develops shortness of breath. The patient is alert and speaking in complete sentences. Her respiratory rate is 20 breaths per minute, pulse is 90 beats per minute and blood pressure is 115/75 mmHg. Oxygen saturations have decreased from 98% on 2 litres of oxygen per minute to 92%. On examination of the chest, there is decreased expansion of the right hemithorax and ipsilateral reduced air entry and hyper-resonance. From the list below, choose the most appropriate step to take in this patient's management.

     A.   Increase the oxygen delivery to 4 litres/min via a nasal cannula
     B.   Request a chest radiograph
     C.   Increase the oxygen delivery to 12–15 litres/min via a non-rebreathe facemask
     D.   Re-open the collar incision to evacuate the haematoma
     E.   Insertion of a right-sided chest drain

(it is not tension pneumothorax)

X **4. Postoperative acute confusion**

An otherwise well 57-year-old male is 45 minutes post transurethral resection of the prostate gland for benign prostatic hyperplasia. The procedure was
performed under general anaesthesia and lasted one and a half hours. You are
asked to see the patient due to the fact that he has become acutely confused
and drowsy. Initial observation showed an oxygen saturation of 98% on 2
litres of oxygen per minute, respiratory rate of 18 breaths per minute, pulse
rate of 40 beats per minute, blood pressure of 90/70 mmHg and temperature
of 37.3 °C. From the list below, choose the most likely cause for this patient's
deterioration.

hypotension
bradycardia

A.   Sepsis
B.   Hypervolaemia
C.   Hypovolaemia
D.   Microcytic anaemia
E.   Hyperthermia

* Complication of TURP.
TURP Syndrome : absorption of
Irrigation fluid (glycine)

* Hypervolemia, bradycardia
dyspnea, ↑ confusion

5. Abdominal aortic aneurysm repair

You are asked to see a 67-year-old man who is 10 hours post open abdominal
aortic aneurysm repair. His oxygen saturations are 97% on 3 litres of oxygen,
respiratory rate is 20 breaths per minute, pulse rate is 115 beats per minute, blood
pressure is 105/78 mmHg and body temperature is 37.2 °C. On assessment of his
fluid balance chart, you notice that the patient's urine output is low at 20 ml in
the last hour. From the list below, choose the most appropriate next step in this
patient's management.

A.   Increase the oxygen flow rate
B.   Speak with the Surgical Registrar in light of taking the patient back
     to theatre
C.   Administer an intravenous fluid bolus of 500 mls of normal saline
D.   Perform an arterial blood gas investigation
E.   Request an urgent mobile chest radiograph

6. Shortness of breath

You are asked to see an 80-year-old female patient who is 2 days post insertion
of a right dynamic hip screw following an extracapsular right neck of femur
fracture. She has become acutely short of breath with a respiratory rate of 28
breaths per minute. The oxygen saturations are 96% on 5 litres of oxygen per
minute. Her pulse rate is 120 beats per minute, blood pressure is 110/70 mmHg
and body temperature is 37 °C. Examination of the chest is normal. You perform an arterial blood gas investigation. From the list below, choose the most
likely type of acid–base disturbance you expect to see from the arterial blood
gas results.

* tachycardia
tachypnea → ↑ RR → ↑ CO_2 washed out.

    A.   Metabolic acidosis
    B.   Respiratory acidosis
    C.   Metabolic alkalosis
    D.   Respiratory alkalosis
    E.   Lactic acidosis

7. Tension pneumothorax

A 39-year-old lady is having a diagnostic laparoscopy to investigate her symptoms of right iliac fossa pain. The procedure lasts 50 minutes and following
the removal of the endotracheal tube, the patient is taken to the recovery room
where she develops sudden onset shortness of breath, tachycardia and hypotension. Following rapid assessment, she is found to have a tension pneumothorax
which is decompressed by needle thoracocentesis. From the list below, choose the
clinical sign which is not a feature of tension pneumothorax.

    A.   Tracheal deviation away from the affected side
    B.   Increased expansion on the affected side
    C.   Decreased breath sounds on the affected side
    D.   Hyper-resonance on the affected side
    E.   Distended neck veins

8. ASA grading

You see a 48-year-old man in the theatre admission lounge who is due for an
open abdominal incisional hernia repair. The anaesthetist tells you that a high
dependency unit bed has been booked for the patient owing to his co-morbidities
and will therefore require close monitoring following surgery. The anaesthetist
tells you that the patient falls under ASA 3. From the list below, choose the definition that best describes an ASA grading of 3.

    A.   A moribund patient who is not expected to survive without an
        operation
    B.   A patient with mild systemic disease
    C.   A normal healthy patient
    D.   A patient with severe systemic disease that is a constant threat to life
    E.   A patient with severe systemic disease

9. Head injury

You are asked to see a 35-year-old man who sustained a head injury during
a road traffic accident. The patient was stable upon arrival to the emergency
department, but over the last hour, his GCS has fallen from 15/15 to 13/15 and he
is now drowsy and complaining of a headache. From the list below, choose the
most appropriate next step to take in this patient's management.

    A.   Repeat the GCS score in an hour
    B.   Speak with the Neurosurgical Registrar on-call with a view to take
        the patient to theatre

C. Prescribe analgesia
D. Request an urgent CT scan of the head
E. Prescribe an intravenous infusion of mannitol

10. Preoperative starvation

You see an 18-year-old lady in the theatre admission lounge who is due to have a removal of a right breast fibroadenoma under general anaesthesia. You ask her whether she has had anything to eat or drink after midnight on the same day as the operation. From the list below, which of the following correctly applies to preoperative starvation in adults?

A. Patients should not eat solid food for 6 hours prior to a general anaesthetic
B. Patients may eat solid food up to 4 hours before a general anaesthetic
C. Patients should not eat solid food for 12 hours prior to a general anaesthetic
D. Patients may eat solid food up to 2 hours before a general anaesthetic
E. None of the above

11. Thyroid storm

A 56-year-old lady is having a total thyroidectomy for Graves' disease. During the operation she develops thyroid storm and the anaesthetist informs you that the patient has developed a tachycardia. From the list below, please choose a feature not likely to be associated with thyroid storm.

A. Hypothermia
B. Pyrexia
C. Cardiac arrhythmias
D. Cardiac failure
E. Coma

12. Hypokalaemia

You are reviewing the blood test results of a 50-year-old man who has been admitted following a crush injury to his right leg. His serum potassium is found to be low at 2.9 mmol/L following earlier correction of hyperkalaemia. You request an ECG for this patient. Which one of the following ECG changes is not characteristic of hypokalaemia?

A. Small and inverted T-waves
B. Small P-waves   → hyper kalemia
C. Prolonged P-R interval
D. S-T segment depression
E. Presence of U-waves

13. Disseminated intravascular coagulation

You review the coagulation blood investigations for a patient who has sustained 18% body surface area third-degree burns. PT and APTT are both prolonged. Your Consultant informs you that the patient has disseminated intravascular coagulation (DIC) and to request urgent blood products from Pathology. From the list below, please choose the most appropriate blood product that you would request from Pathology for the management of this clotting abnormality.

    A.   Albumin
    B.   Platelets
    C.   Protein C concentrate
    D.   Antithrombin III concentrate
    E.   Immunoglobulins

14. The oxygen dissociation curve

You are discussing basic oxygen physiology with the Intensive Care Consultant. He explains the physiology of the oxygen dissociation curve and the Bohr effect. From the list below, choose the answer that is characteristically seen in the Bohr effect.

    A. $\downarrow pCO_2$
    B. $\downarrow$ 2,3 BPG
    C. $\downarrow$ pH
    D. $\downarrow$ Temperature
    E.   None of the above

15. Cardiac tamponade

You review a patient on the ward who has suspected cardiac tamponade following insertion of a pacemaker. You are asked to perform a rapid initial assessment of the patient. Which one of the following clinical signs from the list below would you expect to see in a patient with cardiac tamponade?

    A.   Prominent first heart sound
    B.   Muffled heart sounds
    C.   Prominent second heart sound
    D.   Low jugular venous pressure
    E.   Hypertension

16. Acute respiratory distress syndrome

A 40-year-old man is admitted to the Intensive Care Unit following a diagnosis of severe pancreatitis. The patient develops acute respiratory distress syndrome. Which of the following is associated with the diagnostic criteria for ARDS?

A. Slow onset of symptoms
B. White cell count of $>9 \times 10^9$/L
C. Pulmonary capillary wedge pressure ≤ 18 mmHg
D. $PaO_2:FIO_2 >200$
E. Presence of bilateral pulmonary infiltrates on chest radiograph or CT

17. Acute hypocalcaemia

You are asked to see a patient one day post total thyroidectomy who has a serum calcium of 2.0 and is complaining of muscular cramps. Which of the following is the most appropriate next step in this patient's management?

A. Prescribe a bisphosphonate infusion
B. Prescribe calcitonin
C. Establish cardiac monitoring
D. Administer high dose steroids
E. Contact the Surgical Registrar in light of taking this patient back to theatre

18. Nutrition

You are assessing the nutritional status of a patient in the Intensive Care Unit who has been admitted with polytrauma. The Consultant has advised the team that this patient will require a period of total parenteral nutrition (TPN). You are discussing the essential elements which the TPN feed should contain. Which of the following is referred to as a fat-soluble vitamin involved in cell membrane stabilisation and retinal function?

A. Vitamin D
B. Vitamin B_1
C. Vitamin C
D. Vitamin A
E. Vitamin K

19. Gram negative bacteria

You are reviewing the blood culture results of a patient who was admitted to the Intensive Care Unit after developing septic shock post laparotomy for a diverticular perforation. The blood results reveal the presence of Gram negative bacteria. Which of the following is a Gram negative bacteria?

A. *Streptococcus pneumoniae*
B. *Neisseria meningitidis*
C. *Staphylococcus aureus*
D. *Streptococcus viridans*
E. *Clostridium botulinum*

20. Sepsis

You are asked to review a 45-year-old man who has been admitted following acute onset of epigastric pain. His initial observations reveal a pulse of 108 beats per minute, a blood pressure of 95/80 mmHg, a respiratory rate of 32 breaths per minute and a body temperature of 38.5 °C. You are asked to take a set of blood cultures. Which of the following is correct concerning blood cultures?

A. Aerobic and anaerobic blood cultures will only be positive in approximately 20% of patients with sepsis
B. Blood cultures should not be taken through in-dwelling central venous catheters
C. Antibiotic therapy should commence prior to taking blood cultures
D. Results from blood cultures can be obtained is less than an hour from time of analysis
E. None of the above

21. Lactic acidosis

You perform an arterial blood gas investigation on the patient in Question 20. The results show a pH of 7.31, pO_2 11.5, pCO_2 4.1 kPa, bicarbonate 24 mmol/L and lactate 6.0. Which of the following is not a cause of lactic acidosis?

A. Pancreatitis
B. Excessive exercise
C. Pyloric stenosis
D. Septic shock
E. Biguanides

22. Respiratory failure

You are asked to review a 30-year-old man who has sustained chest trauma. He has a pO_2 of 7.9 kPa and a pCO_2 of 7.0 kPa. From his arterial blood gas reading (taken on 5 L O_2 per minute), this patient has type 2 respiratory failure. Which of the following is not associated with type 2 (hypercapnic) respiratory failure?

A. Pulmonary embolism
B. Raised intracranial pressure
C. Poliomyelitis
D. Phrenic nerve injury
E. Myaesthenia gravis

23. Local anaesthetic

A 25-year-old lady, weighing 65 Kg, is having a sebaceous cyst excised from her mid back. You are asked to infiltrate local anaesthetic around the area before the sebaceous cyst can be removed. Which of the following is the maximum safe dose of lidocaine that can be used before it reaches toxic levels?

A. 250 mg
B. 200 mg
C. 195 mg
D. 160 mg
E. 120 mg

24. Aortic dissection

You are asked to review a chest radiograph of a 67-year-old lady who has been admitted with suspected aortic dissection. Which of the following chest radio-graph procedures is not associated with aortic dissection?

A. Widened mediastinum
B. Depression of the left main bronchus
C. Displacement of the 'aortic knuckle'
D. Haemothorax
E. Loss of the right heart border — indicates pathology in R middle lobe of Lung.

25. Intraoperative complication

A 45-year-old lady is having an elective wide local excision of a right breast carcinoma followed by right axillary sentinel node biopsy under general anaes-thesia. After 2–3 minutes of injecting the blue dye at the breast tumour site, you notice that the skin overlying the patient's chest has become erythematous. The anaesthetist alerts the surgeon that the patient has become tachycardic. Which of the following is the most appropriate next step to take in the anaesthetised patient?

A. Administer intravenous chlorpheniramine → stabilize first *
B. Maintaining intravascular volume with intravenous fluids
C. Endotracheal tube removal and waking the patient
D. Continue with the surgery as this is not a serious condition
E. Administer intravenous hydrocortisone

Stabilize patient first

no need → It is elective

ANSWERS

Stages of anaesthesia

1 D 4

There are four stages of anaesthesia (classified by Arthur Ernest Guedel):

Stage 1 refers to induction of anaesthesia whereby patients begin to slowly lose consciousness.

Stage 2 is called the excitement stage where there is complete loss of consciousness, but there may be uncontrolled movement.

Stage 3 is call the surgical anaesthesia phase whereby the skeletal muscles begin to relax and eye movement stops. The patient is now ready for surgery.

Stage 4 is the overdose phase, whereby the patient has received too much medication resulting in severe brain stem or medullary depression leading to subsequent hypotension or circulatory failure. Stage 4 can be fatal and requires prompt clinical support and close monitoring.

Uses of a central venous cannula

2 B Total parenteral nutrition

The short-term uses of a central venous cannula include CVP measurements, pulmonary artery catheterisation, fluid resuscitation, drug administration (e.g. inotropes, potassium amiodarone, etc.), haemodialysis and transvenous cardiac pacing.

The long-term uses include feeding by total parenteral nutrition, long-term venous blood sampling using, for example, a Hickman line and cytotoxic drug administration.

Difficulty breathing

3 C Increase the oxygen delivery to 12–15 litres/min via a non-rebreathe facemask

From the clinical history and examination, this patient is having an acute onset of shortness of breath secondary to a right pneumothorax. This is not a tension pneumothorax because there are no signs of haemodynamic compromise. Furthermore, the airway is patent because the patient is able to speak in complete sentences and therefore an upper airway obstruction secondary to a surgical wound haematoma is unlikely here.

The immediate management of an acutely ill surgical patient should follow a sequence of

- Airway (A) assessment and treatment
- Breathing (B) assessment and treatment
- Circulation (C) assessment and treatment
- Dysfunction (D) of the CNS; neurological status can be assessed rapidly by examining the pupils as well as using the 'AVPU' system (A – alert, V – responds to verbal stimulus, P – responds to pain and U – unresponsive to any stimulus)
- Exposure (E) of the patient sufficient for full assessment and treatment

Although the definitive treatment for this patient is to insert a chest drain, using the 'ABCDE' system, the patient has decreased oxygen saturations despite receiving 2 litres of oxygen per minute. She therefore requires high flow oxygen in aid of increasing oxygen saturations. Nasal cannula are used to deliver oxygen at low flow rates of up to 5 litres per minute. In the initial stages of her management this patient requires high flow oxygen delivery and this will be achieved using 10–15 litres of oxygen per minute using a non-rebreathe facemask.

Postoperative acute confusion

4 B   Hypervolaemia

The clinical history, combined with the nature of the surgical procedure and the onset of symptoms, point towards TURP syndrome, which occurs following absorption of excess irrigation fluid (mostly glycine). This condition is characterised by an increase in intravascular volume, dilutional hyponatraemia, intracellular oedema and metabolism of glycine to ammonia. Clinical signs include bradycardia or arrhythmias, hypertension followed by hypotension, dyspnoea, visual disturbance, and mental irritation leading to reduced levels of consciousness.

In summary, following initial resuscitation protocol, the management of TURP syndrome involves slow correction of the hyponatraemia with diuretics; the use of hypertonic saline is controversial. In addition, close patient monitoring (for coagulopathy, electrolyte disturbances, hypothermia and arrhythmias) is required and therefore, the intensive care and surgical teams should be involved as soon as possible.

Sepsis is possible, but unlikely given the history. The patient is not hyperthermic owing to a normal body temperature and it is unlikely for the patient to have a microcytic anaemia causing his acute deterioration.

Abdominal aortic aneurysm repair

5 C   Administer an intravenous fluid bolus of 500 ml of normal saline

Hypovolaemia is not uncommon in elderly patients who have had major surgical procedures. The elevated pulse rate coupled with a reduced blood pressure and low urine output suggests that the patient is hypo-volaemic. Following the 'ABCDE' system (please refer to Question 3 in this chapter for further information), increasing this patient's supplemental oxygen flow rate is not an unreasonable step to take; however, the patient is maintaining adequate oxygen saturations on 3 litres of oxygen per minute. This question points towards a 'C' (circulation) problem which requires treatment and re-evaluation.

Calling the Surgical Registrar, performing an arterial blood gas and requesting an urgent mobile chest radiograph are steps which may need to be taken in the future, but initially this patient requires an intravenous fluid challenge to ascertain whether the urine output increases. In most cases this type of problem can be corrected with adequate intravenous fluid resuscitation but care must be taken in patients who have cardiac and pulmonary co-morbidities. The use of fluid balance charts is imperative in patients who have undergone major surgery.

Shortness of breath

6 D Respiratory alkalosis

This patient is suffering from an acute pulmonary embolism owing to the acute onset of shortness of breath, low oxygen saturations and normal chest examination. The electrocardiogram shows a sinus tachycardia, which is more frequently seen in pulmonary embolism than the traditionally taught prominent S wave in lead 1, Q wave and an inverted T wave in lead 3 ('S1Q3T3'). → not usually seen.

The patient is tachypnoeic which will result in a decreased blood concentration of carbon dioxide leading to hypocapnia. The decreased levels of carbon dioxide will lead to a decreased concentration of hydrogen ions resulting in an alkalosis. In addition, the level of bicarbonate is usually normal in the acute phase. Respiratory alkalosis is therefore the acid–base disturbance which would occur in this scenario.

Tension pneumothorax

7 B Increased expansion on the affected side

Clinical features of tension pneumothorax include respiratory distress, a rise in the jugular venous pressure (which manifests as distended neck veins), tracheal deviation away from the affected side, ipsilateral decreased breath sounds, ipsilateral decreased expansion and ipsilateral hyper-resonance.

ASA grading

8 E   A patient with severe systemic disease

The ASA grading system, created by the American Society of Anaesthisologists, has been adopted to stratify patients' preoperative physical status. There are six grades:

ASA – 1: A normal healthy patient
ASA – 2: A patient with mild systemic disease
ASA – 3: A patient with severe systemic disease
ASA – 4: A patient with severe systemic disease that is a constant threat to life
ASA – 5: A moribund patient who is not expected to survive without the operation
ASA – 6: A declared brain-dead patient whose organs are being removed for donor purposes

If there is an addition of an 'E' next to the grade, this implies that the patient is having emergency surgery. The 'E' is not used for ASA grade 6.

Head injury

9 D   Request an urgent CT scan of the head

This patient has sustained a head injury causing a decrease in the level of his consciousness. This scenario warrants concern and the patient requires urgent attention. Before the patient can be discussed with the Neurosurgery team, urgent imaging of the head would be required in order to ascertain whether this patient has an intracranial bleed. Situations where a CT head scan would be performed are (1) persisting neurological signs following resuscitation, (2) persisting headache or vomiting, (3) falling level of consciousness, (4) suspicion of a base of skull fracture and (5) suspected penetrating injury.

Repeating the GCS in an hour and prescribing analgesia for the patient are not appropriate here and just unnecessarily delay the time for the patient to receive definitive management.

Prescribing an intravenous mannitol infusion could be performed once a diagnosis is made of elevated intracranial pressure secondary to a mass-effect-causing intracerebral bleed.

Preoperative starvation

10 A   Patients should not eat solid food for 6 hours prior to a general anaesthetic

The American Society of Anaesthesiologists (ASA) and the Association of Anaesthetists of Great Britain and Ireland (AAGBI) have recommended that for adults solids and liquids should not be consumed by patients undergoing elective surgical procedures involving general anaesthesia or sedation for 6 and 2 hours respectively, prior to their surgical procedure. In addition, patients having regional or local anaesthetic procedures should follow the same 'nil by mouth' policy as those scheduled for a general anaesthetic.

For patients undergoing emergency surgical procedures that involve a general anaesthetic, nasogastric aspiration is usually performed to decrease gastric contents and hence reduce the risk of pulmonary aspiration.

Thyroid storm

11 A   Hypothermia

Thyroid storm, also known as thyrotoxic crisis, is an acute rare manifestation of hyperthyroidism, which may be precipitated by stress, surgery and infection. There is a sudden release of thyroid hormones such as thyroxine (T4) and/or triiodothyronine (T3) into the systemic circulation. This leads to an exaggerated thyrotoxicosis manifestation, the features of which include hyperventilation, tachycardia, fever, agitation, dehydration, shock, cardiac arrhythmias, cardiac failure and coma; it can be fatal if not managed promptly. This condition is seen most commonly in patients who have thyrotoxicosis secondary to Graves' disease.

Hypokalaemia

12 B   Small P-waves

Hypokalaemia is a serum potassium level of less than 3.5 mmol/L. ECG characteristics include S-T segment depression, a prolonged P-R interval, small and inverted T-waves and U-waves, which are seen following the T-wave.

ECG changes associated with hyperkalaemia include wide QRS-complexes, small P-waves and tall, tented T-waves.

Disseminated intravascular coagulation

13 B   Platelets

DIC occurs as a result of pathological activation of the coagulation pathway by damaged tissues (e.g. in trauma, sepsis, burns, hypothermia) which release tissue factors and cytokines leading to activation of the fibrinolytic pathway. This results in widespread intravascular occlusion in small and large vessels. Vascular occlusion by fibrin causes shock and end organ failure whilst high consumption of clotting factors and platelets increases the bleeding tendency.

From this list of answers platelets (Answer B) would be the most appropriate blood product to request. In DIC the platelet count may fall due to rapid consumption of the latter as well as fresh frozen plasma (which contains factors II, V, VII, IX, X and XI).

Albumin and immunoglobulins are not clotting substitutes and therefore would not be required in this clinical scenario.

Protein C concentrate is given to patients who are predisposed to venous thrombotic disease and have a congenital protein C deficiency.

Antithrombin III is usually administered to patients with a congenital antithrombin III deficiency which is associated with recurrent venous thrombosis and pulmonary embolism.

The oxygen dissociation curve

14 C ↓pH

The Bohr effect is a shift of the oxygen dissociation curve to the right as a result of a reduction in the oxygen affinity of haemoglobin. This leads to a greater tendency of haemoglobin to offload oxygen into the tissues. A shift of the oxygen dissociation curve to the right is caused by an increase in temperature, acidity (i.e. a decrease in pH), 2,3 BPG (2,3-Bisphosphoglycerate; an organophosphate which is produced as a product of glycolysis in erythrocytes) and in the circulating partial pressure of carbon dioxide.

↑ Temp
↑ 2,3 BPG } *at level of cells*
↓ pH } *facilitates offloading of O_2 from Hb to the tissues*

Cardiac tamponade

15 B Muffled heart sounds

Cardiac tamponade (which can be traumatic or non-traumatic) occurs as a result of pericardial sac being filled with inflammatory fluid or blood leading to a pericardial effusion. As the effusion increases in volume, this in turn results in a decrease in cardiac contractility which ultimately leads to (obstructive) shock.

Beck's triad
→ muffled heart sounds
→ distended neck veins
→ hypotension

Traumatic causes of pericardial effusion include blunt or penetrating trauma to the chest. Cardiac tamponade can also occur during cardiac catheterisation, central line insertion or insertion of a pacemaker. Some non-traumatic causes include hypothyroidism, pericarditis, invasive neoplastic disease and high exposure of the chest to radiation.

On assessment of the patient with cardiac tamponade the following signs may be seen (the first three of which are referred to as Beck's triad):

- Hypotension (due to obstructive shock)
- Increased jugular venous pressure

- Muffled heart sounds
- Kussmaul's sign; a paradoxical rise in JVP on inspiration
- Electromechanical dissociation arrest

Acute respiratory distress syndrome

16 E **Presence of bilateral pulmonary infiltrates on chest radiograph or CT**

ARDS is characterised by reducing lung compliance and hypoxaemia due to a combination of acute respiratory failure (due to acute lung injury) with the formation of non-cardiogenic pulmonary oedema. The condition is refractory to oxygen therapy and can be diagnosed if the following three are present:

(handwritten margin note: • Acute onset • Infiltrates on CXR • Refractory to O₂)

- Chest radiographs or CT imaging confirms bilateral pulmonary infiltrates
- Acute onset; within 1 week of a known clinical insult
- Refractory hypoxaemia: PaO_2:FIO_2 <200

The pulmonary artery capillary wedge pressure (PCWP) being ≤ 18 mmHg was part of the diagnostic criteria but has now been removed.

Acute hypocalcaemia

17 C **Establish cardiac monitoring**

The most common surgical cause of hypocalcaemia is inadvertent removal or damage to the parathyroid glands during thyroid surgery.

Clinical features associated with hypocalcaemia include (1)neuromuscular irritability which may manifest as peripheral and circumoral parathesia, (2) tetany, (3) muscular cramps, (4) twitching of the facial muscles on tapping of the facial nerve (Chvostek's sign) and (5) tetanic spasm of the hand following blood pressure cuff-induced arm ischaemia (Trousseau's sign).

This patient is experiencing symptomatic hypocalcaemia and requires close monitoring and correction of the low serum calcium. Following initial assessment using the ABCDE system (refer to Question 3 in this chapter), the most appropriate next step to take is to establish cardiac monitoring to monitor for cardiac arrhythmias. In addition, an ECG trace may show intermittent QT prolongation.

Prescribing bisphosphonates or calcitonin or administering high dose steroids are measures which are usually taken in the management of hypercalcaemia.

The patient does not need to be taken back to theatre and hence contacting the Surgical Registrar would not be indicated.

Nutrition

18 D Vitamin A

Vitamins A, D, E and K are fat soluble. Vitamin A is a fat soluble vitamin which is important for the stabilisation of cell membranes as well as retinal function. Vitamin D is required for calcium homeostasis and mineralisation of bone. Vitamin K is required for blood coagulation through the γ-carboxylation of glutamic acid residues of the clotting factors, namely II, VII, IX and X.

The family of Vitamin B (B_1/B_2/B_3/Biotin/B_6/B_{12}) and Vitamin C are water soluble vitamins. Vitamin C, as well as possessing antioxidant functions, plays an important role in hydroxylation of proline and lysine residues during collagen synthesis, absorption of iron from the gastrointestinal system and the synthesis of epinephrine from tyrosine. Vitamin B1 (riboflavin) deficiency leads to Weinicke's encephalopathy or beri-beri.

Gram negative bacteria

19 B *Neisseria meningitides*

Neisseria meningitidis is a Gram negative bacteria. *Streptococcus pneumoniae*, *Staphylococcus aureus*, *Streptococcus viridans* and *Clostridium botulinum* are all Gram positive bacteria.

Characteristics of Gram negative bacteria include a cytoplasmic lipid membrane, a thick peptidoglycan layer (forming rigid cell walls) and the presence of lipoteichoic acids (which are chelating agents and are involved in adherence) within the cell wall.

Gram negative bacteria possess a cytoplasmic membrane, a thin pep-tidoglycan layer and an outer cell membrane containing lipopoly-saccharide. They do not contain lipoteichoic acids.

Sepsis

20 A Aerobic and anaerobic blood cultures will only be positive in approximately 20% of patients with sepsis

Blood cultures are taken in patients with signs of systemic sepsis. Two blood culture bottles (anaerobic and aerobic blood culture bottles) should always be taken and sent to the pathology laboratory promptly. The blood culture analysis usually takes a minimum of 3 days, however in some cases, owing to high amounts of bacteraemia and higher bacterial proliferation rates, results may be relayed to you in 2 days. Antibiotic therapy should start after a blood culture investigation is performed.

An in-dwelling central venous catheter could be the source of sepsis and blood cultures should be taken through them to isolate the offending organism.

Generally the following measures should be taken within the first 6 hours from onset of symptoms in patients with suspected sepsis:

- Administer high flow oxygen
- Take blood cultures
- Administer intravenous antibiotics
- Commence intravenous fluid resuscitation
- Measure and check haemoglobin and lactate levels
- Accurate measurement of hourly urine output and fluid balance

For further information, please refer to the Surviving Sepsis Campaign at www.survivingsepsis.org.

Lactic acidosis

21 C   Pyloric stenosis

The features of lactic acidosis include the presence of a metabolic acidosis, a varying degree of respiratory compensation and an elevated serum lactate >5 mmol/L (normal range <2 mmol/L). The causes of lactic acidosis include shock, pancreatitis, liver impairment/failure, renal impairment/failure, excessive exercise, leukaemia and biguanides.

Excessive vomiting (e.g. as seen in pyloric stenosis) is associated with loss of gastric contents. Since gastric fluids are low pH this leads to decreased levels of hydrogen, chloride and potassium ions, resulting in a hypokalaemic-hypochloraemic metabolic acidosis. *alkalosij*

Respiratory failure

22 A   Pulmonary embolism

Pulmonary embolism is associated with type 1 (hypoxic) respiratory failure (pO_2 <8kPa and pCO_2 may be low or normal). In pulmonary embolism, there is an associated ventilation/perfusion mismatch leading to hypocapnia due to hyperventilation (please refer to Question 6). Raised intracranial pressure, poliomyelitis, phrenic nerve injury and myasthenia gravis are common causes of type 2 (hypercapnic) respiratory failure (pO_2 <8 kPa and pCO_2 >6.5 kPa).

Local anaesthetic

23 C   195 mg

The maximum safe dose of lidocaine is 3 ml/kg and therefore, the latter value multiplied by the patient weight (65 × 3 mg/kg = 195 mg) gives the maximum safe dose of lidocaine that can be administered to the patient. Bupivacaine has a maximum dose of 2 mg/kg, lidocaine with adrenaline is 5 mg/kg and prilocaine is 6 mg/kg.

Furthermore, local anaesthetics and vasoconstrictors (e.g. lidocaine and adrenaline) should not be administered together to pedicled structures with end arteries (e.g. ear lobes, digits, the nose, penis, etc.) as this can lead to ischaemia and necrosis.

Aortic dissection

24 E **Loss of the right heart border**
Chest radiographs taken from patients with aortic dissection are normal in 80% of cases. Rare radiographic signs which may present are (1) widened mediastinum, (2) haemothorax, (3) displacement of the 'aortic knuckle' and (4) depression of the left main bronchus.

Loss or obscurity of the right heart border usually implies that there is an abnormality/disease of the right middle lobe of the lung.

Intraoperative complication

25 B **Maintaining intravascular volume with intravenous fluids**
The patient is experiencing anaphylaxis from the blue dye. This is a rare complication and occurs at an incidence rate of 0.1%, but can be fatal if not managed promptly. Patients who develop intraoperative anaphylaxis may show signs of tachycardia, hypotension, laryngeal oedema and bronchospasm.

The mainstay of treatment involves maintaining intravascular volume through intravenous fluid resuscitation to anticipate the ensuing hypotension. Administering intravenous adrenaline is also required to maintain systemic vascular resistance. Once the patient is stable, intravenous antihistamine (e.g. chlorpheniramine) and hydrocortisone are administered.

From the list of answers, maintaining intravascular volume with intravenous fluids would be the most appropriate step in the first instance followed by administering intravenous adrenaline to maintain systemic vascular resistance. Removal of the endotracheal tube and waking the patient would be fatal due to the fact that the endotracheal tube is maintaining the airway and its removal would lead to loss of the airway secondary to anaphylaxis inducing laryngeal oedema. Intravenous antihistamines and steroids are used once the patient is resuscitated and stable.

Since the procedure being performed is an elective case, continuing with the operation is not indicated. Anaphylaxis is a life threatening condition and needs to be attended to first.

SECTION 5: TRAUMA

Questions

1.	Trauma and its management	77
2.	Resuscitation of the injured patient	77
3.	Primary survey	77
4.	Initial assessment	77
5.	Assessing ventilation	78
6.	Airway protection	78
7.	Airway adjunct selection	78
8.	Shock	78
9.	Estimating blood loss	79
10.	Peripheral access	79
11.	Chest trauma (1)	79
12.	Flail chest	80
13.	Chest trauma (2)	80
14.	Complications of chest drain insertion	80
15.	Diagnosis of intra-abdominal injury	80
16.	Explorative laparotomy	81
17.	Splenic trauma	81
18.	Focused assessment with sonography for trauma (FAST) scan	81
19.	Evaluation of Glasgow Coma Scale score (1)	82
20.	Evaluation of Glasgow Coma Scale score (2)	82
21.	Brain injury	82
22.	Intracranial haemorrhage	83
23.	Management of severe head injury	83
24.	Head injury	83
25.	Cervical spine trauma	83

26. Burns management   84
27. Early burns management   84
28. Management of a burn victim   84
29. Management of burn injury   84
30. Hypothermia   85

Answers   86

QUESTIONS

1. Trauma and its management

A 25-year-old man is blue-lighted into the emergency department following an accident at work. A pan of hot cooking oil had spilled over half of his back and over both his legs and he has sustained extensive burns in this distribution. He weighs 70 kg. Calculate the additional volume of crystalloid this patient will require in the first 8 hours (from the time of his burn) of his treatment using the Parkland formula and the Wallace Rule of Nines.

A.   250 mL
B.   3,150 mL
C.   6,300 mL
D.   12,600 mL
E.   None, only patients with a percentage burn more than 15% require admission

[handwritten:] $= \dfrac{\%45 \times 4 \times 70\,kg}{2}$

[handwritten:] * Back of trunk is 18%

2. Resuscitation of the injured patient

A patient is admitted following a motorcycle accident. He has fractured his left femur, tibia, fibula and pelvis. His blood pressure is 70/35 mmHg, pulse is 140 beats/min, respiratory rate is 35 breaths/min and the Glasgow Coma Scale score is 9/15. You wish to resuscitate the patient. Which one of the following procedures may be contraindicated in such a patient?

A.   Motorcycle helmet removal
B.   Urinary catheterization
C.   Neck line insertion
D.   Nasogastric tube insertion
E.   Intubation

3. Primary survey

[handwritten:] will notice all except

An initial primary survey of the chest is intended to quickly identify the following causes of cardiorespiratory compromise, except

A.   Flail chest
B.   Cardiac tamponade
C.   Tension pneumothorax
D.   Haemothorax
E.   Pulmonary contusion

[handwritten:] • Chest may look normal but may be injured from within !!

4. Initial assessment

A patient is admitted following an assault. On assessment, he has a stab wound to his chest. Clinically, he has a massive haemothorax and his Glasgow Coma

[handwritten:] die because of

Scale score is 4/15. Without further management this patient will succumb to which cause of death first?

  A. Haemorrhagic shock
  B. Respiratory failure
  C. Airway compromise
  D. Intracranial haemorrhage
  E. Multiorgan failure

5. Assessing ventilation

As well as measuring oxygen saturation, a pulse oximeter also gives useful information regarding what other factor, used in initial assessment of the traumatized patient?

  A. Blood pressure
  B. Partial pressure of oxygen
  C. Partial pressure of carbon dioxide
  D. Peripheral perfusion
  E. Acid–base balance

6. Airway protection

naso
oro
surgical

Which of the following techniques does not provide a definitive airway?

  A. Cricothyroidotomy   *— surgical*
  B. Tracheostomy
  C. Nasotracheal tube
  D. Laryngeal mask airway   *→ sits on top of larynx → doesnt protect from aspiration.*
  E. Endotracheal tube

7. Airway adjunct selection

A patient is admitted following a road traffic accident. He has sustained significant blunt injury to his head, chest and abdomen and has a Glasgow Coma Scale score of 8/15. His saturations are poor at 89% on 15 L of oxygen via a rebreathing mask. You note bruising around both eyes and blood-stained fluid issuing from his left ear, which forms concentric circles when dripped on a white sheet. You wish to support his airway to improve oxygenation. The first choice of airway adjunct would be

  A. Oropharyngeal airway   *★ basal skull fracture*
  B. Nasopharyngeal tube   *airway?*
  C. Laryngeal mask
  D. Intubation
  E. Positive pressure ventilation (continuous positive airway pressure)

8. Shock

A 35-year-old man is admitted after severing his arm on industrial machinery. His airway is patent and there is no identifiable hindrance to breathing. His pulse is 110 beats/min, blood pressure is 130/105 mmHg, and respiratory rate is 25 breaths/min. Which stage of shock is this patient in?

A. Class I
B. Class II
C. Class III
D. Class IV
E. Impossible to say from given information

9. Estimating blood loss

A 35-year-old butcher is admitted after stabbing himself with a knife inadvertently. His airway is patent and there are no identifiable hindrances to breathing. His pulse is 110 beats/min, BP is 130/105 mmHg, and respiratory rate is 25 breaths/min. Assuming a body mass of 70 kg, what is the best estimated volume of blood lost?

A. 400 mL
B. 1000 mL
C. 1800 mL
D. 2500 mL
E. Impossible to say from given information

10. Peripheral access

A patient is admitted in haemorrhagic shock following a road traffic accident. A final year medical student places an intravenous cannula; they have inserted a pink (20 G) cannula in the antecubital fossa. What rate of flow into the patient will this allow?

A. 250 mL/min
B. 170 mL/min
C. 55 mL/min
D. 25 mL/min
E. 10 mL/min

11. Chest trauma (1)

A patient is admitted to the emergency department following an assault. You note a penetrating wound on the anterior chest wall. On examination, his blood pressure is 80/65 mmHg, pulse is thready and respiratory rate is 38 breaths/min. His jugular venous pulse is unrecognizable as the neck veins are grossly distended. Breath sounds are equal bilaterally. During your evaluation the patient's output becomes undetectable. The next course of action should be

A. Thoracocentesis
B. Plain chest radiograph
C. Pericardiocentesis

    D.   Resuscitative thoracotomy
    E.   Echocardiogram

12. Flail chest

A 42-year-old construction worker is admitted following a crush injury. The patient is in great distress and complaining of chest pain. The patient is working hard to breathe, however there is some paradoxical movement of her chest wall. Arterial blood gases show hypoxia with pO_2 7.5 and pCO_2 8.2. A chest radiograph shows multiple rib fractures. The life-saving intervention is *RespF II*

    A.   High-flow oxygen   *Flial chest*   *Flial chest c̄*
    B.   Cricothyroidotomy   *RespF II ?*
    C.   Endotracheal tube insertion
    D.   Aggressive fluid resuscitation
    E.   Adequate analgesia to allow effective respiration

13. Chest trauma (2)

A male patient is admitted following a fall from height. On arrival his Glasgow Coma Scale score is 5/15 and he is therefore intubated. During primary resuscitation a chest film is taken which shows a widened mediastinum and right-sided deviation of the trachea. The diagnosis is

    A.   Tension pneumothorax
    B.   Ruptured oesophagus
    C.   Cardiac tamponade
    D.   Right lobe collapse
    E.   Aortic rupture

14. Complications of chest drain insertion

A 20-year-old woman was resuscitated in the emergency department and required the insertion of a chest drain. The drain was removed 2 days later before she was discharged. She re-presents 10 days later complaining of chest pain associated with high fever and sweats. An empyema is suspected and a chest radiograph confirms a collection. The most appropriate next course of action is

    A.   Intravenous antibiotics for 6 weeks
    B.   Needle tap and aspiration : *fluid is thick*
    C.   Chest drain reinsertion : *Yes but aft localizing it*
    D.   Computed tomography scan of the thorax
    E.   Ultrasound scan

15. Diagnosis of intra-abdominal injury

Which one of the following statements regarding diagnostic peritoneal lavage is not true?

(A.) A positive test would follow injury to spleen, liver, pancreas or intestine : nonspecific

B. It is more sensitive than computed tomography and focused assessment with sonography for trauma (FAST) scanning

C. It is the technique of choice when attempting to confirm the hollow viscus injury

D. Urinary catheterization and nasogastric tube insertion is required prior to diagnostic peritoneal lavage

E. - Diagnostic peritoneal lavage is contraindicated in the presence of an indication for explorative laparotomy

16. Explorative laparotomy

Which of the following is not an independent indication for laparotomy following trauma?

A. Evisceration of healthy bowel
B. Evisceration of omentum
(C.) Stab wound to anterior abdomen : fail to reach peritonium
D. Gunshot to abdomen
E. Blunt abdominal trauma with free intraperitoneal air on erect chest radiograph

17. Splenic trauma

A 35-year-old man was involved in a motor vehicle collision where he was thrown against the steering column. He sustained a blunt trauma injury to his left upper abdomen. On arrival at the emergency department, he complains of abdominal pain, but is haemodynamically stable. Computed tomography (CT) scanning shows a splenic tear and retained intra-abdominal haematoma. The tear extends through the splenic capsule, but not to the hilum. Which one of the following treatment options is not indicated in this case?

III ?
II | conservativ
I

A. Cross-match, group and save
B. Pneumovax
(C.) Explorative laparotomy   IV = laprotomy
D. Serial CT scanning
E. 24-hour monitoring in the high-dependency/intensive care setting

18. Focused assessment with sonography for trauma (FAST) scan

The following factors detract from the diagnostic sensitivity of FAST scanning, except

A. Surgical emphysema
B. A patient with high body mass index
C. Operator inexperience

D. Previous surgery

E. Large-volume intraperitoneal blood loss

19. Evaluation of Glasgow Coma Scale score (1)

A patient is admitted to the emergency department with a reduced level of consciousness, smelling of alcohol. A boggy haematoma is noted on the posterior aspect of his skull. The patient's eyes open to voice, but he makes no attempt to vocalize. A sternal rub causes the patient to open his eyes, moan and extend his arms and legs. His Glasgow Coma Scale score is

A. 4/15
B. 5/15
C. 6/15
D. 7/15
E. 8/15

handwritten notes:
- eye = 3
- speech = 2
- motor = 2 extensi

20. Evaluation of Glasgow Coma Scale score (2)

A patient is admitted into the emergency department following a head injury at work. He is resuscitated and stabilized, but a computed tomography scan shows significant brain contusion. He is intubated and cared for on the intensive care unit. You attempt to evaluate his Glasgow Coma Scale score; there is no response to voice, but pressing a pen into his fingernail causes the patient to open his eyes and attempt to withdraw his hand from you. His Glasgow Coma Scale score is therefore

handwritten notes: 4 ; So speech is discounted

A. 5/10
B. 6/10
C. 5/15
D. 6/15
E. 7/15

21. Brain injury

A 31-year-old man is admitted following an assault outside a nightclub. During the fight, he was hit by a blunt object across the side of the head. On admission his Glasgow Coma Scale score is initially 12/15 but falls to 8/15 during his evaluation. The decision is taken to perform a computed tomography head scan, which identifies a lens-shaped space-occupying lesion within the cranial vault. The diagnosis is

A. Extradural haematoma
B. Subdural haematoma
C. Subarachnoid haemorrhage
D. Cerebral contusion
E. Intracerebral haemorrhage

22. Intracranial haemorrhage

Of the following options, which is not a risk factor for subdural haematoma?

    A. Pregnancy
    B. Alcoholism
    C. Dementia
    D. Old age
    E. Schizophrenia

23. Management of severe head injury

The following are the treatment options available for the management of the patient with severe head injury. Which of the following does not have an effect on reducing intracranial pressure?

    A. Corticosteroids
    B. Mannitol
    C. Barbiturates
    D. Hyperventilation
    E. Furosemide

24. Head injury

A female patient is admitted following a domestic assault during which she sustained an isolated head injury. On admission she had a Glasgow Coma Scale score of 13/15 but remained confused. She was therefore admitted overnight for observations. You are called to see her by the high-dependency unit nurses who have noticed a drop in her Glasgow Coma Scale score to 8/15. On examination you note her left pupil is now fixed and dilated. The most likely cause of this is

    A. Transient ischaemic attack/cerebrovascular accident
    B. Basal skull fracture
    C. Isolated III nerve palsy
    D. Uncal herniation
    E. Previously undocumented eye trauma

25. Cervical spine trauma

A patient is admitted following a fall from 4 m. He has sustained an injury to the posterior aspect of his head and has a Glasgow Coma Scale score of 12/15. On primary and secondary survey you identify a fracture of the left tibia but no focal neurology. You wish to remove the cervical spine collar and spinal board and so you review the cervical spine films; they show no abnormalities, but the lateral and swimmer's view films do not show the C7–T1 junction. Which one of the following is the most appropriate next step?

    A. Clear the cervical spine clinically, asking whether neck pain is felt and assessing for neurology
    B. Flexion and extension views

C. Continue management on a spinal board and collar until clinical assessment is possible

D. Ask senior clinician/radiologist to review films

E. Clear the cervical spine using computed tomography

26. Burns management

Which of the following is not a recognized complication of severe burn injury?

A. Renal failure

B. Pancreatitis

C. Liver failure

D. Gastric ulceration

E. Carbon monoxide poisoning

27. Early burns management

A patient is admitted following a house fire. He has extensive partial and full thickness burns over his arms, upper torso and neck. You note black carbon deposits around his nostrils and oropharynx. Which of the following is the immediate priority?

A. Adequate analgesia

B. Sterile water irrigation

C. Intubation

D. Fluid resuscitation

E. Immediate transfer to a specialist burns centre

28. Management of a burn victim

A 32-year-old woman is admitted following a house fire. She has no obvious injuries save for some partial thickness burning to her back and legs. On initial assessment she appears confused, Glasgow Coma Scale score 14/15, and complains of nausea and headache. Her blood pressure is 165/110 mmHg, pulse rate is 105 beats/min and respiratory rate is 23 breaths/min. Oxygen saturation is 98% on room air. Arterial blood gases reveal respiratory alkalosis and a normal PO_2. The next stage of management is

A. High-flow oxygen via non-rebreathable mask

B. Intubate and ventilate

C. Computed tomography head scan

D. Focused assessment with sonography for trauma (FAST) scan of the abdomen

E. 100% oxygen via rebreathing bag

29. Management of burn injury

A 48-year-old man is admitted with a burn over his arm and anterior chest. The involved tissue includes the entire circumference of his upper arm. Following initial resuscitation, he is admitted for observation. You are called to assess him as he is beginning to complain of increasing pain and tightness in his forearm. On examination you note weak peripheral pulses, paraesthesia and pain on active movement of the fingers, hand and wrist. The next stage in management is

    A.   Angiography
    B.   Fasciotomy
    C.   Fluid resuscitation
    D.   Electrolyte assay and replenishment
    E.   Escharotomy

30. Hypothermia

A homeless man is admitted unresponsive after being found by police on a park bench. He has no external signs of injury. An oesophageal temperature probe records his core body temperature to be 34 °C. Which of the following management options is not routinely indicated in this case?

    A.   Cardiac monitoring
    B.   Warmed peritoneal lavage
    C.   Warmed intravenous fluids
    D.   Intravenous dextrose
    E.   Blood alcohol and toxin screen

ANSWERS

Trauma and its management

1 C 6,300 mL

Burn victims lose a lot of fluid following their injury and their treatment is notoriously difficult. The current ATLS guidelines quote the
Parkland formula as the preferred method by which fluid replacement
should be calculated. The formula is as follows:

Weight (kg) × % Burn × 4 = Volume of crystalloid required over
24 hours

The percentage burn is best calculated using the Wallace Rule of
Nines:

- Head = 9%
- Arm = 9%
- Leg = 18%
- Trunk front = 18%
- Back = 18%

Therefore, this patient has a percentage burn of 45%. Using this percentage in the formula gives a volume of 12,600 ml. Half of this should
be given in the first 8 hours, the rest over the subsequent 16 hours.
Obviously this is a rough guide and local practice will differ. All
patients with this extent of injury should be managed in a specialist
centre, typically in an intensive care unit. The take home message is
that large volumes of fluid are required.

Resuscitation of the injured patient

2 B Urinary catheterization

This patient has sustained severe injuries and has developed an
advanced degree of haemorrhagic shock. Circulatory support is
paramount and therefore central line insertion is justifiable. Intubation
may not be urgently required; however, his low GCS at presentation
identifies him as a patient at risk of further deterioration, and intubation
in these cases certainly is not contraindicated. Severely traumatized
patients can develop gastric distension and with an obtunded conscious
state they are at risk of aspiration, therefore NG tube insertion is
advocated. Helmet removal is not recommended at the scene of injury;
however removal in the emergency department is advised to allow
appropriate assessment and airway protection.

Urinary catheterization is desirable in shock patients to guide fluid management. However, any suspicion of urethral disruption is an absolute

contraindication for urethral catheter insertion. You should have a high index of suspicion in the following circumstances:

- Blood at the penile meatus
- Perineal bruising
- Blood in the scrotum
- High-riding prostate
- Pelvic fracture

Conformation of the integrity of the urinary tract is required by retrograde urethrógram prior to catheter insertion. If urethral injury is confirmed, suprapubic catheterization is indicated.

Primary survey

3 E **Pulmonary contusion**
The ATLS guidelines teach a method of rapid assessment of the traumatized patient divided into a primary survey, which is aimed at the identification of immediate threats to life, and a secondary survey, which aims to identify more minor injuries. Thoracic injuries which are an immediate threat to life include flail chest, tension pneumothorax, open pneumothorax, massive haemothorax and cardiac tamponade. Pulmonary contusion is not an immediate threat to life, and therefore is not of initial concern during the primary survey. However, it can complicate recovery as the injured lung can impair gas exchange and may be more susceptible to fluid overload.

Initial assessment

4 C **Airway compromise**
The ATLS primary survey follows an ABCDE format so that those injuries which most rapidly threaten life are identified and dealt with first.

- A = Airway (+ cervical spine support)
- B = Breathing
- C = Circulation
- D = Disability
- E = Exposure

This patient has a GCS of 4, rendering him unable to maintain his own airway, which will therefore be the first factor to lead to his death. Consequently, his airway must be managed before addressing his other injuries.

Assessing ventilation

5 D **Peripheral perfusion**
Many factors may influence the accuracy of the oximetry trace; the majority are a hindrance, such as methaemoglobinaemia, nail

varnish and the presence of a blood pressure cuff on the arm in question. Another factor is poor peripheral perfusion; an oximetry trace which is low compared with the values gained from arterial blood gas sampling indicates that the patient is peripherally shut down, a consequence of low circulating volume and shock. Pulse oximetry gives no indication of pO_2, pCO_2, blood pressure or acid–base balance.

Airway protection

6 D Laryngeal mask airway

The definition of a definitive airway is a tube in the trachea with an inflatable cuff. Definitive airways are of three types: nasotracheal, orotracheal and surgical. A laryngeal mask airway has an inflatable cuff, but this sits on top of the larynx and does not intubate the trachea. It therefore provides no airway protection from aspiration or laryngeal oedema.

Airway adjunct selection

7 A Oropharyngeal airway

This patient has sustained a significant head injury which complicates your choice of airway. Candidates should be aware that any suspicion of a basal skull fracture is an absolute contraindication to nasopharyngeal airway and nasogastric tube insertion. This is because of the risk of penetrating through the damaged cribriform plate and intubating the brain.

The signs suggestive of basal skull fracture include periorbital ecchymosis (panda eyes/raccoon eyes), retroauricular ecchymosis (battle sign), CSF leakage from the nose or ears and VII/VIII cranial nerve dysfunction. The internal carotid artery may also be injured resulting in dissection or pseudoaneurysm. CSF leakage can be differentiated from blood by dripping the fluid on a white sheet; CSF will form concentric circles whereas blood will simply make a spot.

With nasopharyngeal tube placement contraindicated, the first option in this patient would be Guedel oropharyngeal airway placement. A patient with a GCS score of 8 may still gag on the Guedel airway, although with a patient thus obtunded, it is possible it will be tolerated without sedation. An endotracheal tube may well be required later in the resuscitation because this patient has a severe head injury; however, endotracheal intubation requires an anaesthetist and significant time. Guedel airway placement should still be considered the first choice adjunct as it is quick, allowing further assessment of the patient to continue, and it acts as a bridge to intubation.

Shock

8 B   Class II

Shock is classified into classes I–IV and its clinical evaluation is judged on the derangement of vital signs. Each class of shock can be considered to be equivalent to an estimated percentage loss, and this percentage may be used to calculate volume loss (see Question 9). The following table illustrates the clinical signs of the different stages of hypovolaemic shock.

	Class I	Class II	Class III	Class IV
Per cent blood loss	Up to 15	15–30	30–40	>40
Pulse rate	<100	>100	>120	>140
Blood pressure	Normal	Normal	↓	↓
Pulse pressure	Normal	↓	↓	↓
Respiratory rate	14–20	20–30	30–40	>35
Urine output (mL/h)	>30	20–30	5–15	<5
Mental status	Slight anxiety	Mild anxiety	Anxious, confused	Confused

(handwritten annotations above the columns: 750 above Class I; 1500 above Class II; 2000 above Class III)

Estimating blood loss

9 B   1000 mL

Circulating volume accounts for approximately 7% of body mass. Therefore, a 70 kg adult has a circulating volume of 5 L. This rough guide is less reliable in children, in whom the circulating volume accounts for 8%–9% of body mass, or in obese people, in whom calculation should be based on their ideal body weight to avoid gross overestimation of blood loss.

Once the total volume has been calculated, estimate blood loss by assessing the class of shock. Class I shock (see Question 8) corresponds to a blood loss of up to 15% (750 mL in a 70 kg man). Class II shock equates to 15%–30% blood loss (750–1500 mL) and class III to 30%–40% (1500–2000 mL). Class IV shock accounts for blood loss of over 40%. Therefore, in this scenario, with the patient in class II shock, the best answer would be B (1000 mL blood loss).

Peripheral access

10 C   55 mL/min

Flow rates through a hollow tube are dependent on two factors: the radius and the length of the tube. Poiseuille's law states that flow rate is proportional to the fourth power of the radius of the cannula and inversely proportional to the length. Therefore the most effective way of giving fluids is through a short fat peripheral cannula, and not, as commonly believed, through a central line. Other factors affecting flow rate include the viscosity of the fluid and the pressure difference across the tube.

- Brown/orange (14 G) cannula – may deliver 250 mL/min
- Grey (16 G) cannula – 170 mL/min
- Green (18 G) cannula – 90 mL/min
- Pink (20 G) cannula – 55 mL/min
- Blue (22 G) cannula – 25 mL/min

Chest trauma (1)

11 C Pericardiocentesis

Beck's triad consists of venous pressure elevation, reduced arterial blood pressure and muffled heart sounds. These three features are the classic identifying features of cardiac tamponade. In addition, an exaggerated pulsus paradoxus (a fall in arterial blood pressure >10 mmHg on spontaneous inspiration) and Kussmaul's sign (rising venous pressure on spontaneous inspiration) are also signs of tamponade. Knowing this, candidates can correctly identify tamponade as the likely diagnosis in this scenario.

The next thing to recognize is that this patient is peri-mortem. There are two methods used to confirm the diagnosis of tamponade: echocardiography in the form of a FAST (a focused assessment with sonography for trauma) scanner is less invasive, but has a false negative rate of 10% even in experienced hands. In a patient as compromised as the scenario suggests, with a convincing history of penetrating chest injury, pericardiocentesis is both diagnostic and therapeutic, and should not be delayed by other diagnostic adjuncts. Resuscitative thoracotomy may be required, but is the reserve of surgeons experienced enough to perform such a procedure. Pericardiocentesis should be attempted first to allow time for a more controlled surgical management. Thoracotomy or a pericardial window procedure should be reserved for cases where pericardiocentesis fails.

Flail chest

12 C Endotracheal tube insertion

Flail chest is a term used to describe an injury to the chest wall which results in a section losing continuity with the remainder. This loose segment is therefore sucked in by the negative pressures implicit in inspiration, preventing effective respiration and causing significant damage to the underlying lung parenchyma. These two factors combined result in significant impairment of gas exchange and respiratory failure.

Analgesia will improve the patient's pain but since the respiratory failure is not due to pain restricting breathing it will not save this patient's life. Fluid resuscitation is a complicated issue in these patients; a careful balance must be struck as the injured lung is vulnerable to fluid overload, which only exacerbates the poor gas exchange. High-flow oxygen will partially reverse the hypoxia, but is only a holding measure and will not affect the carbon dioxide retention. This patient requires mechanical ventilation and therefore the placement of a definitive airway. Both endotracheal intubation and cricothyroidotomy will provide this, but surgical airways are reserved for cases in which intubation fails or is impossible due to severe facial injury. Therefore, endotracheal intubation is the best option in this case.

Chest trauma (2)

13 E Aortic rupture

Aortic rupture is a common cause of sudden death following sudden-deceleration injuries occurring in traffic collisions or after falls from height. The point of disruption in the wall of the aorta is at the ligamentum arteriosum, across which the aorta may kink or twist, causing dissection or rupture.

Rupture into the left side of the chest is nearly universally fatal, unless it occurs in the emergency department itself. In those who survive, the haematoma is retained either within the adventitia or within the mediastinum. Features on a chest radiograph include the following:

- Widening of the mediastinum
- Loss of the aortic knuckle
- Deviation of the trachea to the right
- Obliteration of the space between the aorta and pulmonary artery (the AP window)
- Depression of the left main bronchus
- Left-sided haemothorax

It is rare for there to be no signs evident on plain radiographs following great vessel disruption; however, it can occur in in 1%–2% of cases.

Complications of chest drain insertion

14 E Ultrasound scan

Empyema typically occurs at around 10 days after chest drain insertion. It is a common and potentially fatal complication of this procedure. Like all abscesses and collections, there is little scope for conservative therapy, and empyema requires invasive drainage. The fluid collection is typically thick and loculated, making needle aspiration an inappropriate method of therapy. Definitive management is with chest drain re-insertion; however, this should be guided by appropriate imaging. Computed tomography may be helpful; however, ultrasound is perfectly adequate in assessing loculations and can also be used to guide drain insertion. As it does not involve exposure to ionising radiation, ultrasound should be the first choice technique.

Diagnosis of intra-abdominal injury

15 A A positive test would follow injury to spleen, liver, pancreas or intestine.

Diagnostic peritoneal lavage (DPL) is a useful technique for the identification of intra-abdominal bleeding and hollow organ rupture. Its use is more common in blunt injury as penetrating injury with significant likelihood of viscus injury is managed with explorative laparotomy. A litre of Hartmann's solution is instilled into the peritoneal cavity through a catheter and then drained. The fluid is sent to the laboratory, examined for blood and food fibre and Gram stained for bacteria.

Although non-specific, it is 98% sensitive, making it more reliable than CT and FAST scanning. In addition, it is able to identify hollow organ injury more reliably in the immediate post-injury setting than CT or ultrasound. However the use of DPL is declining in favour of the less invasive techniques and because the procedure requires insertion of a catheter into the peritoneal cavity decompression of the bladder and stomach is required to minimize risk of injury to these organs. The disadvantage of DPL is that it is unable to identify retroperitoneal injury i.e. damage to the kidneys, ureters, duodenum and pancreas. Therefore option A is the correct answer in this case.

Explorative laparotomy

16 C Stab wound to anterior abdomen

Although opinions among trauma surgeons vary, studies show that 33% of anterior abdominal stab wounds fail to penetrate the peritoneum and only 30% of stabbing injuries cause visceral injuries. Therefore, the current ATLS guidance does not advocate explorative laparotomy in all such cases. A haemodynamically stable patient with no evidence of peritonism may be managed conservatively with regular observations and serial clinical examinations over a 24-hour period. Where doubt remains, local exploration of the wound under local anaesthesia may clarify the extent of the injury. Other options include DPL and diagnostic laparoscopy.

A laparotomy is automatically indicated if evisceration of bowel or omentum occurs following penetrating injury or if the patient is haemodynamically unstable or has peritonism. In addition, if penetration of the peritoneum is confirmed, the majority of trauma surgeons advocate explorative laparotomy in the absence of clinical evidence of haemodynamic instability or peritonitis. In contrast to stab wounds, gunshots to the abdomen carry a 90% risk of visceral injury, and therefore all such patients are candidates for laparotomy. Blunt trauma carries a risk of diaphragmatic injury as well as injury to solid and hollow viscus. Hypotension, peritonism or free air or fluid evident on abdominal radiographs or an erect chest radiograph following blunt abdominal trauma are all indications for surgical exploration.

Splenic trauma

17 C Explorative laparotomy

Splenic injury is the most common organ injury sustained as a consequence of blunt trauma to the abdomen. Complications in trauma patients who require splenectomy are significantly greater than in similar patients who do not require splenectomy; causes of death include sepsis, pneumonia and meningitis. All splenic injury patients should receive vaccines against pneumococcus and meningococcus immediately, regardless of the extent of injury.

In modern surgical care, every effort is made to retain the spleen. Haemodynamically, stable patients require investigation utilizing both ultrasound and CT scanning. Injury is graded 1–4, according to the extent of the capsule laceration and involvement of the hilum. Grades 1–3 are widely considered to be suitable for conservative therapy. Grade 4 injuries extend into the hilum; as such they are at greater risk of major haemorrhage and devascularisation of the spleen. Significant controversy has existed regarding the management of this group of patients, although evidence suggests surgery can be safely avoided in haemodynamically stable patients using conservative measures. Splenic artery embolization using interventional radiographic techniques can be used if bleeding should continue in such cases.

In patients being managed conservatively, close monitoring is required in a high-dependency setting as a minimum. There is a risk of major haemorrhage and serial examination supplemented with regular CT scanning should be implemented. Patients should, of course, be crossmatched according to the centre's major bleeding protocol. Clinicians must be aware that in 5% of cases of presumed isolated solid organ injury, there exists an unrecognized concomitant hollow viscus injury. Deterioration, peritonism or haemodynamic compromise indicates the need for laparotomy, but in the case described above this is not yet required.

Focused assessment with sonography for trauma (FAST) scan

18 E Large-volume intraperitoneal blood loss

FAST is a non-invasive technique that can be performed in the emergency department, advantages which mean it is increasingly preferred to DPL and CT scanning in the assessment of the traumatized abdomen. In experienced hands, this technique is equivalent in sensitivity and specificity to DPL and CT; however as with all ultrasound scanning techniques this is operator-dependent and an experienced individual is required.

Four views are taken:

- The pericardium and the three sites within the abdomen where free fluid most commonly collects:
  - Hepatorenal fossa
  - Splenorenal fossa
  - Pouch of Douglas

Scanning is difficult to achieve in obese patients and subcutaneous free air makes ultrasound imagery impossible, as air does not transmit sound waves to deeper tissues. Previous surgery distorts normal anatomy and increases the likelihood of adhesions which prevent the free movement of blood within the peritoneal space and therefore its collection in the normal areas. This has a predictable effect on the sensitivity of FAST scanning.

The primary aim of FAST scanning is not to achieve a diagnosis, but to confirm the presence of peritoneal free fluid. Therefore a large-volume haematoperitoneum will be easier to detect on FAST scanning, although finding its source might not be. Therefore, option E is the most appropriate answer in this case.

Evaluation of Glasgow Coma Scale score (1)

19 D 7/15

The Glasgow Coma Scale is a commonly used method of assessing and monitoring consciousness level. It is frequently assessed in both written and practical exams and should therefore be well known to candidates. It consists of three parts with a fully conscious patient scoring 15/15, and a completely unresponsive patient scoring 3/15 (Table 5.1).

Table 5.1 The Glasgow Coma Scale

	Score
Motor	
Obeys commands	6
Localizes to pain	5
Flexor withdrawal	4
Abnormal flexion	3
Abnormal extension	2
No response	1
Eyes	
Open spontaneously	4
Open to verbal command	3
Open to pain	2
No response	1
Verbal	
Orientated	5
Confused	4
Inappropriate words	3
Incomprehensible sounds	2
No response	1

Evaluation of Glasgow Coma Scale score (2)

20 B 6/10

Rarely examiners will attempt to confuse candidates by asking how assessment of GCS in intubated patients differs. Put simply, assessment of motor and eyes is exactly the same. Assessment of vocalization is impossible and therefore discounted entirely. Therefore a fully conscious intubated patient scores 10/10, and an unresponsive intubated patient scores 2/10. The level of sedation obviously is a compounding factoar and mention should be made of this in a viva.

Brain injury

21 A **Extradural haematoma**

Haemorrhage within the cranial vault is commonly classified according to the layer of meninges in which the bleeding collects. The three layers of membranes which make up the meninges are the tough fibrous dura, the arachnoid and the pia mater. The dura is firmly adherent to the undersurface of the skull; within the folds of dura run the venous sinuses which drain to the internal jugular veins. Between the dura and the skull run the meningeal arteries, whose branches penetrate the dura to supply the brain substance. The arachnoid lies beneath the dura but does not adhere to it which leaves a potential space, the subdural space, for blood to collect (see Question 22). Between the arachnoid membrane and the pia mater flows the CSF. Bleeding into the subarachnoid space causes signs of meningism and puts the patient at increased risk of hydrocephalus, because blood may occlude the arachnoid granulations and prevent CSF reabsorption (post-traumatic communicating hydrocephalus).

This case is a classic description of extradural haemorrhage; bleeding is most commonly, but not exclusively, from a meningeal artery. The most commonly involved vessel is the middle meningeal artery, as it under-lies the weakest point in the cranial vault, the temporal bones. Although the temporal bone is protected somewhat by the temporalis muscle, a blow to the side of the head may cause a fracture, with consequential rupture of the underlying vessel. Because the dura is adherent to the bone, blood spread is restricted and therefore collects in a lens shape. In subdural and subarachnoid haemorrhage the blood is free to spread out over the surface of an entire cerebral hemisphere due to the lack of membrane adherence to overlying or underlying structures.

Intracranial haemorrhage

22 A Pregnancy

A subdural haematoma is a collection of blood between the dura and arachnoid membrane (see Question 21). Because these two membranes are not adhering to one another, this allows shearing forces which damage vessels traversing the subdural space. Veins, with their thin-ner walls, are more susceptible to such damage and therefore the vast majority of subdural haematomas are venous. They occur more com-monly than other forms of intracranial haemorrhage, complicating approximately 30% of severe head injuries.

Factors which predispose to subdural haemorrhage include all causes of cerebral atrophy, namely old age, alcohol, dementia and schizophrenia. Pregnancy does not predispose to it.

Management of severe head injury

23 A Corticosteroids

Injury to the head following trauma can be divided into primary (i.e. damage sustained as a direct result of the injury itself) and secondary. Minimization of secondary brain injury should be the main aim of man-agement of the injured patient and maintenance of cerebral perfusion is paramount. Patients usually require ventilation and should be managed on ITU/HDU and kept normotensive with a normal pO_2 and pCO_2.

This management is complicated by the presence of increased ICP. Mechanical hyperventilation has been used extensively as a technique to effectively reduce ICP; the resulting hypocapnia results in cerebral vasoconstriction and therefore reduced CSF and vascular volume within the cranial vault. However, vasoconstriction results in hypoxic brain injury, so prolonged hyperventilation must be discouraged and, ideally, pCO_2 should be maintained above 4.5 kPa. In the normotensive patient, diuretics such as mannitol with or without furosemide may be used to reduce ICP. These agents can cause hypotension, which should be avoided, and therefore they are not used in patients with low blood pressure. When raised ICP proves refractory to other measures, barbiturates can be used, but are associated with a high risk of inducing hypotension and are therefore avoided in the acute resuscitative phase. Steroids have been shown to have no effect on ICP and no beneficial effect on short-term or long-term outcome following brain injury; therefore their use is in decline and is not advocated in current guidelines.

Head injury

24 D Uncal herniation

This patient presented with a moderate brain injury. Up to 20% of such patients can be expected to deteriorate or become comatose. The first thing to consider is an expansion of an intracranial haemorrhage with subsequent raised ICP. The Monro–Kellie concept is useful in explaining why intracranial bleeding may initially be compensated for but, once the threshold for compensation is exceeded, eventually results in rapid decompensation unless intervention supervenes. The cranial vault has a fixed volume; bleeding within the skull has a mass effect and therefore some of the existing volume must be sacrificed. This is initially possible since venous volume and CSF volume can be lost, hence the initial period of compensation. However, once haematoma volume exceeds approximately 150 mL, the ability for the venous and CSF compartments to compensate is overwhelmed and ICP rises exponentially with further added volume. With increased ICP, arterial flow is compromised and brain matter is under pressure, leading to herniation.

Most commonly, the result is uncal herniation; the uncus is the medial part of the temporal lobe, which may be pushed against the edge of the tentorial notch. This puts pressure on the III cranial nerve, which runs along the edge of the tentorial notch, resulting first in loss of parasympathetic supply, then complete oculomotor palsy. The motor tracts are also vulnerable, positioned superficially at that level of the midbrain. Therefore the typical signs of uncal herniation include ipsilateral parasympathetic ± motor oculomotor nerve palsy with motor weakness. Confusion can arise when considering the motor signs of uncal herniation; hemiparesis can be contralateral or ipsilateral (Kernohan's phenomenon) to the lesion depending on the severity of herniation. Therefore, all head injury patients with altered consciousness, third nerve and motor signs should be referred for immediate emergency neurosurgical consultation.

Cervical spine trauma

25 E Clear the cervical spine using computed tomography

Cervical spine support is of primary importance when managing a trauma patient. Because of this the vast majority of accident victims will be brought to the emergency department with a collar in place, and candidates will need to know when it can be removed, and when they must not do so. It is acceptable to clear a cervical spine on clinical grounds when a patient is fully awake, sober, alert and neurologically intact with no neck pain. If the patient complains of neck pain, or if their consciousness is impaired, it is obligatory to perform plain film examination as a minimum. If the patient does not complain of neck pain, but has a distracting injury, such as in this case, cervical spine films may be taken despite a normal level of consciousness.

For plain films to be adequate, both AP and lateral views of the entire cervical spine should be taken, inclusive of the base of the skull and T1 vertebrae. In addition a view through the mouth visualizing the C1 and C2 vertebrae (also called a 'peg view') is required. Failure to meet these requirements, or identification of areas of suspicion, indicates the need for CT scanning. Flexion–extension films should only be attempted in patients who are fully conscious with normal AP, lateral and peg views; they are used to identify areas of occult instability. They are contraindicated in patients with an altered level of consciousness.

Leaving a patient on a backboard for over 2 hours puts them at risk of development of decubitus pressure ulceration. The risk is particularly high in patients with a reduced level of consciousness, therefore clearance of the cervical spine and avoidance of unnecessary immobilization is advisable.

Burns management

26 B Pancreatitis

Severe burns are best regarded as systemic insults. The fluid loss from extensive burns is considerable and will cause hypovolaemic shock. This is commonly undertreated and often results in acute renal and liver failure. An added insult to the kidneys is deep tissue damage releasing myoglobin, a nephrotoxin, into the circulation. Carbon monoxide poisoning is obviously a common cause of death in industrial and domestic fires and can exacerbate respiratory distress secondary to inhalation injury. The systemic stress response may lead to gastric and duodenal ulceration known as Curling's ulcers. Pancreatitis is not caused by burn injuries, but may be associated with hypothermia.

Early burns management

27 C Intubation

The subglottic airway is protected from thermal injury by the larynx. However, the supraglottic airway is susceptible to such injury and upper airway occlusion is a common consequence of inhalational injury or extensive burns to the neck. Signs of inhalation injury include singed nasal hair, facial burns, carbon deposits around the nose and oropharynx, hoarseness of voice, carbonaceous sputum and history of confinement in a burning environment.

This patient is at high risk of complicating his airway, with evidence of inhalational injury combined with external injury to the neck. Securing his airway is of highest priority as delay may lead to laryngeal oedema and need for surgical airway placement. This patient will also require fluid resuscitation and transfer to a specialist burns centre. Water irrigation and removal of all clothing is required to ensure removal of all burning material from the site of injury; only warmed fluid should be used to avoid hypothermia. Excessive analgesia should be avoided in the acute stages of burn resuscitation, as such medications mask signs of hypoxia and hypotension, which are used to guide fluid therapy.

Management of a burn victim

28 A **High-flow oxygen via non-rebreathable mask**
Carbon monoxide poisoning is a common consequence of being trapped in an enclosed space during a fire. It should be considered in all patients with such a history as it is easily treated and failure to do so may have serious consequences. However, if confusion continues despite appropriate treatment, or if there is evidence of head injury or focal neurology, further investigation such as CT scanning may be warranted.

Carbon monoxide's affinity for haemoglobin is 240 times that of oxygen. Its half-life is 4 hours while a patient breathes room air; this is reduced to 40 minutes if appropriate oxygen therapy is instituted. Symptoms depend on the percentage haemoglobin saturation by carbon monoxide; saturations less than 20% are typically asymptomatic, 20%–40% saturation causes nausea, headache and confusion. Saturations of 40%–60% result in coma and death occurs once levels exceed 60%. Appropriate management is high-flow oxygen via a non-rebreathing mask. Intubation and ventilation is only rarely required.

Because of its high affinity for haemoglobin, carbon monoxide saturates haemoglobin at low partial pressures; therefore normal arterial pO_2 does not exclude a high carbon monoxide saturation. Pulse oximetry does not differentiate between haemoglobin saturated with oxygen and that saturated with carbon monoxide, and therefore saturations will appear normal. Carboxyhaemoglobin levels are used to confirm the diagnosis; some arterial blood gas machines are able to provide these measurements.

Management of burn injury

29 E Escharotomy

Skin is inherently elastic and allows expansion and relaxation of underlying tissues. When skin is lost due to burns or other causes, fibrotic scarring occurs. When such injuries are circumferential, as in this case, healing can constrict underlying tissues, blood vessels and nerves. Limbs are vulnerable, as is the neck and even the chest, where extensive injury can restrict chest expansion and impair breathing.

The patient in this case is clearly exhibiting the signs of muscle compartment compromise secondary to restricted blood supply. There is concomitant paraesthesia, which may be as a result of ischaemia or a direct result of nerve compression. Fluid resuscitation is not required and although an electrolyte imbalance should be ruled out it is unlikely to be causative. Angiography is not indicated. This patient requires urgent escharotomy (incision of scar tissue to release constricting pressure). Fasciotomy is rarely required in such cases, but may be indicated if vascular supply remains compromised for a prolonged period and true compartment syndrome develops.

Hypothermia

30 B Warmed peritoneal lavage

Hypothermia is classified into mild (35–32°C), moderate (32–30°C) and severe (less than 30°C). The clinical manifestations of hypothermia include decreased consciousness, decreased respiratory rate and decreased heart rate. Cardiac output also falls proportional to the severity of hypothermia, and a patient who initially lacks any signs of life may make a full recovery with appropriate supportive therapy.

The main cause of death is cardiac arrhythmia; the myocardium becomes increasingly irritable below a temperature of 33°C and patients are at particular risk of fibrillation. Because of this, all hypothermia patients require cardiac monitoring and should be rewarmed using 'passive external warming techniques' including blankets, external heat sources and warmed IV fluids. The possibility of confounding causes of unresponsiveness should not be overlooked, and evidence of alcohol, drug use or sepsis should be excluded. Hypoglycaemia is another cause of reduced responsiveness that also frequently occurs secondary to hypothermia; therefore blood glucose monitoring and IV dextrose should be initiated as standard.

'Active core rewarming methods' are the reserve of severe hypothermia or hypothermia in high-risk patients (i.e. in conjunction with other injuries) and would not therefore be indicated in this scenario. Such techniques include warmed peritoneal lavage, warmed pleural lavage, warmed bladder irrigation, arterio-venous rewarming and cardiopulmonary bypass.

SECTION 6:
ABDOMEN: UPPER GASTROINTESTINAL AND HEPATOBILIARY SURGERY

Questions

1.	Anatomy	103
2.	Gastric cancer	103
3.	Oesophageal cancer	103
4.	Surgical anatomy of the oesophagus	103
5.	Dysphagia (1)	104
6.	Dysphagia (2)	104
7.	Acute pancreatitis	104
8.	Scleroderma and CREST syndrome	104
9.	Gastro-oesophageal sphincter	105
10.	Oesophagitis	105
11.	Abdominal surgery	105
12.	Gastrointestinal haemorrhage	105
13.	Variceal bleeding	106
14.	Abdominal emergency	106
15.	Abdominal wall anatomy	106
16.	Upper gastrointestinal bleeding	107
17.	Upper gastrointestinal haemorrhage	107
18.	Duodenal ulcers	107
19.	Gastric outflow obstruction	107
20.	Gastro-oesophageal reflux disease	108
21.	Gallstone disease	108
22.	Cholelithiasis	108
23.	Complications of cholelithiasis	108
24.	Obstructive jaundice	109
25.	Complicated gallstones	109
26.	Oesophagitis	109
27.	Cholangiocarcinoma	109

28. Upper gastrointestinal surgery   110
29. Hyposplenism   110
30. Splenectomy (1)   110
31. Splenectomy (2)   110
32. Pancreas   110
33. Pancreatitis (1)   111
34. Pancreatitis (2)   111
35. Complications of acute pancreatitis   111

Answers   112

QUESTIONS

1. Anatomy

The epiploic foramen of Winslow is an important anatomical landmark as it is the only communication between the greater and the lesser sac. Of the five structures listed below, which one is not a border of the epiploic foramen of Winslow?

A. Inferior vena cava *(posterior)*
B. First part of the duodenum *(inferior)*
C. Hepatoduodenal ligament *→ contains the portal triad* *(anterior)*
D. Gallbladder
E. Caudate lobe of the liver *(superior)*

Borders:
Anterior: free edge of lesser omentum (hepatoduodenal ligament)
Posterior: peritoneum covering the IVC.
Superior: peritoneum covering the caudate lobe of liver
Inferior: peritoneum covering beginning of duodenum and hepatic. a.
Portal Triad
1. proper hepatic a.
2. Hepatic portal v. 3. Bile ducts

2. Gastric cancer

Of the following, which is not a risk factor for gastric cancer?

A. Pernicious anaemia
B. Helicobacter pylori
C. Partial gastrectomy *→ need to discuss with pt before surgery*
D. Blood group O
E. Dried fish
↳ high in nitrosamines

* Blood group A
↳ higher risk

3. Oesophageal cancer

Which of the following investigations are not used in staging of oesophageal malignancy?

A. Mediastinoscopy
B. High-resolution computed tomography scanning
C. Endoscopy *→ used for diagnosis not staging*
D. Endoluminal ultrasound
E. Laparoscopy

• 75% have metastases by the time of diagnosis
• 5 year survival is 5%.
• Choice of investigation depends on site of 1° tumor.

4. Surgical anatomy of the oesophagus

The blood supply to the oesophagus is derived from which three vessels?
→ first ½ *→ middle ⅓* *lower ⅓*
A. Inferior thyroid artery, descending aorta, left gastric artery
B. Internal carotid, descending aorta, oesophageal artery
C. Lateral thoracic artery, phrenic artery, right gastric artery *← no br.* *outside cranial vault*
D. Pharyngeal artery, long thoracic artery, phrenic artery *↳ does not exist*
E. Ascending aorta, common hepatic artery, left gastric artery

Esophagus
Upper ⅓: Striated muscles
Middle: Mixed
Lower ⅓: Smooth muscle

5. Dysphagia (1)

A 58-year-old patient presents with a 6-week history of increasing difficulty swallowing. He first noticed problems when eating meat which became stuck 'behind his heart', but this gradually began to include other foods. The patient is currently worried because he is now struggling with thick fluids and has noticed some involuntary weight loss. What is the most appropriate investigation?

- A. Staging computed tomography → need to confirm first
- B. Barium meal
- Ⓒ Upper gastrointestinal endoscopy → gold standard
- D. Barium swallow → for neuro muscular causes of dysphagia
- E. Electrocardiography

6. Dysphagia (2)

A 27-year-old patient presents with a 3-month history of increasing difficulty in swallowing. He first noticed the problem when drinking fluids, but is now commonly experiencing it when eating food as well. He has presented as regurgitation of food is becoming a problem and he has noticed unintentional weight loss. A chest radiograph shows a widened mediastinum. What is the most likely diagnosis?

Acholasia: degeneration of Auerbach plexus. failure of LES to relax

- A. Thoracic aortic aneurysm
- B. Oesophageal malignancy → starts with solids then liquids
- C. Plummer–Vinson syndrome → risk of malignancy
- Ⓓ Achalasia → starts with liquids then food
- E. Oesophageal spasm → chest pain similar to MI

webs, IDA

7. Acute pancreatitis

The severity of acute pancreatitis can be assessed using the Glasgow criteria. Which of the following is not used in the calculation?

- Ⓐ Serum amylase
- B. White cell count   > 15
- C. Serum calcium   < 2.0
- D. Alanine aminotransferase   > 200
- E. Serum urea   > 16

8. Scleroderma and CREST syndrome

CREST syndrome is an autoimmune condition which is associated with atrophy and fibrosis of the oesophageal musculature resulting in dysphagia and reflux-type symptoms. Which of the following is not a feature of CREST syndrome?

systemic sclerosis
↳ diffuse
↳ limited (CREST)

- A. Raynaud's phenomenon
- Ⓑ Erythematous malar rash

Handwritten margin notes:
- C — Calcinosis
- R — raynaud's phenomenon
- E — Esophageal disorders.
- S — Sclerodactyly.
- T — telengiectacia

C. Sclerodactyly
D. Soft tissue calcification
E. Telangiectasia

9. Gastro-oesophageal sphincter

The gastro-oesophageal sphincter is not a true sphincter in that it does not rely on a ring of contractile muscle to maintain patency. It therefore relies on several other mechanisms to prevent reflux. Which of the following does not contribute to gastro-oesophageal sphincter function?

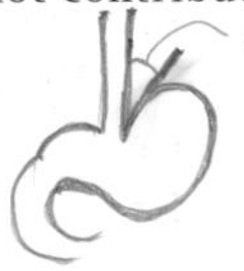

A. Left crus of diaphragm
B. Smooth muscle of the lower oesophageal sphincter
C. Angle of His
D. Right crus of diaphragm
E. Intra-abdominal pressure

Handwritten: angle of His

Handwritten: gastro esophageal sphincter
3 parts :. LOS
. Extrinsic sphincter (support by R.crus of diaphragm)
. physiological sphincter

10. Oesophagitis

A 58-year-old builder is referred to outpatients with a long history of retrosternal chest pain associated with food. Oesophagogastroduodenoscopy was performed which showed grade 2 oesophagitis with a hiatus hernia. The stomach and duodenum were normal. What is the most appropriate management?

A. Triple eradication therapy
B. Proton pump inhibitor
C. Nissen's fundoplication
D. Yearly endoscopic surveillance and biopsy
E. Supportive gusset

Handwritten: Esophagitis grading
Grade1: Small mucosal breaks limited to 2 mucosal folds
2: Mucosal breaks >5mm long limited to 2 mucosal folds
3: mucosal breaks more than 2 mucosal folds but <75% of esophageal circumference
4: Circumferential mucosal breaks involving >75% of Circumference

11. Abdominal surgery

Which one of the following is not a recognized long-term complication of partial/total gastrectomy?

A. Gastric malignancy
B. Obstruction
C. Folate deficiency
D. Iron deficiency
E. Vitamin B$_1$ deficiency

12. Gastrointestinal haemorrhage

A 45-year-old man presents to the emergency department with a history of coffee-ground vomiting. He also reports that for 2 days his stool appeared darker than usual. Which of the following gives the most sensitive guide as to the severity of his gastrointestinal haemorrhage?

A. Haemoglobin
B. Systolic blood pressure
C. Pulse rate
D. Volume of vomitus/melaena
E. Lying and standing blood pressure

13. Variceal bleeding

A 51-year-old patient is brought into the emergency department following a large-volume haematemesis. The patient is a known cirrhotic and previously survived variceal haemorrhage. The patient is haemodynamically stabilized and an emergency endoscopy is performed which identifies actively bleeding varices, and banding is attempted. Shortly following the procedure the patient again has a large-volume haematemesis and becomes haemodynamically compromised. The next step is

A. Oesophageal transection
B. Transjugular intrahepatic portal–systemic stent shunting
C. Sengstaken–Blakemore tube
D. Repeat endoscopy
E. Angiographic arterial embolisation

applies traction on GTE junction → reducer blood flow to varices.
Can inflate esophageal balloon to tamponade bleeding if traction alone is not enough.

14. Abdominal emergency

A 45-year-old patient presents in shock complaining of sudden-onset general-ized upper abdominal pain radiating to the right iliac fossa and the tip of his right shoulder. He reports one episode of vomiting, but none since. He has no past medical problems. On examination, his abdomen is rigid and bowel sounds are absent. The diagnosis is

A. Caecal volvulus → *not much vomiting.*
B. Pancreatitis → *radiation to back*
C. Perforated duodenal ulcer
D. Ascending cholangitis → *no fever or jaundice*
E. Appendicitis
    ↘ RIF → starts periumbilical

15. Abdominal wall anatomy

Which of the following is not encountered when making Kocher's (right subcos-tal) incision during an open cholecystectomy?

A. Anterior rectus sheath
B. Superior epigastric vessels
C. Eighth intercostal nerve
D. Falciform ligament
E. External oblique

Anterior rectus
sup. epigastric vessels (sacrificed)
lateral ab. wall muscles
Eight n. sacrificed
posterior rectus
peritoneum

16. Upper gastrointestinal bleeding

A patient is admitted from the emergency department following a large-volume haematemesis. Oesophagogastroduodenoscopy is performed, which identifies a posteriorly positioned duodenal ulcer that is actively bleeding. The vessel responsible is

    A. Gastroduodenal artery
    B. Abdominal aorta
    C. Right gastric artery
    D. Left gastric artery
    E. Right gastroepiploic artery

17. Upper gastrointestinal haemorrhage

A patient is admitted to hospital following referral by his GP for melaena. An oesophagogastroduodenoscopy identifies an actively bleeding gastric ulcer. Haemostasis is achieved. You are called to see the patient 48 hours later by nursing staff concerned that the patient has again passed black stool. On examination the patient is comfortable, blood pressure is 120/80 mmHg lying and 115/85 mmHg standing, pulse rate is 70 beats/min and respiratory rate is 16 breaths/min. Rectal examination reveals black stool on the glove. The next best course of action should be   * Hemodynamically Stable.

    A. Urgent endoscopy
    B. Repeat full blood count
    C. Intravenous fluids and colloid
    D. Intravenous terlipressin
    E. Nothing, this is normal following upper gastrointestinal bleeding

18. Duodenal ulcers

Which of the following syndromes is associated with multiple duodenal ulcers not amenable to conventional medical therapy?

    A. Hereditary non-polyposis colon cancer (HNPCC)
    B. Plummer–Vinson syndrome
    C. Gardiner's syndrome
    D. Zollinger–Ellison syndrome
    E. CREST syndrome

19. Gastric outflow obstruction

A patient presents with a short history of perfuse, projectile vomiting without bile staining. He has a history of peptic ulceration and chronic dyspepsia and has noticed increased bloating over the preceding 9 months. On examination, there is distension in the epigastric region and a succession splash. The abdominal radiograph shows a grossly distended stomach and collapsed bowel. The most likely cause is

→ second most common cause → difficult to distinguish from stricturing on clinical examination

A. Carcinoma of the pylorus
B. Carcinoma of the head of pancreas

history of peptic ulcer ← C. Fibrotic stricture *most common cause of outflow obstruction*

D. Compression by malignant nodes
E. Chronic pancreatitis

20. Gastro-oesophageal reflux disease

Which of the following is not a lifestyle change which might reduce the occurrence of reflux-type symptoms?

A. Smoking cessation
B. Abdominal exercise
C. Avoid tight clothing
D. Eat smaller portions more often
E. Raise the head of the bed at night

21. Gallstone disease

4 Fs:
fat
female
forty
fertile

Which one of the following statements regarding gallstone disease is incorrect?

A. Gallstones occur in 15% of all people over 65 in Western countries
B. 85% of gallstones are asymptomatic
C. 10% are identifiable using plain film radiography
D. Gallstones are more common in males
E. Gallstone disease is the most common cause of acute pancreatitis

22. Cholelithiasis

Which of the following is not a risk factor for gallstone formation?

A. Smoking
B. Pregnancy
C. Crohn's disease
D. Diet high in fats
E. Contraceptive pill

23. Complications of cholelithiasis

A 29-year-old patient presents with a short history of right upper quadrant pain. She is jaundiced with dark urine and pale stool. She has a fever of 38.9 °C. Abdominal examination gives no suggestion of a palpable gallbladder. The diagnosis is

A. Ascending cholangitis
B. Acute cholecystitis
C. Biliary colic with duct obstruction
D. Pancreatitis
E. Mirizzi's syndrome

24. Obstructive jaundice

A 62-year-old patient is admitted with jaundice. His stool is pale and urine dark red. On examination he has a palpable gallbladder. The most likely cause is

⤷ Courvoisier's sign.

A. Ascending cholangitis
B. Impacted stone in the common bile duct (choledocholithiasis)
C. Tumour of the head of pancreas (more common than Cholangiocarcinoma)
D. Impacted stone in the neck of the gallbladder
E. Cholangiocarcinoma

Courvoisier's law

25. Complicated gallstones

A 63-year-old patient is admitted with intermittent, colicky right upper quadrant pain and jaundice. Abdominal ultrasound shows a thickened gallbladder, but no identifiable stones. He is treated for biliary colic with fluids and analgesia but fails to improve. His serum bilirubin continues to rise and after 24 hours his C-reactive protein level and white cell count become elevated. Two days after initial presentation he develops a pyrexia of 39.2 °C and his pain is now constant. The next step in management is

A. Cholecystectomy
B. Endoscopic retrograde cholangiopancreatography ⟶ diagnostic and therapeutic
C. Open stone removal with T-tube drainage
D. Magnetic resonance cholangiopancreatography
E. Lithotripsy ⟶ if ERCP fails

26. Oesophagitis

A 65-year-old patient presents with symptoms of oesophagitis. Endoscopy is performed and biopsies taken from the patients lower oesophagus which demonstrates Barrett's oesophagus with low grade dysplasia. What is the next best course of action?

, rebiopsy at 6-12 wks
after high dose suppression
• then endoscopic surveillance 6 monthly

A. Referral for oesophagectomy
B. Staging CT chest abdomen and pelvis
C. Oesophageal ablation
D. High dose PPI and repeat endoscopy
E. Triple eradication therapy

if Barrett but no dysplasia
⟶ Endoscopic surveillance every 2 years.

27. Cholangiocarcinoma

Which of the following is not a risk factor for the development of cholangiocarcinoma?

A. Primary sclerosing cholangitis ⟶ associated with UC
B. Choledochal cysts
C. Hepatitis B/C infection
D. Primary biliary cirrhosis
E. Lynch syndrome II

28. Upper gastrointestinal surgery

Whipple's procedure is an operation used in the management of pancreatic cancer and, more rarely, in chronic pancreatitis. Which of the following structures is not resected during the classical procedure?

    A. Duodenum
    B. Head of pancreas
    C. Gallbladder
    D. Common hepatic duct
    E. Pylorus

29. Hyposplenism

Which of the following abnormal findings on peripheral blood film is not typical of changes associated with hyposplenism?

→ in G6PD deficiency, heinz bodies are recognized by spleen and removed.

    A. Bite cells
    B. Howell–Jolly bodies → *DNA remnants normally removed by spleen*
    C. Target cells   *↑ membrane abnormalities → also normally*
    D. Ecchinocytes   *removed by spleen.*
    E. Pappenheimer bodies → *seen in iron loaded cells normally removed by spleen.*

30. Splenectomy (1)

Which is the most common early complication following splenectomy?

    A. Pancreatitis
    B. Gastric dilatation
    C. Atelectasis → *most common complication of any surgery involving organs close to diaphragm*
    D. Thrombosis
    E. Overwhelming post-splenectomy sepsis

31. Splenectomy (2)

Splenectomy patients should be immunized against all the following organisms, except

    A. *Haemophilus influenzae*
    B. *Clostridium tetani*
    C. *Meningococcus C*
    D. *Streptococcus pneumoniae*
    E. Influenza virus

32. Pancreas

Which of the following is not secreted by the endocrine or exocrine pancreas?

    A. Chymotrypsinogen
    B. Glucagon

α: glucagon
β: insulin
D: somatostatin
F: pancreatic polypeptid

• amylase
• lipase } *PH*
• Trypsinogen : activated by enterokinase

C. Somatostatin Paracrine
D. Lipase certain plt
E. Gastrin present in fetal life
    ↳ by G cells in stomach (?)

33. Pancreatitis (1)

Of the following, which is not a clearly recognized cause of acute pancreatitis?

A. 5-acetyl salicylic acid
B. Furosemide
C. Coxsackie B virus
D. Hyperlipidaemia
E. Magnetic resonance cholangiopancreatography MRCP

34. Pancreatitis (2)

A 48-year-old patient is admitted into hospital with acute-onset abdominal pain and perfuse vomiting. Serum amylase is 2500 IU/mL, C-reactive protein is 250 mg/L. The patient is managed conservatively, but 48 hours later you are called to see him as the nursing staff has become concerned. On examination the patient is distressed and combative. His blood pressure is 125/65 mmHg, pulse rate is 130 beats/min and respiratory rate is 38 breaths/min. Arterial blood gases show pH 7.20, pO$_2$ 7.9 and pCO$_2$ 5.8. The most likely cause of his deterioration is

A. Septic shock
B. Acute respiratory distress syndrome
C. Pancreatic pseudocyst
D. Acute alcohol withdrawal
E. Disseminated intravascular coagulation

·hypovolemic shocks
· CVF
· ARF
· ARDS: atelectasis, sepsis
· cerebral Ischen
· liver damage
· DIC
· thrombosis adjacend vessels

35. Complications of acute pancreatitis

A patient was admitted for acute pancreatitis secondary to alcohol misuse. He was treated conservatively and discharged for outpatient follow-up. He presents to your clinic after 8 weeks complaining of continued abdominal pain in the epi-gastrium radiating into the back. Serum amylase is 7800 IU/L. On examination, he is tender over the epigastrium. Blood pressure, pulse rate and temperature are all unremarkable. The diagnosis is

A. Pancreatic pseudocyst : 6-8w aft acute pancreatitis, persistan↑amylase, alcoholism
B. Cholecystitis
C. Chronic pancreatitis : Possible DD, but cyst   pseudo has to be rolled gst
D. Recurrent acute pancreatitis ·normal vitals
E. Pancreatic abscess : normal vitals

A ·abcess, duodenal - biliary obstructi, Rupture into Pleural, Peritoml space,
     vessel erosion (complication)
  · small resolve spont , ↑6cm CT/US percutaneous drainage

ANSWERS

Anatomy

1 D Gallbladder

Anatomy is taught to a greater or lesser degree in all medical schools. However, if a candidate is doing well in a viva or PACES format exam, he or she *will* be asked basic anatomy. Some schools also include anatomy questions in their written papers, so it is worth knowing, even if surgery is not your chosen career pathway. Of the above options, the gallbladder is the only structure which does not border the foramen of Winslow. Of note is that the portal triad is contained within the hepatoduodenal ligament. Candidates should know the three structures that make up the portal triad.

Gastric cancer

2 D Blood group O

The incidence of gastric cancer in the UK is declining, although incidence is still approximately 16:100 000. It is more common in Japan, where it is such a problem that national screening programmes are in place. It affects males twice as commonly as females. Dried fish and cured meats are associated with increased risk, due to the high quantities of nitrosamines in them. Pernicious anaemia, an autoimmune disorder with antibodies produced against intrinsic factor, also predisposes to gastric cancer as does chronic *H. pylori* infection – which carries a 1% risk of malignancy. Previous gastrectomy is a risk factor for malignancy, something which must be discussed with the patient prior to their operation.

Blood group A is a risk factor for gastric cancer, but blood group O is not. Other risk factors include atrophic gastritis, low social status and smoking.

Oesophageal cancer

3 C Endoscopy

Over 75% of cases of oesophageal carcinoma will have metastasis at the time of diagnosis and overall 5-year survival is just 5%. The spread is initially by direct invasion, then by lymphatics. Haematogenous spread occurs late. Appropriate choice of staging investigations depends on the positioning of the primary tumour. Endoscopy is not a staging investigation, although it is a diagnostic investigation and is the means through which tissue diagnosis is made.

Surgical anatomy of the oesophagus

4 A Inferior thyroid artery, descending aorta, left gastric artery

The first reaction to a question of this type is typically panic as the majority of candidates will not know the blood supply to the oesophagus. However, candidates should be able to rule out most of the options using more basic knowledge. The internal carotid has no branches outside the cranial vault, and therefore option B can be discounted. The lateral thoracic artery runs in the mid-axillary line supplying the lateral chest wall and the long thoracic artery is fictitious, therefore options C and D can be discounted. Option E should be similarly discounted: neither the common hepatic nor the ascending aorta are likely to supply the oesophagus. By applying such an analytical approach candidates will be able to answer such questions without in-depth knowledge of the relevant anatomy.

The anatomy of the oesophagus is complex, primarily because of its length and passage through several anatomical regions. The first third is composed of striated muscle and is supplied by the inferior thyroid artery and drained by the inferior thyroid veins and the deep cervical lymph vessels. The second third is a blend of striated and smooth muscle fibres. It is supplied by the descending aorta, and drains via the azygos vein and the posterior mediastinal lymph vessels. The lower third is made up of smooth muscle fibres, and is supplied by the oesophageal branches of the left gastric artery and drained via the left gastric vein into the portal venous system and the lymph vessels surrounding the coeliac plexus.

Dysphagia (1)

5 C Upper gastrointestinal endoscopy

This patient has a history which is highly suggestive of oesophageal cancer. The rapid progression from solid food to liquids, weight loss and age should all raise the possibility of malignancy in the mind of the clinician. However, this should not tempt one to move straight to staging CT, however certain one might be. It is still necessary to confirm the diagnosis prior to staging, the gold standard investigation being endoscopy as it allows histological examination as well as direct visualization of pathology. Barium meal has little role in the investigation of dysphagia. Barium swallow has largely been replaced by endoscopy for mechanical causes of dysphagia, although it remains invaluable when investigating neuromuscular causes such as achalasia and in the evaluation of swallowing deficits following cerebrovascular accidents.

Dysphagia (2)

6 D Achalasia

Achalasia is a neuromuscular disorder caused by degeneration of Auerbach's plexus, which results in a failure of the lower oesophageal sphincter to relax. Its cause is idiopathic although infection with *Trypanosoma cruzi* (Chagas' disease) causes a similar problem. The characteristic presentation is with problems swallowing fluids initially, followed by food. Chest pain and weight loss are also common. This conflicts with mechanical causes such as malignancy and compression, as these will initially cause problems with large food boluses, progressing to fluids. The spectre of malignancy is raised by the history of weight loss and mediastinal mass; however, the pattern of symptoms and the patient's age count against this as an answer. The mass seen on the chest radiograph is a dilated oesophagus loaded with food.

The principal symptom associated with oesophageal spasm is chest pain, which may closely mimic that caused by myocardial infarction and is relieved by GTN. Dysphagia does occur, but is almost never associated with weight loss. Plummer–Vinson syndrome is a disorder characterized by severe iron deficiency and hyperkeratinization of the upper third of the oesophagus, which causes web formation and obstructive dysphagia. It is, therefore, presented in a similar fashion to other mechanical causes such as malignancy. Both achalasia and Plummer–Vinson syndrome are associated with an increased incidence of oesophageal cancer and require long-term endoscopic monitoring.

Acute pancreatitis

7 A Serum amylase

The Glasgow criteria are the most commonly applied prognostic scoring system in the UK. There are other criteria – the Ranson scoring system is preferred in the USA and the Balthazar score is based on the findings on CT scanning. It is important to know one of these, and for simplicity's sake the authors' suggest the Glasgow criteria for use by junior doctors. The score is based on the following findings: 1 point is awarded for each, and a score of 3 points within 48 hours of onset indicates severe disease. The score can be remembered using the mnemonic 'PANCREAS'.

- P – pO_2 <8 kPa
- A – age >55 years
- N – neutrophil count >15 × 10^9/L
- C – calcium <2 mmol/L
- R – raised urea >16 mmol/L
- E – enzymes; LDH >600 IU/L, AST >300 IU/L
- A – albumin <32 g/L
- S – sugar (glucose) >10 mmol/L

Scleroderma and CREST syndrome

8 B   Erythematous malar rash

The scleroderma spectrum of disorders are a group of connective tissue diseases inclusive of localized scleroderma (affects skin only), Raynaud's (vasospastic involvement of the fingers) and systemic sclerosis which is itself divided into diffuse cutaneous systemic sclerosis (DCSS) and limited cutaneous systemic sclerosis (also known as CREST syndrome). The two conditions vary in their symptom pattern and onset, but both involve the internal organ systems, including the renal tract and lungs (causing failure and pulmonary fibrosis). Skin involvement in DCSS is severe and widespread, but organ involvement is maximal at around 3 years and then typically improves. In CREST skin involvement is confined to the face and extremities; however, organ involvement tends to be progressive and more severe. CREST syndrome is typified by the following features: calcinosis, Raynaud's, esophageal disorders, sclerodactyly and telangiectasia.

Diagnosis is clinical and backed by identification of certain auto-antibodies. Anti-nuclear antibodies are usually present, anti-Scl-70 is positive in 40% of scleroderma, the presence of anti-centromere antibody occurs in 80%–90% of CREST and is suggestive of the diagnosis. However, auto-antibody testing is non-specific, and either antibody or both antibodies may occur in both conditions.

Gastro-oesophageal sphincter

9 A   Left crus of diaphragm

The gastro-oesophageal sphincter comprises three separate components, which work in tandem to prevent reflux. The LOS is a 4 cm section of hypertrophied smooth muscle, which is continuous with the smooth muscle wall of the oesophagus. It maintains a tonic contraction of 25 cmH$_2$0 above the resting intra-gastric pressure. The LOS requires support, however, when intra-gastric pressure rises above the baseline. The second component of the gastro-oesophageal sphincter is the extrinsic sphincter formed by the skeletal muscle fibres of the right crus of the diaphragm that sling around the oesophagus. The extrinsic sphincter supports the LOS at rest but also contracts with the diaphragm during inspiration and abdominal straining, preventing reflux.

The third component of the gastro-oesophageal sphincter is the 'physiological sphincter'; the oesophagus projects 2–3 cm into the abdominal cavity and therefore a rise in intra-abdominal pressure leads to compression of the abdominal portion of the oesophagus, preventing reflux. In addition the angle of His provides a flap valve which also protects against reflux. Knowledge of this mechanism is important when considering the effects of hiatus hernia on the integrity of the gastro-oesophageal sphincter, which leaves the LOS completely without support and therefore prone to severe reflux.

Oesophagitis

10 B   Proton pump inhibitor

Hiatus herniation is common, occurring in 30% of the population aged over 50, and 50% of those with a hiatus hernia complain of symptomatic GORD. Eight per cent of hiatus hernias are sliding hernias and do not require surgery in the majority of cases; rolling hiatus hernias, however, may necessitate repair due to the risk of strangulation.

Severity of oesophagitis is graded according to the Los Angeles classification:

- Grade 1 = small mucosal breaks, limited to less than two mucosal folds
- Grade 2 = mucosal break >5 mm long, limited to less than two mucosal folds
- Grade 3 = mucosal breaks extending beyond two mucosal folds, but involving < 75% of the oesophageal circumference
- Grade 4 = circumferential mucosal breakdown involving > 75% of the mucosal circumference

Complications include bleeding (usually small volume and chronic), stricture, Barrett's and oesophageal malignancy. Surgery should be avoided unless symptoms are severe and life-altering, refractory to optimal lifestyle and medical management and 24-hour pH monitoring confirms severe reflux. The best option in this patient is a trial of acid suppression therapy such as a proton pump inhibitor (e.g. omeprazole, lansoprazole) or an H_2 antagonist (e.g. ranitidine). Endoscopic surveillance is not indicted in this mild disease.

Abdominal surgery

11 E   Vitamin B_1 deficiency

Gastrectomy (partial or total) is a procedure which has been falling out of favour as medical and endoscopic therapy for ulceration and upper gastrointestinal bleeding have proved their effectiveness. Currently, the most common indication for gastrectomy is resection of gastric carcinoma, however procedural rates are rising as endemic obesity becomes more of a problem and the demand for bariatric surgery increases.

As such, it is important for surgical trainees to be aware of the potential complications of such surgery. There is a lifelong increased risk of malignancy in patients treated with partial gastrectomy, and as with all intra-abdominal surgery, there is an increased risk of obstruction, either from anastomotic strictures or adhesions. Malabsorption syndromes following gastric surgery include B_{12}, iron and folate deficiencies; vitamin B_{12} uptake is dependent on intrinsic factor normally produced by gastric parietal cells and bypassing of the duodenum and jejunum causes deficiency in iron and folate as they are chiefly absorbed in the proximal small bowel. Thiamine (vitamin B_1) deficiency is not associated with gastrectomy.

Other common complications following gastrectomy include reduced gastric capacity, causing abdominal discomfort and early satiety, and dumping syndrome, which results from uncontrolled release of large volumes of chyme into the proximal bowel. The sugars from the chyme are rapidly absorbed and promote an exaggerated insulin response. This results in hot flushes, palpitations and syncope, similar to a hypoglycaemic attack.

Gastrointestinal haemorrhage

12 E   Lying and standing blood pressure
The above scenario is strongly suggestive of a diagnosis of gastrointestinal bleeding. This patient will require an endoscopy, but the timing of such will be determined by his haemodynamic status. Systolic blood pressure and heart rate can be difficult to interpret in patients with a good cardiopulmonary reserve; the most sensitive way of identifying decompensation following haemorrhage is to dynamically test the cardiovascular reserve by assessing for postural drop. Equally, vital signs can be difficult to interpret in patients with pre-existing co-morbidities such as hypertension. A blood pressure of 110/80 mmHg in an individual with a baseline systolic pressure of 180 mmHg indicates profound shock; however, this relative hypotension will be easily missed. Similarly, medications such as β-blockers or digitalis will prevent a normal tachycardic response to hypovolaemia. Decompensation in these patients is also most accurately identified by comparing lying and standing blood pressures.

A patient's haemoglobin level may indicate the need for transfusion (aim for haemoglobin >8.0 g/dL), but it is a poor marker of severity of haemorrhage in the absence of a baseline level. Furthermore, following an acute haemorrhage the haemoglobin level may be normal if the dilutional effect of fluid replacement has not had time to affect the result. Volume of melaena and vomit is an extremely unreliable marker and is seldom worth consideration.

Variceal bleeding

13 C   Sengstaken–Blakemore tube
Oesophageal varices account for 7% of upper gastrointestinal bleeds, with 80% of these occurring in people with cirrhosis. Peptic ulceration accounts for 40% of upper GI bleeds, oesophagitis/gastritis accounts for 20% and Mallory–Weiss tears for 15%. Without treatment, 30% of varices will bleed, and once bleeding has occurred 80% will re-bleed within 2 years. The most effective management is a combination therapy with propranolol and repeat endoscopic monitoring and banding.

In the acute stage, first line therapy is haemodynamic stabilization and urgent endoscopy with sclerotherapy or banding. This can be performed in the emergency department in most major hospitals. Intravenous infusion with a PPI and terlipressin is also required along with correction of any co-existent clotting abnormalities. If this fails to control bleeding, then passage of a Sengstaken–Blakemore tube is the next line of therapy; remember only the gastric balloon is inflated to tamponade the bleeding – inflation of the oesophageal balloon is unnecessary and hazardous. A repeat endoscopy after a failed attempt is less likely to achieve haemostasis and is therefore avoided if the patient is haemodynamically compromised. Repeat endoscopy may have a role in the stable patient.

Oesophageal transection is an outdated emergency surgical technique rarely employed. This patient will probably require TIPSS to prevent further re-bleeding, but it is not the 'next step' in the acute scenario. It carries long-term consequences following insertion, namely increased risk of sepsis (as portal blood bypasses the liver), the precipitation of encephalopathy and risk of re-occlusion. Angiographic embolisation is inappropriate as bleeding is from the portal venous system, not from arterial vessels.

Abdominal emergency

14 C   Perforated duodenal ulcer

To correctly derive the answer from the given information try to exclude options to leave the single best fitting answer. The history is of sudden-onset pain and minimal vomiting, which makes caecal volvulus unlikely. This history also fails to fit with ascending cholangitis as there is no mention of fever or jaundice.

On examination the patient has signs of generalised peritonitis; this is not typical of acute pancreatitis, the early stages of which are characterized by pain which radiates through to the back and associated vomiting, with peritonism localised to the epigastrum. The presentation of appendicitis can be variable the rapid-onset pain and generalized peritonitis should not suggest a diagnosis of appendicitis to most candidates. The location of the pain, the severity of the shock and the scanty vomiting are all typical of perforated duodenal ulcer. Do not be put off by the radiation of pain to the right iliac fossa; this commonly occurs as fluid tracks down the peritoneal gutter.

Perforated peptic ulcer is an important diagnosis to arrive at quickly as it carries 5%–10% mortality. Approximately 50% of those affected give a history of previous ulcer symptoms or risk factors for ulcer disease; however, 50% have no such history. A high index of suspicion is therefore required.

Abdominal wall anatomy

15 D   Falciform ligament

Depending on what emphasis a candidate's medical school places on surgical teaching and applied anatomy, he or she may be asked simple questions regarding the more common or classic surgical incisions in the written or viva examination. Candidates should therefore know the surgical anatomy of Kocher's incision, Lanz incision, mid-line laparotomy incision and open hernia repair (i.e. the inguinal canal).

Kocher's incision may be made on the left or the right side, but it is most commonly used in open biliary tree surgery. The incision is made 3–5 cm below the costal margin. The anterior rectus sheath is exposed and divided along the line of incision exposing the rectus muscles which may then be divided with care taken to ensure haemostasis when branches of the superior epigastric vessels are sacrificed. The incision is extended through the lateral abdominal wall muscles which are split to allow better access. The eighth and ninth intercostal nerves lie between the internal oblique and transverse muscles; the eighth nerve is often sacrificed, but effort is made to preserve the larger ninth nerve. The incision is deepened through the posterior rectus sheath and peritoneum.

The falciform ligament inserts in the midline into the lina alba; this structure is not crossed in Kocher's incision and therefore should not be encountered.

Upper gastrointestinal bleeding

16 A   Gastroduodenal artery

Detailed knowledge of the arterial supply of the stomach is not required for undergraduate exams, however certain facts should be remembered. All the blood supply to the stomach is derived from the coeliac plexus, which branches from the abdominal aorta at the level of T12. The lesser curve is supplied by the right and left gastric vessels, the greater curve of the right and left gastroepiploic vessels. The right gastroepiploic artery is a branch of the gastroduodenal artery. The gastroduodenal artery passes underneath the first part of the duodenum, closely associated with its posterior wall; it is this vessel which classically causes major haemorrhage in the event of posterior erosion by a duodenal ulcer.

Upper gastrointestinal haemorrhage

17 B   Repeat full blood count

This patient is not in shock as evidenced by his observations and postural blood pressure; therefore the possibility of ongoing major haemorrhage is unlikely and options A, C and D can all be discounted. Melaena can continue for up to 3 days after cessation of bleeding from an upper gastrointestinal source, or even longer in the presence of constipation. Therefore the statement in option E is absolutely correct; reassure the patient that his continued passing of melaena is not necessarily a sign of continued bleeding, and also repeat the patient's FBC to exclude occult haemorrhage. There would be concern if the patient had had a normal bowel motion since his melaena initially started, then returned to passing melaena stool; this would more strongly indicate re-bleeding and if accompanied by a drop in haematocrit would necessitate a repeat endoscopy.

Duodenal ulcers

18 D Zollinger–Ellison syndrome

Rare diseases, including eponymous syndromes, are numerous and therefore take up an amount of revision time entirely disproportionate to their clinical or examinational importance. Candidates are advised against spending excessive time revising their clinical presentations and treatments. Instead, they should concern themselves only with those syndromes linked to cancer or severe illness or common symptomatology such as dysphagia, as these will typically be the only ones in the minds of examiners.

Zollinger–Ellison syndrome is caused by a non-insulin secreting tumour of the pancreas, which releases high levels of gastrin-like hormone. This causes hyperacidity of the stomach and therefore predisposes to severe and extensive duodenal ulceration.

Gastric outflow obstruction

19 C Fibrotic stricture

This form of question is particularly difficult to answer as all of the above options are potential causes of gastric outlet obstruction. However, candidates should be aware that the most common causes in an adult are fibrotic structuring secondary to duodenal ulceration and cancer of the pylorus. Other causes are more unusual, particularly in the absence of preceding suggestive history.

The distinction between duodenal ulcer disease and cancer of the pylorus may be more difficult; both present with painless projectile vomiting, which is free from bile, but contains stale food and often smells faeculent. Profound weight loss is also common to both conditions. However, the long history of peptic ulcer disease in this case suggests fibrotic stricturing to be the most likely cause. Also the gross distension described suggests that this process has been ongoing over the years with compensatory gastric hypertrophy; cancer typically presents more acutely, and distension is therefore less marked. Caution is advised when applying this maxim in clinical practice as duodenal ulceration may also cause acute obstruction if associated oedema is severe enough to prevent gastric emptying; therefore the only reliable way of distinguishing cause is by endoscopy.

Gastro-oesophageal reflux disease

20 B Abdominal exercise

Gastro-oesophageal reflux is a common symptom suffered by the majority of the population; its serious sequelae oesophagitis, anaemia, fibrotic stricture and Barrett's oesophagus are thankfully less common. Nevertheless Barrett's oesophagus afflicts approximately 2% of the adult population of the United Kingdom, and 2% of these individuals will develop malignant change.

The majority of reflux can be managed with conservative therapies and lifestyle changes; these include cessation of smoking, weight loss, avoidance of tight clothing, avoidance of large meals and raising the head of the bed at night. Abdominal exercises have no role and may exacerbate reflux. Consideration must be given to whether a patient requires further investigation; failure to respond to conservative management and a PPI may require endoscopy to exclude a hiatus hernia or other causative factor. New dyspepsia in patients over 55 or the presence of certain 'red flag' signs should precipitate urgent endoscopic investigation to exclude the possibility of a serious underlying cause; these include signs that can be remembered using the 'ALARMS' mnemonic:

- Anaemia
- Loss of weight
- Anorexia
- Recent onset of rapidly progressive symptoms
- Melaena
- Swallowing difficulty

Gallstone disease

21 D Gallstones are more common in males

Gallstones are found in around 15% of the population over 60 years of age, but are only symptomatic in 15% of those. There are three types of stone: cholesterol stones (15%), pigment stones (5%), seen in haemolytic anaemias, and mixed stones (80%). Pigment stones are typically small, black, irregular, multiple and fragile. Cholesterol stones often form as a single large stone (solitaire) but can form as multiple stones termed mulberry stones. Pure cholesterol stones contain crystals when cut in cross-section. Mixed stones are often multiple; they are laminated in cross-section and approximately 15% of these are radio-opaque due to the variable extent to which they become calcified.

Gallstone pancreatitis accounts for 45% of all acute pancreatitis in Western countries, its nearest rival being alcohol (25%). The incorrect statement is that gallstones occur more commonly in males; there is a slight female predominance overall, although this is more marked in the younger age ranges (see Question 22).

Cholelithiasis

22 A   Smoking

Factors predisposing to gallstone formation include sepsis within the biliary tree, anatomical variants which predispose to stasis and changes in the composition of bile which make it lithogenic. Amirand's triangle is a diagrammatic representation of how changes in bile composition can predispose to stone formation. Put simply, if the percentage composition of cholesterol increases, or the percentage composition of bile salts or phospholipids (lecithin) decreases, then the bile is more likely to form gallstones.

When taking a focused history and examination, candidates should aim to elicit/exclude the following risk factors for gallstone formation:

- Race (higher incidence in black and Asian populations)
- High-fat diet/history of hypercholesterolaemia
- Obesity
- High oestrogen states (CCP, pregnancy, PCOS; hence the slight female predominance)
- Haemolytic states

The loss of the terminal ileum following surgery or as a consequence of Crohn's disease also predisposes to gallstone formation as the terminal ileum is the site of re-absorption of bile salts. Smoking is not known to directly influence the risk of gallstone formation.

Complications of cholelithiasis

23 A   Ascending cholangitis

The high pyrexia is not typical of biliary colic, pancreatitis or Mirizzi's syndrome without supervening infection. Most candidates should therefore quickly narrow down the options to a choice between ascending cholangitis and acute cholecystitis. Acute cholecystitis is inflammation within the gallbladder most commonly due to long standing presence of gallstones. It presents with right upper quadrant pain and signs of sepsis. Jaundice may complicate cholecystitis if a gallstone migrates into the common bile duct; however, it is more usual for cholecystitis to present without jaundice. In addition, the fact the patient does not have Murphy's sign makes acute cholecystitis less likely, although it is not a reliable sign and therefore cholecystitis is a possible answer.

However, this patient is jaundiced with high fever and right upper quadrant pain – these three symptoms constitute Charcot's triad, the classic description of the presentation of ascending cholangitis. Therefore A is the single best answer, although in reality, both A and B would be on your differential list.

Obstructive jaundice

24 C Tumour of the head of pancreas
Dark urine and pale stool is the classic presentation of obstructive jaundice; one would also expect this patient to be complaining of pruritus as itching is a common symptom of conjugated hyperbilirubinaemia. The causes of obstructive jaundice are multiple and may be divided into obstructions within the lumen (stones, parasites) or within the wall (stricture, inflammation, tumour) or external pressure (lesions of the head of the pancreas, vascular aneurysms, local lymph nodes, Mirizzi's syndrome).

The key to answering this question is recognizing that a palpable gallbladder makes stone-related disease unlikely. Courvoisier's law states that 'in obstructive jaundice, the presence of a palpable gallbladder precludes the diagnosis of stones'. This is because the presence of gallstones irritates the gallbladder, resulting in wall fibrosis and thickening, a feature used when ultrasound scanning to confirm the presence of stones and a feature which prevents gallbladder distension in the presence of obstruction. Therefore answers A, B and D may all be discounted. The answer therefore relies on the candidate knowing the relative incidence of pancreatic cancer and cholangiocarcinoma, the former being the more common of the two.

Complicated gallstones

25 B Endoscopic retrograde cholangiopancreatography
This patient has obstructive jaundice. The likely culprit is gallstones, as his gallbladder is thickened on ultrasound. On admission there were no clear signs of cholecystitis as his pain was intermittent and colicky. The majority of biliary colic may be successfully managed with fluids and analgesia in the absence of superseding infection or pancreatitis. All patients should subsequently be offered cholecystectomy 6–12 weeks following recovery to avoid recurrence.

Escalation of acute management is required when jaundice fails to resolve or when acute cholecystitis or ascending cholangitis supervenes, as has occurred in this case. The immediate priority is to treat the sepsis with intravenous antibiotics and fluids. However, this is not an option in this question. The next step in the management of such patients is the decompression of the biliary tree and the release of the stagnating bile.

MRCP is not an appropriate option, and nor is lithotripsy which is reserved for renal calculi lying within the renal pelvis; ERCP is the single best procedure as it is minimally invasive, and allows confirmation of diagnosis and therapeutic intervention. In young patients, or in patients where ERCP fails, open stone removal with T-tube placement is a viable alternative to ERCP, however percutaneous cholecystostomy is more frequently used as it is a lower risk procedure.

Cholecystectomy risks leaving the obstructing stone in place and is best avoided in patients with an obstructed biliary tree. Cholecystectomy is commonly deferred and performed as an elective day case procedure following resolution of the life-threatening sepsis.

Oesophagitis

26 D High dose PPI and repeat endoscopy
This patient has Barrett's oesophagus with low grade dysplasia. As such, he is at high risk of developing oesophageal malignancy. Such patients require high dose acid suppression and surveillance endoscopy until the dysplasia resolves. Initially this patient will require extensive re-biopsy following 8–12 weeks of high dose acid suppression. Thereafter endoscopic surveillance should continue 6 monthly until the dysplasia resolves. Barrett's without dysplasia requires surveillance every 2 years, and lifelong acid suppression.

Patients with high grade dysplasia have a 30%–40% incidence of invasive adenocarcinoma. These patients should be referred for consideration of oesophagectomy. In patients unfit or unwilling to undergo surgery, ablation may be an alternative. Triple eradication is only indicated in the presence of Helicobacter pylori.

Cholangiocarcinoma

27 D Primary biliary cirrhosis
Cholangiocarcinoma is a rare primary tumour of the intrahepatic or extrahepatic bile ducts. It accounts for approximately 20% of primary liver tumours. Although detailed knowledge of all risk factors associated with this disease is beyond the level of final examinations, finals candidates should be aware that 20%–30% of those with primary sclerosing cholangitis (PSC) will develop cholangiocarcinoma and that no similar relationship is seen in primary biliary cirrhosis. Therefore, answering this question correctly requires a basic level of knowledge and good exam technique.

The other factors mentioned all predispose to cholangiocarcinoma. In addition, inflammatory bowel disease is also associated, although it is unclear how much this association is attributable to the increased rate of PSC in patients with IBD. Age positively correlates with incidence of cholangiocarcinoma, the peak age of presentation being between 50 and 70 years. However, patients with PSC or choledochal cysts typically develop a malignant change up to two decades before the unaffected populous.

Upper gastrointestinal surgery

28 D   Common hepatic duct

Whipple's procedure is indicated in cancer of the pancreatic head, distal bile duct, ampulla or duodenum, and can also be undertaken in patients with chronic pancreatitis. The standard procedure provides a greater level of clearance as it involves removal of gastric antrum, pylorus and proximal duodenum, but despite this there is no difference in survival rates compared with pylorus-sparing techniques. Pylorus-sparing surgery is easier and quicker to perform, but there is a greater risk of gastric outlet obstruction. There is no difference in morbidity between the two operations.

Both procedures involve the resection of the gallbladder, cystic duct, common bile duct, head of the pancreas and distal duodenum. Whipple's procedure requires the preservation of the common hepatic duct which is then anastomosed to a blind loop of jejunum. The jejunum is also anastomosed to the remnant pancreas and stomach.

Hyposplenism

29 A   Bite cells

The spleen's functions are numerous and include immune function, erythropoiesis and the identification of abnormal or damaged red cells and their clearance from the circulation. Hyposplenism due to iatrogenic removal or innate disease (sickle cell disease, haematological malignancy, coeliac disease, IBD, amyloidosis) therefore causes a variety of changes on the blood film. Howell–Jolly bodies are DNA remnants which are normally removed by a functional spleen. Their presence in peripheral blood cells is the classic hyposplenic abnormality. Pappenheimer bodies are granules seen in iron-loaded cells, also usually removed by a functioning spleen. Target cells and echinocytes are red cells with membrane abnormalities, and normally these would also be removed by the spleen.

Bite cells are red blood cells in which a piece of the membrane has been removed. This occurs in glucose 6-phosphate dehydrogenase deficiency, in which oxidative stress causes oxidized denatured haemoglobin to aggregate into Heinz bodies on the RBC membrane; these Heinz bodies are detected and removed by the spleen. Therefore, for bite cells to exist, the spleen must be functional.

Splenectomy (1)

30 C Atelectasis

Splenectomy may be a laparoscopic or open procedure; the open technique is performed through either a left subcostal (Kocher's) incision or through a mid-line laparotomy. Candidates should be aware of the major postoperative complications which may occur.

Atelectasis is the most common complication and is a risk of any procedure which involves operating adjacent to the diaphragm. Post-splenectomy patients are at increased risk of thrombosis due to a paradoxical increase in platelet count; this risk typically lasts for 3 weeks postoperatively in the majority of patients, but persists in around 30%. Thromboembolic complications are best avoided by early mobilization and prophylactic treatment with aspirin ± dipyridamole. Gastric dilatation is also a common complication with potentially serious consequences; it occurs due to gastric ileus and the danger is major haemorrhage following disturbance of ligatures on the vessels over the greater curve. Therefore all post-splenectomy patients must have an NG tube *in situ* following the procedure. Pancreatitis may follow splenectomy as the tail of the pancreas shares a common blood supply with the spleen which may occasionally become compromised during surgery. Overwhelming post-splenectomy sepsis is a well-documented long-term issue with all post-splenectomy patients and is described in greater detail in Question 31.

Splenectomy (2)

31 B Tetanus

The spleen's functions are various and include haemopoiesis, filtration of blood cellular components, storage of platelets and endocrine effects. In addition, the spleen is a major constituent of the lymphoreticular system functioning as a processor of antigens and the presentation of such to immune cells. In particular the spleen is vital in the defence against encapsulated organisms such as streptococcus, meningococcus and *Haemophilus*.

Therefore it is advisable for all patients who are having an elective splenectomy to receive vaccines against all these organisms prior to the procedure. In addition, all patients admitted following traumatic splenic injury which does not require an immediate operation are also immunized in case their condition deteriorates and they require splenectomy. Post-splenectomy patients typically receive seasonal flu vaccines for life as well as prophylactic antibiotics, most commonly penicillin V.

Option B is the correct answer in this case as vaccination against tetanus is not required.

Pancreas

32 E Gastrin

The functions of the pancreas are both exocrine and endocrine. The exocrine pancreas is a compound alveolar gland similar in structure to the salivary glands. The digestive enzymes are secreted into the alimentary tract via the pancreatic duct (duct of Wirsung) which usually joins the common bile duct to form the ampulla of Vater. Around 1500 mL of pancreatic juice is secreted every day, which contains various pro-enzymes including trypsinogen and chymotrypsinogen, the activation of which requires exposure to specialist enzymes secreted by the brush boarder of the small bowel. Various intact enzymes are also secreted, including pancreatic lipase and amylase, which are activated by the change in pH.

The endocrine pancreas produces four peptide hormones; insulin and glucagon are well known, somatostatin is produced by the D cells of the islets and serves a paracrine auto-regulatory function, and pancreatic polypeptide is produced by the F cells; its function is uncertain but it is thought to regulate gut motility.

Gastrin is a hormone produced by the G cells in the gastric wall and influences acid secretion, gut motility and mucosal growth in the stomach and small bowel. It is produced by the pancreas in fetal life, but not in adulthood. Therefore although gastrinomas may occur within the pancreas, they are not tumours of pre-existing physiological endocrine glands.

Pancreatitis (1)

33 E Magnetic resonance cholangiopancreatography

This question is a blatant trick which intends to highlight the importance of paying attention to the question and also to emphasize that the causes of pancreatitis are numerous and varied, and not confined to those included in the 'GET SMASHED' mnemonic. Of course MRCP does not cause acute pancreatitis; it is a non-invasive investigation which avoids the risks of ERCP.

The causes of acute pancreatitis, according to the famous mnemonic, include:

- Gallstones – the most common cause, accounting for 45% of acute pancreatitis.
- Ethanol – the second most common cause, accounting for 25% of acute pancreatitis.
- Trauma – contusion or laceration of the gland precipitates a generalized inflammatory reaction.

- Steroids – a common pharmacological cause (see below for more detail).
- Mumps – and other viral infections affecting exocrine glands (Coxsackie B).
- Autoimmune – rarely in isolation; usually occurs in the presence of PSC, PBC, Sjögren's.
- Scorpion sting – a species of Trinidadian scorpion (*Tityus trinitatis*), the poison of which is a powerful pancreatic secretagogue that causes pancreatic injury.
- Hyperlipidaemia (types I and IV), hypothermia, hypercalcaemia, hypotension.
- ERCP – accounts for 5% of all pancreatitis.
- Drugs – collectively the third most common cause; causative agents include thiazide diuretics, furosemide, azathioprine, 5-aminosalicylate, 6-mercaptopurine, metronidazole, tetracycline and oestrogens.

Pancreatitis (2)

34 B Acute respiratory distress syndrome

Acute pancreatitis is a systemic insult; do not be falsely reassured by a patient who appears relatively well on admission! A patient will continue to deteriorate for several days and mortality remains at 10% despite optimal management. Cardiovascular collapse secondary to hypovolaemia is common and requires aggressive fluid resuscitation with central monitoring advisable. Gastrointestinal bleeding may occur secondary to stress ulceration or vessel erosion by the inflammatory process. Thrombosis may also occur in vessels adjacent to the sites of inflammation, causing viscus ischaemia, infarction and perforation. Renal failure is a common cause of death and carries a poor prognosis. Coagulation derangement is common but rarely severe.

The patient described in this scenario is in respiratory failure. Respiratory complications of pancreatitis include atelectasis and acute lung injury/ARDS. The latter may be a consequence of primary lung injury or systemic inflammatory response to sepsis or inflammatory insult. It carries a poor prognosis with patients often requiring intubation, respiratory support and ITU admission.

Complications of acute pancreatitis

35 A Pancreatic pseudocyst

This scenario describes the classic presentation of a pancreatic pseudocyst, which is a common late complication of pancreatitis occurring in approximately 20% of cases, more commonly in alcoholism. The time frame of 6–8 weeks following the acute episode is typical and the persistently raised amylase is characteristic. The lack of systemic upset and pyrexia makes recurrent acute pancreatitis unlikely and precludes the diagnosis of a pancreatic abscess. Chronic pancreatitis and cholecystitis may be in the differential, but should only be entertained after exclusion of a pseudocyst.

A pancreatic pseudocyst is a collection of pancreatic juices enclosed by a non-epithelialized wall of fibrous and granulomatous tissue. It is this wall which distinguishes it from a simple fluid collection. These pseudocysts can occur within the pancreas itself, but more commonly collect in the lesser peritoneal sac. Complications include infection (when it becomes known as a pancreatic abscess), vessel erosion, duodenal obstruction, biliary obstruction or rupture into the peritoneal or pleural space. Smaller cysts may resolve spontaneously without complication and therefore such patients are admitted for observation. Management of large cysts (> 6 cm) or cysts at risk of complication may be by CT/ultrasound-guided percutaneous drainage, endoscopic drainage or open pancreatectomy, although the latter is technically difficult, poorly tolerated and tends to be avoided.

SECTION 7:
ABDOMEN: LOWER GASTROINTESTINAL SURGERY

Questions

1. Per-rectal bleeding   133
2. Hospital-acquired infection   133
3. Colonic carcinoma (1)   133
4. Colonic resections   134
5. Change in bowel habit   134
6. Stomas   134
7. Constipation   134
8. Volvulus   135
9. Inflammatory bowel disease (1)   135
10. Diverticular disease   135
11. Abdominal pain   135
12. Inflammatory bowel disease (2)   136
13. Appendix mass   136
14. Diagnosis of perianal disease   136
15. Perianal anatomy   137
16. Perianal pathology   137
17. Treatment of fistula *in ano*   137
18. Anal fissure   138
19. Abdominal wall anatomy   138
20. Appendicitis   138
21. Right iliac fossa mass   138
22. Hereditary colon carcinoma   139
23. Colonic carcinoma (2)   139
24. Management of colonic carcinoma   139
25. Lower gastrointestinal haemorrhage   139
26. Bowel obstruction   139

27. Obstruction   140

28. Meckel's diverticulum   140

29. Carcinoid tumours   140

30. Inflammatory bowel disease (3)   140

Answers   141

QUESTIONS

1. Per-rectal bleeding

A 50-year-old man presents to the outpatient clinic with an 8-week history of bleeding from his back end. This is typically bright red and copious during or following a stool. The patient has had no change in his bowel habit, no weight loss, and has no family history of bowel cancer. What is the most appropriate course of action?

A. Perform rubber band ligation of haemorrhoids
B. Perform injection sclerotherapy of haemorrhoids
C. Blood tests including CEA
D. Examination under anaesthetic +/- proceed to treat haemorrhoids
E. Flexible sigmoidoscopy

2. Hospital-acquired infection

A postoperative patient has been moved to a side room after developing diarrhoea following the start of a course of antibiotics. Faecal samples test positive for *Clostridium difficile* toxin and metronidazole is started. After 10 days the antibiotic course is finished and nursing staff repeat the toxin assay on a formed stool sample, which is again positive. What is the most appropriate next management step?

A. No further action required
B. Continue metronidazole for a further 10 days
C. Start intravenous vancomycin
D. Start oral vancomycin
E. Urgent colonoscopy as this patient is at significant risk of pseudo-membranous colitis

3. Colonic carcinoma (1)

A 60-year-old patient is being treated for colonic carcinoma. The primary lesion has been excised and chemotherapy started. However, computed tomography (CT) scanning identifies a 1 cm metastasis in the right lobe of the liver. The patient has no history of alcohol misuse or viral hepatitis. CT chest and CT brain show no abnormalities. The most appropriate next stage of management would be:

A. Liver resection
B. Gadolinium-enhanced liver magnetic resonance imaging
C. CT/ultrasound-guided biopsy
D. Referral to a palliative care setting with appropriate counselling and support
E. Monitor lesion – If size exceeds 1.5 cm, add irinotecan to 5-fluorouracil and folinic acid chemotherapy

4. Colonic resections

On colonoscopy a malignant lesion is identified 5 cm proximal to the splenic flexure. There are no contraindications to resection and the decision is made to operate with curative intent. The most appropriate procedure would be

    A. Right hemicolectomy
    B. Total colectomy
    C. Sigmoid colectomy
    D. Anterior resection
    E. Extended right hemicolectomy

5. Change in bowel habit

A 32-year-old female patient presents with a 6-week history of bloody bowel motions. She has noticed significant weight loss over the preceding 6 weeks with increasing lethargy and fatigue. She has previously had constipation and admits to regular laxative use. What is the most likely diagnosis?

    A. Bowel cancer
    B. Irritable bowel syndrome
    C. Diverticular disease
    D. Inflammatory bowel disease
    E. Anal fissure

6. Stomas

Which one of the following statements regarding stomas is the most correct?

    A. Hartmann's procedure results in a defunctioned rectum and loop colostomy
    B. An abdominoperineal resection may be reversed by formation of an ileal J-pouch
    C. A mucus fistula functions to decompress residual distal bowel
    D. Small bowel obstruction is a common early complication and indicates need for revision
    E. Positioning of the stoma is not important

7. Constipation

You are called to see an 85-year-old female patient as the nursing staff is concerned that the patient has not passed stool for 4 days. The patient has been admitted after family members became increasingly concerned regarding her general deterioration in health and level of function. She is orientated but frail and complains of increasing abdominal discomfort. On examination bowel sounds are increased. The abdomen is distended with generalized tenderness, but no rebound or guarding. There is a firm palpable mass in the left iliac fossa. Digital rectal examination shows an empty rectum. What diagnosis must be excluded?

A. Simple constipation
B. Paralytic ileus
C. Sigmoid volvulus
D. Peritonitis secondary to diverticular disease
E. Neoplasia

8. Volvulus

An 85-year-old male patient with a history of chronic constipation presents with acute severe colicky abdominal pain and absolute constipation. Plain abdominal film shows a grossly dilated oval of large bowel arising from the left lower quadrant. A diagnosis of sigmoid volvulus is made. The next step in management is:

A. Laparotomy
B. Sigmoidoscopy with flatus tube insertion
C. Sigmoid colectomy with colostomy
D. Barium swallow
E. Computed tomography

9. Inflammatory bowel disease (1)

Which one of the following does *not* occur as a systemic manifestation of inflammatory bowel disease?

A. Amyloidosis
B. Pyoderma gangrenosum
C. Scleritis
D. Cardiomyopathy
E. Sclerosing cholangitis

10. Diverticular disease

Which one of the following statements regarding diverticular disease is the most correct?

A. Colonic diverticula are true diverticula
B. Diverticular disease describes the outpouching of colonic mucosa between the muscle layers of the colonic wall
C. The most common site of diverticula is the rectum, where the highest pressures occur
D. Saint's triad consists of diverticular disease, cholelithiasis and inguinal herniation
E. 95% of complications from diverticula occur at the sigmoid colon

11. Abdominal pain

A 78-year-old patient is admitted with a short history of sudden onset colicky abdominal pain and bleeding per rectum. On assessment his blood pressure is

110/55 mmHg, respiratory rate is 30 breaths/min and he is in atrial fibrillation with a ventricular response of 130 beats/min. He is known to you as he has previously presented in the outpatients department and been investigated for intermittent abdominal pain associated with food associated with a 2 stone weight loss. He had a colonoscopy and upper GI endoscopy 3 months ago which was normal. Whilst you are investigating his pain, it changes to a constant central ache. The diagnosis is

   A. Obstruction secondary to neoplasia
   B. Inflammatory colitis
   C. Ischaemic colitis secondary to embolus
   D. Angiodysplasia
   E. Mesenteric atherosclerosis

12. Inflammatory bowel disease (2)

A 27-year-old patient is seen in outpatients, as part of the follow-up for his ulcerative colitis. His current maintenance drugs include mesalazine and azathioprine, but he has not been tolerating azathioprine, and complains of malaise, nausea and vomiting. The next treatment option is

   A. Long-term oral steroids
   B. 6-mercaptopurine
   C. Ciclosporin
   D. Infliximab
   E. Methotrexate

13. Appendix mass

An 18-year-old patient presents with a 12-day history of abdominal pain and pyrexia. On examination bowel sounds are present and the abdomen is soft with no rebound. A mass in the right iliac fossa is palpable. Abdominal computed tomography confirms the diagnosis of an appendix mass with an associated abscess. The patient is started on cefuroxime and metronidazole and admitted for observation and conservative management. After 2 days the mass has not reduced in size and the temperature remains raised. The next stage in management is

   A. Continue antibiotics for further 14 days (antibioticoma)
   B. Proceed to appendicectomy hazardus? abcess spellage
   C. Percutaneous drainage
   D. Colonoscopy if cecal carcinoid suspected
   E. Laparoscopy if there is doupt

14. Diagnosis of perianal disease

A 60-year-old homosexual man presents with a 6-month history of passing fresh blood per rectum and anal pain. His presentation has been precipitated by the recent loss of continence to faeces. The blood coats the stool and he had noticed it on the paper after wiping. On rectal examination the patient has an empty rectum. You identify a third-degree haemorrhoid in the 11 o'clock position, as well as two further second-degree haemorrhoids. No other masses are palpable. The diagnosis is

A.   Anal squamous carcinoma
B.   Haemorrhoids
C.   Sigmoid adenocarcinoma
D.   Diverticular disease
E.   Anal fissure

15. Perianal anatomy

Which of the following statements regarding the anatomy of the anal canal is false?

A.   There is no touch or pain sensation above the dentate line
B.   The anal canal below the dentate line drains lymph to the inguinal nodes
C.   The anorectal ring is made up of the blended fibres of the puborectal muscle and internal anal sphincter
D.   The superior rectal vein drains into the portal system
E.   The pelvic diaphragm delineates the point at which the rectum becomes the anal canal

16. Perianal pathology

A 60-year-old diabetic patient presents with an 8-hour history of being unable to pass urine. On taking his history, he reports a 3-day history of pyrexia and throbbing pain around the back passage. He is also concerned as he has also noticed he has been passing urine increasingly frequently and worries that his diabetes is getting worse since increased urinary frequency was how his condition was initially diagnosed. On examination of his abdomen there is no evidence of peritonism. On digital rectal examination there are no abnormalities visible in the perianal area; the procedure is extremely painful. However, the prostate feels normal and is in the normal position. The diagnosis is

A.   Ischiorectal abscess
B.   Acute prostatitis
C.   Urinary tract infection
D.   Invasive pelvic malignancy
E.   Supralevator abscess

17. Treatment of fistula *in ano*

A patient with a previous anal abscess presents with persistent discharge from the anus and perianal discomfort. On examination a sinus is identifiable at the 6 o'clock position with the patient in the lithotomy position. A fistula is diagnosed and the patient is booked for theatre. What procedure is the surgeon most likely to perform?

    A. Diversion loop colostomy
    B. Plug insertion
    C. Open exploration of tract
    D. Endoanal ultrasound
    E. Examination under anaesthetic +/- proceed

18. Anal fissure

Which of the following is *not* an option when treating an anal fissure?

    A. Propranolol
    B. Botulinum toxin A injections
    C. Glyceryl trinitrate cream
    D. Diltiazem cream
    E. Laxatives

19. Abdominal wall anatomy

Which of the following is *not* encountered when making a Lanz incision during an open appendicectomy?

    A. External oblique aponeurosis
    B. Rectus abdominis
    C. Peritoneum
    D. Internal oblique muscle
    E. Transversus abdominis

20. Appendicitis

Which of the following is *not* a sign associated with acute appendicitis?

    A. Murphy's sign   *acute cholecystitis*
    B. Cope sign   *obturator, appendix in pelvis near obturator internus*
    C. Psoas sign   *+ve in retrocecal app.*
    D. Rovsing's sign   *low lying app. ... to ... int*
    E. Pain on rectal examination   *(low lying appendix or pus in Douglas pouch.)*

21. Right iliac fossa mass

All of the following may cause a right iliac fossa mass that is palpable on abdominal examination, except

    A. Mucocele
    B. Ulcerative colitis
    C. Tuberculosis
    D. Appendicitis
    E. Ovarian cancer

22. Hereditary colon carcinoma

Which of the following is *not* a syndrome associated with an increased risk of colonic adenocarcinoma?

A. Congenital hypertrophy of retinal pigment epithelium
B. Familial adenomatous polyposis coli
C. Hereditary non-polyposis colon cancer
D. Multiple endocrine neoplasia syndrome II
E. Gardner's syndrome

23. Colonic carcinoma (2)

Which of the following is the most common site for colorectal adenocarcinoma?

A. Rectum
B. Sigmoid colon
C. Caecum and ascending colon
D. Descending colon
E. Transverse colon

24. Management of colonic carcinoma

Which of the following is not an indication for radiotherapy or chemotherapy in colonic cancer?

A. Dukes' stage A
B. Intraoperative peritoneal contamination during resection
C. Dukes' stage C
D. Rectal adenocarcinoma threatening the resection margin
E. Dukes' stage D

25. Lower gastrointestinal haemorrhage

An 85-year-old patient is admitted to the emergency department in shock with a short history of large-volume fresh bleeding per rectum. You resuscitate the patient with blood and fluids. There is no identifiable source on rectal examination. However, the patient continues to be unstable and you suspect continued bleeding. Her bowels open and pass an additional large volume of blood. Your next stage of management is

A. Laparotomy
B. Radionucleotide red cell scanning
C. Oesophagogastroduodenoscopy
D. Mesenteric angiography
E. Colonoscopy

26. Bowel obstruction

The most common cause of large bowel obstruction in the developing world is

A. Adhesions
B. Intestinal parasites

    C.   Volvulus

    D.   Hernia

    E.   Neoplasia

27. Obstruction

A 45-year-old woman with a history of previous gynaecological surgery is admitted through the emergency department with central colicky abdominal pain, vomiting and absolute constipation. She is fluid resuscitated and a naso-gastric tube is placed. Abdominal radiograph demonstrates dilated loops of bowel with valvulae conniventes clearly identifiable. Over the next 48 hours she fails to improve. The next stage of management is

    A.   Repeat plain abdominal film

    B.   Barium meal

    C.   Diagnostic laparoscopy

    D.   Gastrografin via a nasogastric tube

    E.   Radio-opaque contrast enema

28. Meckel's diverticulum

Which of the following is not a recognized complication of a Meckel's diverticulum?

    A.   Volvulus

    B.   Adenocarcinoma

    C.   Peptic ulceration

    D.   Intussusception

    E.   Pancreatitis

29. Carcinoid tumours

Carcinoid tumours occur most commonly in which site?

    A.   Large bowel

    B.   Duodenum

    C.   Appendix

    D.   Stomach

    E.   Lung

30. Inflammatory bowel disease (3)

Which of the following features is *not* characteristic of Crohn's disease?

    A.   Rose thorn abscesses

    B.   Cobblestoning

    C.   Skip lesions

    D.   Lead piping

    E.   Serosal involvement

ANSWERS

Per-rectal bleeding

1 E   Flexible sigmoidoscopy

The most likely diagnosis here is haemorrhoids, however, a left-sided colorectal adenocarcinoma must be excluded, despite the low index of suspicion. Such patients should be reassured, but advised to undergo a flexible sigmoidoscopy to exclude cancer or colonic polyps. Patients with change in bowel habit would need a colonoscopy.

Treating the patient for haemorrhoids without excluding malignancy is not acceptable. An examination under anaesthetic will not allow sufficient visualisation of the left colon unless a flexible sigmoidoscopy was also done as part of the procedure. Blood tests and CEA levels should not be used to diagnose or exclude colonic malignancy.

Hospital-acquired infection

2 A   No further action required

This patient has developed a common complication of broad-spectrum antibiotic therapy, which all graduating foundation year 1 doctors should be able to manage. The key word in the scenario is 'formed'. *Clostridium difficile* toxin assays will remain positive for at least 2 weeks following clearance of the original infection. Therefore, there is no benefit in repeating assays following cessation of treatment. In any case, this patient is asymptomatic and there is no need to continue or escalate antibiotic therapy. Intravenous vancomycin has no role in the treatment of *C. difficile* in this scenario, and colonoscopy on this patient would be entirely inappropriate.

If the patient had remained symptomatic, then oral vancomycin would be the antibiotic of choice. Failure of diarrhoea to resolve following 10 days of metronidazole would be indicative of resistance and therefore continuation for a further 10 days would not be of benefit.

Colonic carcinoma (1)

3 B   Gadolinium-enhanced liver magnetic resonance imaging

Following this patient's initial operative treatment of his colonic cancer, he has been found to have early metastatic disease.

The significance of identifying metastatic deposits is that they impact on prognosis; Dukes' stage C disease carries a 5-year survival of 20%–30%, whereas distant metastasis shorten 5-year survival to <5%. However, aggressive management of metastatic disease isolated to a single lobe of the liver can increase survival from 5% to over 30%. Therefore, this patient would benefit from hepatic resection as long as the disease is truly confined to a single lobe. The gold standard imaging for suspected hepatic malignancy is gadolinium-enhanced MRI and therefore B is the correct answer. Option A is inappropriate as liver resection must only be performed in carefully selected patients, therefore, MRI imaging must be completed prior to planning for resection. Options D or E may well be appropriate if MRI demonstrates more widespread disease, however the possibility of hepatic resection should be considered first.

Histological examination of the lesion using guided biopsy is not necessary in this case as the patient is unlikely to have primary HCC in the absence of identifiable risk factors and in the context of proved gastrointestinal tract malignancy. By biopsying the lesion there is a danger one may seed the biopsy tract; an unnecessary risk in this case.

Colonic resections

4 E Extended right hemicolectomy

This question is simply designed to test candidates' baseline knowledge of common surgical techniques, which are often confused and misunderstood. As with virtually all tumour surgery the aim is to achieve clear resection margins. Therefore the operation is planned to remove the tumour and all mesenteric lymph tissue draining that area.

The choice of operation in this case is either an extended right hemicolectomy or left hemicolectomy; left hemicolectomy is associated with the technical difficulty of forming a large bowel to large bowel anastomosis and the preferred technique for tumours located in the transverse colon is therefore an extended right hemicolectomy. This allows a primary anastomosis between the ileum and descending colon, which avoids the end-to-end anastomosis implicit in left hemicolectomy.

A right hemicolectomy would not excise the area in question and neither would a sigmoid colectomy or an anterior resection. A total colectomy in this patient would be equally inappropriate, as the removal of the entire colon is not necessary to achieve cure.

Change in bowel habit

5 D Inflammatory bowel disease

This is essentially an easy question which will catch out candidates who are aiming for a unifying diagnosis when the question clearly states 'most likely diagnosis'. The key point is the history of weight loss and fatigue, which indicate a systemic illness rather than local disease and therefore makes anal fissure unlikely. Diverticular disease is also unlikely to present in this fashion. The patient's age makes malignancy a less likely diagnosis, but in clinical practice one would have to rule this out.

Inflammatory bowel disease is commonly encountered and is by far the most likely diagnosis in this case; the patient is of the correct age and the history of weight loss and fatigue are very suggestive. The detail of history of constipation is not of any significance. Irritable bowel syndrome is a common misdiagnosis; no clinician should diagnose this condition in a patient with bloody loose stool and weight loss.

Stomas

6 C A mucus fistula functions to decompress residual distal bowel
Care is required when answering this type of question and a systematic approach is essential. Taking each statement in turn

- Hartmann's procedure does result in a defunctioned rectum, but not a loop colostomy. The stoma formed is an end or terminal colostomy which may be reversed in 60%–70% of cases.
- Abdominoperineal resection is not reversible as it leaves the patient without an anus.
- Option C is true. The aim of a mucus fistula is to protect the resection margins of the distal segment by avoiding the potential build-up of mucoid secretions from the defunctioned bowel. More often the distal bowel is sown to the underside of the abdominal wall and left as a 'potential mucus fistula' which may be easily opened if the need arises.
- Small bowel obstruction complicates 10%–15% of stomas in the long term. The majority resolve with conservative measures, however, and they rarely necessitate revision. Early complication of a stoma with mechanical small bowel obstruction is uncommon. The most common post-operative complication is paralytic ileus, which can mimic obstruction.
- Positioning is extremely important, as poorly situated stomas can make it near-impossible for patients to independently manage their stoma, and siting the stoma too near a wound can result in wound sepsis and even dehiscence.

Constipation

7 E Neoplasia
This is a difficult question for many candidates as the information given does not allow a clear distinction between simple constipation and neoplasia. However, the other three options can be excluded relatively easily; ileus is not a viable option as bowel sounds are increased, not absent. Sigmoid volvulus is unlikely as the presentation is over 4 days, and there is no suggestion of the severe pain and systemic upset associated with volvulus. Similarly, peritonitis secondary to diverticular disease would present with peritoneal signs more local to the left iliac fossa. An uncontained

diverticular perforation might result in generalised peritonitis; however, this would certainly be associated with cardiovascular collapse. The absence of rebound and guarding in this age group of patients does not exclude peritonitis, however this patient is described as having a general slower decline rather than an acute deterioration.

Choosing between constipation and neoplasia requires greater consideration. Particular attention must be given to the way in which the question is asked. 'What diagnosis must be excluded?' indicates the examiner is looking for a diagnosis of significance. In this case, the history of general and rapid deterioration in condition and the findings on rectal examination throw sufficient doubt on a diagnosis of simple constipation, making neoplasia the best answer. If the question had asked for 'The most likely diagnosis' then candidates would be justified in considering constipation to be more likely as it is a far more common diagnosis in elderly inpatients.

Volvulus

8   B   **Sigmoidoscopy with flatus tube insertion**
This is a classic presentation of sigmoid volvulus. Volvulus is a condition where a loop of bowel becomes twisted on its mesentery, occluding the blood supply to that section of bowel. Without rapid decompression, ischaemia and subsequent gangrene will occur.

Sigmoid volvulus is more common in men than women (4:1), the elderly and those with a long history of constipation. The radiological appearance on plain radiograph is classically described as the 'coffee-bean' or 'bent inner-tube' sign. These patients require resuscitation and treatment for shock, but definitive management is the decompression of the bowel as soon as possible. The diagnosis in this case is not disputed and sigmoidoscopy with insertion of a flatus tube should not be delayed by further radiological investigations. Following successful decompression at sigmoidoscopy this patient would have to be closely observed for signs suggestive of bowel ischaemia. Laparotomy and colectomy are the reserve of failed attempts at endoscopic decompression and/or proven bowel infarction. Therefore, these options cannot be considered the next step in management. Barium swallow has no place in the management of sigmoid volvulus.

Inflammatory bowel disease (1)

9   D   **Cardiomyopathy**
This is a simple question. The systemic manifestations of inflammatory bowel disease (IBD) are numerous and candidates should familiarize themselves with a comprehensive list from their source reference text. Osteoporosis can occur as a consequence of long-term steroid therapy used to manage IBD. Osteomalacia does occur in direct association with IBD along with other musculoskeletal complaints, most commonly

arthritis, sacroiliitis and ankylosing spondylitis. Sclerosing cholangitis is associated with ulcerative colitis to a greater extent than Crohn's disease and there is also an increased risk of cholangiocarcinoma. Ocular manifestations are common in IBD, and scleritis and iritis are severe and potentially sight-threatening, so require urgent treatment. Episcleritis is more common, but less severe. Pyoderma gangrenosum is a dermatological manifestation of both Crohn's and ulcerative colitis, but is not exclusive to these conditions and may also manifest in PBC, rheumatoid arthritis and neoplasia, particularly haematological malignancies. Amyloidosis is a rare complication of IBD, but nevertheless candidates should be aware that amyloid deposition may complicate *any* chronic systemic inflammatory process.

Cardiomyopathies are not a known systemic manifestation of inflammatory bowel disease.

Diverticular disease

10 E **95% of complications from diverticula occur in the sigmoid colon**
Diverticula are described as outpouchings of the wall of a hollow viscus. They can be congenital, as in Meckel's diverticulum, or acquired, as in the colonic or oesophageal diverticula. A true diverticulum has within its walls all of the components of the viscus from which it originates. Since colonic diverticula are outpouchings of the mucosa between the taenia coli they do not contain all the components of the colon wall and they are not true diverticula. Diverticula occur in approximately 30% of the adult population over the age of 60. Not all these patients have diverticular disease, as this term is reserved for diverticula with complications. The most common site for diverticula to develop is the sigmoid colon. They do not occur in the rectum as within the rectal wall the taenia coli become fused. Saint's triad describes the association between diverticula, cholelithiasis and hiatus herniation, all of which occur with greater frequency in Western societies.

Abdominal pain

11 E Mesenteric atherosclerosis
This patient is presenting with a triad of symptoms classic of mesenteric vascular occlusion: shock, rectal bleeding and colicky abdominal pain which rapidly evolves. The normal colonoscopy 3 months ago makes obstruction secondary to neoplasia virtually impossible. Angiodysplasia presents with painless rectal bleeding. Inflammatory colitis would not explain the history of intermittent pain associated with food.

The key to this question is differentiating the likely cause of bowel ischaemia. This patient has had pain after eating and weight loss, which is typical of intermittent mesenteric ischaemia. So-called intestinal angina is suggestive of the presence of atherosclerotic disease. Atrial fibrillation might suggest embolus as a possible cause, but consider that this patient is in shock, and therefore the AF might be as a consequence of this, rather than an established condition. This patient requires urgent fluid resuscitation and is likely to undergo a CT mesenteric angiogram prior to laparotomy with bowel resection or mesenteric angiography ± angioplasty.

Inflammatory bowel disease (2)

12 B   6-mercaptopurine

The pharmacological management of inflammatory bowel disease is complex and much controversy exists. There are significant differences between the management of remission and acute episodes and in the management of Crohn's disease and ulcerative colitis; the question refers to long-term remission of ulcerative colitis.

Steroids are extremely useful drugs in the acute setting, and topical steroid enema preparations may be used in the maintenance of remission, although oral use is restricted to acute flairs for obvious reasons. Mesalazine is the first line agent in both ulcerative colitis and Crohn's due to its relative low toxicity, although its efficacy in Crohn's is far less than in ulcerative colitis. In those who require additional agents, second line management is with azathioprine; however 33% of patients will not tolerate this drug and in these patients 6-mercaptopurine may be tried next. Although 6-mercaptopurine is the active breakdown component of azathioprine, 50% of those intolerant to azathioprine will respond to this drug without side effects.

Patients intolerant or non-responsive to first and second line management options are candidates for anti-TNF treatments. These should only be instituted by a specialist gastroenterologist. Ciclosporin is typically only used as a salvage drug during acute severe exacerbations. Methotrexate use has declined with the introduction of biological therapies such as the anti-TNF antibody treatments, but still has a role in Crohn's disease.

Appendix mass

13 C   Percutaneous drainage

An appendix mass occurs when an inflamed appendix becomes walled off by adhesions to the omentum. The majority of these cases (80%) are manageable with intravenous antibiotics. Appendicectomy in the presence of an appendix mass is often technically hazardous and should not be attempted in the acute setting. Therefore, B would be an inappropriate answer. Laparoscopy, similarly, is used in the acute setting either to remove the appendix or when the diagnosis of appendicitis is uncertain as it gives the option to proceed. As the diagnosis is not in doubt, and appendicectomy is to be avoided, laparoscopy is not indicated in this scenario. Colonoscopy, similarly, has nothing to add in this case where the diagnosis is not disputed, but an argument could be made to perform a colonoscopy at a delayed point in time to exclude caecal carcinoid or polyp, although no absolute indication exists.

Although 80% of appendix masses will settle with conservative management, 20% will not. Enlargement of the mass or continuation of pyrexia indicates that further intervention is necessary. In these cases, prolonged courses of antibiotics should be avoided as they lead to the development of chronic inflammatory masses laden with abscesses. Appropriate treatment is radiological drainage. Failure to do so may result in perforation of the mass into the abdominal cavity, bladder, rectum or even through the abdominal wall.

Diagnosis of perianal disease

14 A Anal squamous carcinoma

History of blood-coated stool is suggestive of distal disease. Cancer of the sigmoid colon typically manifests with blood mixed into the stool and therefore is less likely in this scenario. Bleeding due to diverticular disease occurs due to erosion of a vessel within the bowel wall. Haemorrhage is typically large volume. Therefore a chronic presentation such as this is not indicative of diverticular disease.

The key point in this history is the loss of continence. Neither haemorrhoids nor anal fissures cause loss of faecal continence although incontinence may complicate attempts to treat these conditions. Carcinoma of the anal canal, however, commonly presents with bleeding and incontinence; 70% of patients have sphincter involvement at presentation. Perianal pain is another common symptom occurring in 50% of cases. Do not be put off making this diagnosis by the absence of a palpable mass – only 25% have a palpable lesion. The relevance of the patient's sexuality is that carcinoma of the anus is closely associated with human papilloma virus, and as such is more common in homosexual men and those with perianal or genital warts.

Perianal anatomy

15 C The anorectal ring is made up of the blended fibres of the puborectal muscle and internal anal sphincter

This question touches on several important concepts regarding rectal and anal anatomy and the application of this knowledge in surgical practice.

- A – True. The anal canal above the dentate line is supplied by nerves of the hypogastric plexus. They are autonomic and therefore are only sensitive to stretch.
- B – True. Anal carcinoma is an increasingly common condition and therefore candidates should familiarize themselves with local drainage, as it impacts on management. The anal canal below the dentate line drains via inguinal nodes, that above drains via internal iliac nodes.
- C – False. The anorectal ring is made up from the combined fibres of the puborectal muscle and the external sphincter. The internal sphincter is hypertrophied smooth muscle.
- D – True. Hence portal hypertensives commonly develop exaggerated haemorrhoids as the anal canal is a site of potential portal–systemic shunting.
- E – True. The pelvic diaphragm is made up from the levator ani and coccygeus muscles, and it divides the pelvis and the perineum, demarcating the division between the rectum and anus.

Perianal pathology

16 E   Supralevator abscess

This patient has an abscess. The short history of sepsis with a throbbing rectal pain are typical and would not be commonly found in malignant disease or uncomplicated UTI. Prostatitis is a possible diagnosis in a patient with fever and painful urinary retention; pain from the prostate is non-specific and may be felt deep within the pelvis, between the legs or in the lower back or from the rectum. However, throbbing pain indicates an abscess and the prostate would feel enlarged and boggy in acute prostatitis.

Answering this question therefore depends on a candidate's ability to differentiate between the sites of perianal abscess formation based on the history provided. The majority of abscesses originates from an infection within one of the glands that lie between the internal and external sphincters. In 65% of cases the infection will then track downwards to form a perianal abscess; these present as a discrete local red swelling close to the anal verge. In 15% of cases, the infection will track through the external sphincters and into the ischiorectal fossa forming an ischiorectal abscess. Because the fossa is full of fat with no natural barriers preventing spread of infection, these abscesses present with systemic illness and extreme pain on palpation/DRE.

In a further 15% of cases the infection remains within the muscle layers, forming an intersphincteric abscess. These present with chronic anal pain and tenderness on DRE.

In 5% of cases the infection extends upwards through the levator ani muscles forming a supralevator abscess. These abscesses cause significant inflammation adjacent to the bladder, and therefore presenting symptoms are those of systemic illness, perianal discomfort and bladder irritation.

Treatment of fistula *in ano*

17 E   Examination under anaesthetic +/- proceed

Over 70% of fistula *in ano* are intersphincteric, that is they do not involve the sphincter muscles. A further 23% do involve the sphincter muscles, but not the anorectal ring. Both these types of fistula are readily identified by passing a probe through the tract while the patient is anaesthetized. Therefore the most appropriate answer is "E"; once the extent of the fistula is known, the surgeon will decide whether it is safe to lay the tract open, or whether a seton is required. Seton insertion is necessary if the anorectal ring is involved with, or closely associated with, the fistula tract. Use of setons carries less risk of permanent incontinence, and is therefore favoured if there is any uncertainty regarding the degree of sphincter involvement, particularly in women. Open exploration of the tract is not an acceptable technique as it risks incontinence. Endoanal ultrasound may be used intraoperatively in cases where doubt remains about the course of the fistula, however, is typically only required in complex perianal Crohn's disease. Diversion colostomy is not a first line treatment for simple fistula *in ano*.

Anal fissure

18 A   Propranolol

Propranolol is the only option not used in the treatment of anal fissure. Of the others, laxatives are commonly used in almost all cases as they treat the major predisposing problem. In conjunction with laxatives, give the patient advice on toilet habits and dietary modification, although this management may still fail in the majority of cases. The most effective medical treatment is 2% diltiazem cream applied twice daily. GTN ointment is a slightly less effective alternative to those who cannot use diltiazem. Such measures, which may allow resolution in up to 75% of cases within the first 8 weeks of therapy. Lidocaine gel is also often co-prescribed to aid symptom relief.

Failing these measures, botulinum toxin A injections can be used, and have been shown to be an effective way of avoiding surgical management, which risks loss of continence.

Abdominal wall anatomy

19 B Rectus abdominis

Depending on what emphasis a medical school places on surgical teaching and applied anatomy, candidates may be asked simple questions regarding the more common or classical surgical incisions in the written or viva examination. Candidates should therefore know the surgical anatomy of Kocher's incision, Lanz incision, mid-line laparotomy incision and open hernia repair (i.e. the inguinal canal).

Appendicectomy may be performed through laparoscopic or open techniques. Open incision is traditionally performed through a gridiron dissection made over McBurney's point at 90° to the line drawn from the umbilicus to the ASIS. However, the current popular practice is to perform a Lanz incision; this cosmetic approach is positioned lower at the level of the ASIS and follows the skin crease transversely. In both incisions, the subcutaneous tissues are divided exposing the external oblique aponeurosis, which is in turn divided along the line of its fibres. This exposes the underlying internal oblique, the fibres of which run at 90° to those of the external oblique. As before, the fibres are split following the line of the muscle fibres; hence the term gridiron, as the divisions occur in 90?° to one another. The transversus abdominis is closely associated with the internal oblique and will usually be split with it exposing the underlying peritoneum. This incision is made lateral to the rectus, which should not be involved. This technique is to be favoured as by splitting structures along the line of their fibres, rather than dissecting across them, the strength of the tissues is maintained. This makes incisional herniation and wound dehiscence rare complications of such operations.

Appendicitis

20 A Murphy's sign

The classic description of appendicitis is peritonitis over McBurney's point, located at two-thirds the distance from the umbilicus to the ASIS. However, this may vary with abnormal anatomical positioning of the appendix, and may occur in the flank (appendix positioned behind the caecum) or even below the right costal margin (sub-hepatic appendix). Therefore, knowledge of the several less-known signs is important.

Rovsing's sign is pain experienced in the right iliac fossa when pressure is placed on the left iliac fossa. Cope sign is pain on flexion and internal rotation of the right hip and indicates the appendix is low lying within the pelvis lying in close association with obturator internus. Psoas sign is pain on extension of the hip and indicates a retrocaecal appendix. Pain on rectal examination indicates either a low-lying appendix or pus in the pouch of Douglas.

Murphy's sign is associated with acute cholecystitis; it is elicited by pal-pating the costal margin with the patient in expiration and then asking the patient to take in a deep breath. The sign is positive if the patient experiences pain and arrests inspiration as the gallbladder moves down onto the examining clinician's hand during inspiration. Murphy's sign can only be considered positive if a similar manoeuvre at the left costal margin fails to arrest inspiration.

Right iliac fossa mass

21 B   Ulcerative colitis

The differential diagnosis of a right iliac fossa mass is a common sub-ject in surgical examinations and candidates should have a comprehen-sive list prepared and be able to differentiate between the most common culprits. Each person will have their own system of remembering the list of differential diagnoses; the authors prefer to divide these into the different surgical specialties as an aide mémoire:

- General: Appendix mass/abscess, colorectal carcinoma, Crohn's, distended gallbladder, lymphadenopathy
- Urological; Pelvic kidney, renal transplant, tumour in an unde-scended testis
- Gynaecological: Ovarian cyst, ovarian tumour, fibroid
- Vascular; Iliac artery aneurysm
- Orthopaedics: Chondrosarcoma or osteosarcoma of the ileum (rare!)
- Infective; Psoas abscess, ileocaecal TB

Hereditary colon carcinoma

22 D   Multiple endocrine neoplasia syndrome II

Familial adenomatous polyposis is an autosomal dominant condition caused by a mutation in the *APC* gene (chromosome 5q21). It results in the development of hundreds of polyps within the colon and carries a 100% lifetime risk of colorectal cancer; these patients are there-fore offered prophylactic proctocolectomy with ileorectal pouch at a young age. Fifty per cent of these patients also develop gastric and duodenal polyps, and therefore require regular endoscopic screening. Gardner's is closely related to FAP, as it is also a consequence of an *APC* gene mutation, but has additional extraintestinal manifestations; it is a syndrome of colonic polyps, epidermoid cysts and osteomas. Similarly, CHRPE is another variant of FAP; CHRPE may be detected on indirect ophthalmoscopy in up to 75% of those with adenomatous polyposis coli.

Hereditary non-polyposis colon cancer is the most common cause of hereditary colon cancer accounting for 3% of all colonic carcinoma.

The genes responsible are various but all function in DNA repair. The MEN syndromes may have gastrointestinal manifestations, including neuroendocrine tumours of the duodenum and pancreas and mega-colon (MEN 2B most commonly, but also 2A) secondary to motility dysfunction. However, adenocarcinoma is not a feature.

Colonic carcinoma (2)

23 A   Rectum

The distribution of colorectal cancer is an extremely common topic in examination and this is a basic question that all candidates should be able to answer. Thirty-three per cent of cancers occur in the rectum, 25% occur in the sigmoid colon, 18% occur in the caecum and ascending colon, 9% occur in the transverse colon and 5% occur in the descending colon. This can be easily remembered by considering the length of time faecal material remains in contact with the part of the colon involved; note that the segments with the longest transit time have the highest incidence of adenocarcinoma.

Management of colonic carcinoma

24 A   Dukes' stage A

Answering this question relies on examination technique as much as knowledge of the subject in question; few candidates will know the intricacies of adjunct chemotherapy and radiotherapy in colorectal car-cinoma, however the majority will know that Dukes' stage A colorectal cancer is treated with surgery alone. This level of knowledge is all that is required in answering this question correctly.

In simple terms, no survival benefit is gained from adjunct therapy in stage A disease. Adjuvant therapy in patients with Dukes B disease is controversial, and the decision to offer such treatments takes into account a range of both tumour-related and patient-related factors. Clear benefit is evident in Dukes C and D disease, however, as once the tumour metas-tasizes to lymph nodes or more distant sites, an increase in survival of 3%–10% can be achieved with adjuvant treatments. Chemotherapy should also be considered if peritoneal contamination occurs intra-operatively or if the tumour has perforated into the peritoneal cavity. Patients with rectal carcinoma undergo pre-operative rectal MRI scanning; in cases where the resection margin is threatened or breached neoadjuvant radio-therapy (+/- chemotherapy) will often be used to 'downstage' the tumour.

Lower gastrointestinal haemorrhage

25 C   Oesophagogastroduodenoscopy

Gastrointestinal haemorrhage is a common clinical problem, account-ing for 1%–2% of acute hospital admissions. It is broadly divided into upper and lower gastrointestinal bleeding, according to whether haemorrhage occurs proximal or distal to the ligament of Treitz. Upper gastrointestinal bleeding accounts for 80% of all gastrointestinal haemorrhage.

Ninety-five per cent of lower gastrointestinal haemorrhage bleeding is from the colon, the small intestine, accounts for less than 5%. The management of lower gastrointestinal haemorrhage relies on the accurate localization of a source; blind emergency hemicolectomy must be avoided as it results in a re-bleeding rate of up to 50%. Initial assessment should aim to exclude anorectal causes as a possible diagnosis by careful rectal examination and rigid proctoscopy/sigmoidoscopy. If no source is found the next stage is to exclude an upper gastrointestinal cause as these are readily treatable at endoscopy; 15% of per-rectal bleeds in haemodynamically compromised patients originate proximal to the ligament of Treitz.

Following a negative OGD further management will depend on the haemodynamic status of the patient. Colonoscopy is possible in mild bleeding, but its diagnostic yield is severely restricted in moderate to severe haemorrhage as the view is compromised. Major haemorrhage in patients who are haemodynamically unstable indicates a need to localise the source of bleeding. CT mesenteric angiography is effective but requires a reasonable rate of blood loss to identify a source. Angiography can localize the lesion to a greater degree of accuracy and has the option of therapeutic intervention, but it takes longer, is more invasive and is more technically demanding. Both techniques require an actively bleeding lesion and a reasonable cardiac output. In severely compromised patients refractory to resuscitation, the decision may be made to perform a laparotomy and isolate the lesion through serial clamping and in-theatre colonoscopy, but this is rarely required.

Bowel obstruction

26 D   Hernia
Adhesions are the most common cause of small bowel obstruction in the developed world due to the greater number of elective procedures performed in Western countries. However in the developing world, the most common cause of obstruction of both small and large bowel is herniae. Other causes of obstruction which occur with greater frequency in the developing world than the developed world include volvulus, due to greater intestinal loading with fibrous matter, and intestinal parasite infection. Neoplastic disease causes obstruction more commonly in developing countries than in Western society as diagnosis is delayed, however hernias still account for a greater overall number of cases.

Obstruction

27 D   Gastrografin via a nasogastric tube

Obstruction may be due to mechanical or non-mechanical causes. Mechanical obstructions may be partial or complete, simple or complicated. A complicated obstruction is one where the bowel shows vascular compromise or is perforated; closed loop obstructions are at particular risk of complications as distension tends to occur rapidly without any possible spontaneous outlet. This patient has generalised small bowel dilatation with a background of previous surgery. The most likely diagnosis is adhesional obstruction.

Initial management of adhesional obstruction includes blood tests, fluid resuscitation and NG tube insertion with aspiration. Complete mechanical obstructions typically require surgery and therefore the role of initial investigations is to exclude mechanical obstruction non-amenable to conservative management. Early investigation is warranted in patients who are unresponsive to resuscitation, those with peritoneal signs, those with a palpable mass and those without a history of surgery in whom obstruction cannot be safely attributed to adhesions. Patients with likely adhesional obstruction can be trialled on non-operative management; however, failure for the obstruction to resolve within 48 hours is an indication for investigation +/- laparotomy.

Gastrografin via the NG tube is a diagnostic investigation as well as a part of therapeutic management since a minority of obstruction secondary to adhesions may spontaneously resolve following oral Gastrografin. Traditionally oral contrast studies consisted of serial plain abdominal radiographs following oral Gastrografin, however the contemporaneous availability of cross sectional imaging means that oral Gastrografin contrast CT scanning is more frequently employed in such patients. Contrast enema is not typically required in cases of small bowel obstruction.

Laparoscopy cannot be considered a first line investigation and use of barium is contraindicated due to the consequences of barium peritonitis should the patients develop a perforation. Repeating a plain abdominal film without oral contrast is unlikely to give you any additional useful information.

Meckel's diverticulum

28 E   Pancreatitis

Meckel's diverticulum is the most common congenital abnormality of the gastrointestinal tract occurring in 2% of the population. It is an embryological remnant of the vitello-intestinal duct and is therefore found within 2 ft of the ileocaecal valve. The diverticulum varies in size in different individuals; large diverticula often have a fibrous cord (the remnant duct) linking them to the umbilicus.

The cells that line the vitello-intestinal duct are pluripotent and may therefore differentiate into any tissue. However, most commonly the diverticulum is lined with heterotrophic gastric epithelium (50%) or pancreatic tissue (5%). The most common clinical presentation of Meckel's is gastrointestinal haemorrhage secondary to peptic ulceration of this abnormal gastric epithelium, which contains a predominance of acid-secreting parietal cells. This is most commonly a childhood presentation causing melaena at around 10 years of age and accounts for over 50% of all symptomatic disease associated with Meckel's. The mucosa is also at risk of malignant change, most commonly adenocarcinoma.

Meckel's diverticula are at risk of mechanical complications. Diverticulitis accounts for 20% of symptomatic presentations with features indistinguishable from acute appendicitis. The abnormal segment is also liable to cause intussusceptions following inversion into the ileum or volvulus caused by the small bowel twisting around on the fibrous band at the diverticulum apex. Other presentations include perforation and umbilical fistulation, which occurs when the entire vitello-intestinal duct remains patent.

Carcinoid tumours

29 C   Appendix
Carcinoid tumours are closely related to neural crest cells and are otherwise known as APUD tumours. They are characterized by their embryological site of origin and may therefore be derived from foregut (respiratory tract, thymus), midgut (stomach, duodenum, jejunum, right colon) or hindgut (left colon and rectum) structures. Foregut and midgut carcinoids secrete serotonin (5-HT) whereas hindgut tumours rarely do. They may also secrete other peptide hormones such as bradykinin, VIP, gastrin, insulin, ACTH, thyroxin, etc. The most common site is the appendix, but they may be found anywhere in the alimentary tract, and 10% occur in the lung.

Carcinoid syndrome is caused by systemically released serotonin, which causes flushing (90%), diarrhoea (70%), abdominal pain (40%), and bronchospasm (10%). In the majority, symptoms are not noticeable because the peptide hormones are delivered via the portal venous system to the liver where they are metabolized. If a patient is symptomatic, this is indicative of metastasis to the liver which allows hormones to escape into the systemic circulation. More commonly patients present with appendicitis or mechanical obstruction and other mass effects.

Inflammatory bowel disease (3)

30 D Lead piping

Comparing and contrasting the histopathological features of ulcerative colitis and Crohn's disease is a classic exam question all candidates should be prepared for. In schools with viva examinations, barium studies may be shown and candidates will be expected to distinguish between the two diseases radiographically.

Ulcerative colitis is a superficial disease and therefore its features are consistent with superficial fibrosis; the colon loses its normal haustra and appears rigid on barium studies, so-called lead piping. Its lesions are confluent and always affect the rectum. Stricturing is rare and fistulae are very rare. Histologically, crypt abscesses are identifiable but the serosa is normal.

Crohn's disease, however, involves all layers of the bowel wall down to the serosa. The mucosal surface is pocketed with deep abscesses, which have a characteristic appearance of rose thorns on barium studies. The mucosa is said to be cobblestoned, strictures are common, as are fistulae. The mucosal involvement is not confluent, that is 'skip lesions', and the rectum is only involved in 50% of cases.

SECTION 8:
ABDOMEN: THE ACUTE ABDOMEN

Questions

1. Haematemesis 159
2. Management of abdominal pain (1) 159
3. Testicular pain 159
4. Investigation of abdominal pain (1) 160
5. Management of abdominal pain and vomiting 160
6. Diagnosis of epigastric pain 160
7. Diagnosis of rectal bleeding 161
8. Murphy's sign 161
9. Management of an abdominal aortic aneurysm 161
10. Antibiotic prophylaxis 162
11. Diagnosis of left iliac fossa pain 162
12. Management of left iliac fossa pain 162
13. Right upper quadrant pain 162
14. Management of an inguinal hernia 163
15. Constipation and abdominal pain 163
16. Acute pancreatitis 163
17. Diarrhoea and abdominal pain 164
18. Bowel obstruction 164
19. Investigation of right upper quadrant pain 164
20. Acute urinary retention 164
21. Management of acute urinary retention 165
22. Vomiting and left upper quadrant pain 165
23. Management of abdominal pain (2) 165
24. Management of intussusception 166
25. Diagnosis of abdominal pain 166
26. Investigation of abdominal pain (2) 166
27. Causes of acute pancreatitis 166

28. Causes of large bowel obstruction   167

29. Lower gastrointestinal infection   167

30. Investigation of a diverticular abscess   167

Answers   168

QUESTIONS

1. Haematemesis

A 55-year-old man, with a 2-year history of dyspepsia, is brought to the emergency department following a sudden onset of severe epigastric pain. The pain is made worse on movement and the patient has also experienced one episode of haematemesis. On examination, the patient is cold, sweating profusely and taking shallow breaths. The abdomen is rigid and bowel sounds are absent. A plain film chest radiograph reveals free air under the diaphragm. The most likely diagnosis is

    A.   Perforated appendicitis
    B.   Acute cholecystitis
    C.   Acute pancreatitis
    D.   Myocardial infarction
    (E) Perforated peptic ulcer

2. Management of abdominal pain (1)

A 26-year-old woman arrives at the emergency department with unbearable intense right iliac fossa pain. Earlier that day, she was experiencing 'on and off' moderate pain in the umbilical area which gradually moved over to the right iliac fossa. Associated symptoms include anorexia, nausea and vomiting. On examination, the patient is pyrexial and there is rebound tenderness and guarding over the right iliac fossa. A beta-human chorionic gonadotrophin test is negative. What should you do next?

    (A) Send the patient to the emergency operating theatre for an
          appendicectomy
    B.   Alert the obstetrics and gynaecology team, suspecting that she may
          have a ruptured ectopic pregnancy
    C.   Manage the patient medically in the emergency department
    D.   Order an ultrasound scan of the abdomen
    E.   Send the patient for a plain film radiograph of the abdomen

3. Testicular pain

A 12-year-old boy is admitted to the emergency department with sudden onset of severe right testicular and lower abdominal pain during athletic training. He has had one episode of vomiting and constantly feels nauseous. On examination, the patient is sweating and in unbearable pain. There is marked tenderness and swelling of the right testicle which is observed to be lying horizontally. What is the most appropriate next step in this patient's management?

    A.   Order a Doppler ultrasound of the testicular arteries
    (B) Send the patient immediately for emergency surgical exploration of
          the scrotum

C. Perform urine dipstick
D. Manage the patient with analgesia and observe
E. Obtain a second opinion from your senior colleague, who will only be able to see the patient in an hour

4. Investigation of abdominal pain (1)

You see a 55-year-old woman in the emergency department, who was admitted with central colicky abdominal pain and multiple episodes of vomiting. She last opened her bowels 4 hours ago. On examination she appears dehydrated and is in pain. The abdomen is generally tender and slightly distended. Bowel sounds are increased. You suspect a bowel obstruction and decide to order some investigations. What is the most valuable initial investigation that will support your suspected diagnosis?

A. Upper gastrointestinal endoscopy
B. Colonoscopy
C. Computed tomography scan of the abdomen
(D.) Plain film radiograph of the abdomen
E. Barium follow-through

5. Management of abdominal pain and vomiting

drip and suck

A 48-year-old woman is admitted with severe epigastric pain and vomiting. The pain is continuous in nature and is made worse on movement. On examination you notice the patient is lying still, taking shallow breaths and sweating. There is marked tenderness in the epigastric and right upper quadrant of the abdomen. Murphy's sign is positive and the patient is slightly pyrexial. You suspect acute cholecystitis. What is the next best step in managing this patient?

(A.) Keep nil by mouth, administer parenteral analgesia and systemic antibiotics
B. Send patient for emergency laparoscopic cholecystectomy
C. Request a plain film abdominal radiograph
D. Administer analgesia and seek the opinion of a superior colleague
E. Request an ultrasound of the abdomen

6. Diagnosis of epigastric pain

A 45-year-old Asian man is brought in with an acute onset of epigastric pain, nausea and severe vomiting. The pain is worse with movement and is only relieved slightly by leaning forward. The patient is an alcoholic and has been admitted to the emergency department on several occasions for alcohol intoxication. On examination the patient is tachycardic, pyrexial and dehydrated. The abdomen is diffusely tender and soft, and bowel sounds are normal. The patient's serum amylase is raised by six times the upper limit of normal. The most likely diagnosis is

A. Perforated peptic ulcer
B. Small bowel obstruction
C. Acute cholecystitis
D. Acute pancreatitis
E. None of the above

7. Diagnosis of rectal bleeding

A 75-year-old man, who suffers from chronic atrial fibrillation, is admitted to the emergency department with a sudden onset of severe central colicky abdominal pain and vomiting. The patient has been bleeding from the rectum. The blood is dark in colour and has an altered consistency. On examination the patient is pale, has cold peripheries and is tachycardic. The abdomen is diffusely tender and bowel sounds are decreased. What is the likely diagnosis?

A. Diverticulitis
B. Small bowel obstruction
C. Acute mesenteric ischaemia
D. Perforated peptic ulcer
E. None of the above

8. Murphy's sign

A 50-year-old woman presents with an acute episode of epigastric pain, vomiting and fever. The registrar, who has already clerked and examined the patient, tells you that 'Murphy's sign is positive'. Despite not having seen the patient, from the information conveyed to you, what is the most likely top differential diagnosis that is running through your mind?

A. Acute appendicitis
B. Acute cholecystitis
C. Peritonitis
D. Biliary colic
E. Cholangitis

✳9. Management of an abdominal aortic aneurysm

A 65-year-old man is admitted to the emergency department following an acute episode of abdominal pain and collapse. The pain is intermittent and radiates to the back and iliac fossae. On examination, the patient appears confused, is sweating and has tachycardia. On inspection, the abdomen appears normal, but on palpation, you discover a pulsatile, expansile swelling in the midline of the abdomen. You suspect a ruptured abdominal aortic aneurysm. What is the most important next step?

A. Establish intravenous access and begin fluid resuscitation with a colloid
B. Send for a computed tomography scan of the abdomen

    C.   Obtain blood to determine haemoglobin and amylase levels
    D.   Request an abdominal plain film radiograph
    E.   Perform electrocardiography

10. Antibiotic prophylaxis

A patient has been sent to theatre for emergency surgery with suspected appendicitis. He is given three doses of intravenous cefuroxime and metronidazole in a timely fashion. When is the best time to administer *the first dose of antibiotics*?

    A.   One hour after the first incision is made
    (B)   One hour before surgery
    C.   One hour postoperatively
    D.   Just before the surgical incision is made
    E.   None of the above

11. Diagnosis of left iliac fossa pain

An elderly man with chronic constipation experiences acute-onset left iliac fossa pain and tenderness. On examination, the patient has fever and is slightly tachycardic. There is marked tenderness and guarding in the left iliac fossa. Full blood count results reveal a raised. What is the most likely diagnosis?

    A.   Diverticular disease
    B.   Diverticulitis
    C.   Diverticulosis
    D.   Perforated diverticulitis
    E.   None of the above

12. Management of left iliac fossa pain

You are asked by your senior colleague to devise the treatment plan for the patient in Question 11. What is the most appropriate treatment plan?

    A.   Keep nil by mouth and send for emergency laparotomy
    B.   Give analgesia and antibiotics
    C.   Keep nil by mouth, administer antibiotics and analgesia
    D.   Keep nil by mouth, administer intravenous fluids, antibiotics and analgesia
    E.   Keep nil by mouth, administer intravenous fluids and analgesia

13. Right upper quadrant pain

You are asked to see a 48-year-old woman who has been admitted to the emergency department with sudden onset of right upper quadrant pain. Your registrar liaises with you, after having seen this patient, and tells you that the patient has 'Charcot's triad'. From the information conveyed to you, what is the most likely diagnosis that you should be thinking of?

A. Biliary colic
B. Acute cholecystitis
C. Cholangitis
D. Gallstone ileus
E. Pancreatitis

14. Management of an inguinal hernia

A 78-year-old African Caribbean man presents to the emergency department with severe pain arising from his hernia in the left groin. The patient is also experiencing central colicky abdominal pain. On examination, the abdomen is generally tender and distended and bowel sounds are raised. Examination of the hernial orifices reveals a left-sided, irreducible, tense and extremely tender inguinal hernia. The overlying skin of the hernia is warm and erythematous. What is the most appropriate course of action in managing this patient?

A. Alert theatre and send patient for emergency surgery
B. Request a computed tomography scan of the abdomen
C. Request an ultrasound
D. Attempt to reduce the hernia
E. None of the above

15. Constipation and abdominal pain

A 57-year-old man presents with acute colicky pain in the suprapubic area. He has been constipated over the last 2 days and has been feeling bloated. He feels nauseous, but he has not vomited. On examination of the abdomen you notice marked abdominal distension, and increased bowel sounds. What is the most likely diagnosis?

A. Small bowel obstruction
B. Irritable bowel syndrome
C. Diverticular disease
D. Large bowel obstruction
E. Appendicitis

16. Acute pancreatitis

What is the least number of factors that must be present from the modified Glasgow criteria for acute pancreatitis to be classified as severe within 48 hours of admission?

A. 2
B. 4
C. 3
D. 5
E. 1

17. Diarrhoea and abdominal pain

A 28-year-old man with a 10-year history of ulcerative colitis presents to the emergency department with an acute severe episode of abdominal pain, nausea and vomiting and blood-stained, watery diarrhoea. On examination you notice that the patient has fever and tachycardia and that the abdomen is markedly distended. An abdominal plain film radiograph shows that the transverse colon is dilated at approximately 6.5 cm. What is the most likely diagnosis?

    A.   Large bowel obstruction
    B.   Toxic megacolon
    C.   Perforated diverticulitis
    D.   Crohn's colitis
    E.   None of the above

18. Bowel obstruction

From the list of options below which one is the most *unlikely* cause of mechanical intestinal obstruction?

    A.   Faecal impaction
    B.   Caecal volvulus
    C.   Paralytic ileus
    D.   Congenital intestinal atresia
    E.   Crohn's colitis

19. Investigation of right upper quadrant pain

A 44-year-old woman presents to the emergency department with acute onset of right upper quadrant pain and fever. On examination, the patient is lying still and has a tachycardia. The abdomen is tender in the right upper quadrant with guarding in that area. Murphy's sign is positive. What is the most useful investigation for this patient?

    A.   Ultrasound
    B.   Colonoscopy
    C.   Barium follow-through
    D.   Upper gastrointestinal endoscopy
    E.   Serum amylase

20. Acute urinary retention

A 75-year-old man is admitted to the emergency department with acute-onset suprapubic pain and inability to pass urine for 2 days. On examination, the patient is in discomfort, neurologically intact, and the abdomen is particularly tender in the suprapubic region. A digital rectal examination reveals a smooth, enlarged prostate. What is the most likely diagnosis?

A.   Bladder outflow obstruction due to prostate cancer
B.   Bladder outflow obstruction due to benign prostatic hypertrophy
C.   Bladder outflow obstruction due to a urethral stricture
D.   Bladder outflow obstruction due to a spinal cord lesion
E.   None of the above

21. Management of acute urinary retention

From the list of options below, select the most appropriate course of action to take in managing the patient in Question 20.

A.   Ask the urology registrar to see the patient
B.   Obtain blood for urea and electrolytes sampling
C.   Request an abdominal plain film radiograph
D.   Urinary catheterization
E.   Request an intravenous urogram

22. Vomiting and left upper quadrant pain

A 55-year-old woman presents to the emergency department with severe epigastric and left upper quadrant pain. Since admission, the patient has vomited. On examination you notice the patient is retching (which is non-productive), tachycardic and hypotensive. There is marked tenderness in the upper abdomen and bowel sounds are slightly raised. There is failure to pass a nasogastric tube. A chest radiograph reveals a dilated stomach and large fluid level behind the heart. Which is the most likely diagnosis?

A.   Small bowel obstruction
B.   Perforated peptic ulcer
C.   Gastro-oesophageal obstruction secondary to a gastric volvulus
D.   Gastro-oesophageal obstruction secondary to an adenocarcinoma
      of the stomach
E.   Sigmoid volvulus

23. Management of abdominal pain (2)

You see an 11-year-old boy in the emergency department who is admitted with an acute onset of abdominal pain, nausea and vomiting. There is diffuse pain around the central abdomen and right iliac fossa and is continuous in nature. On examination, the patient is febrile and there is marked tenderness and rebound in the right iliac fossa. The patient's mother tells you that he has recently had a sore throat. You suspect mesenteric adenitis and request an ultrasound scan which is inconclusive. What is the best next step to take in managing this patient?

A.   Start the patient on analgesia and intravenous antibiotics
B.   Send for a computed tomography scan of the abdomen

C. Observe patient for the next 2 hours and reassess
D. Send for emergency explorative laparotomy
E. None of the above

24. Management of intussusception

A 13-month-old girl is diagnosed with intussusception. She was admitted to the emergency department 2 hours ago with vomiting, passing red mucus-like stools and persistent crying. You are asked by your consultant about the first line treatment for this condition. What is the most likely first line treatment option?

A. Laparotomy and reduction
B. Barium enema per rectum and abdominal plain film radiography
C. Analgesia and observation for 24 hours
D. Intravenous fluids and antibiotics
E. Laparotomy and resection

25. Diagnosis of abdominal pain

A 49-year-old postmenopausal woman is admitted to the emergency department following severe attacks of abdominal pain, nausea and vomiting. The pain is colicky in nature, starts from the left flank of the abdomen and radiates to the left groin. You are unable to take a history from the patient as she is writhing in pain. On examination you notice that the patient is sweating profusely. The abdomen is soft and non-tender and bowel sounds are normal. What is the most likely diagnosis?

A. Diverticulitis
B. Ruptured ectopic pregnancy
C. Renal colic
D. Small bowel obstruction
E. Ruptured abdominal aortic aneurysm

26. Investigation of abdominal pain (2)

From the list below, select the investigation that will be of more diagnostic value of the patient's condition mentioned in Question 25.

A. Computed tomography scan of the abdomen
B. KUB (kidneys, ureters and bladder)
C. Intravenous urogram
D. Ultrasound
E. Abdominal plain film radiography

27. Causes of acute pancreatitis

During a ward round, you are asked by your senior registrar to name the most common causative factor that is responsible for the development of acute pancreatitis. Which option from the list below would you choose as your answer?

A.   Ethanol
B.   Steroids
C.   Gallstones
D.   Drugs
E.   Trauma

28. Causes of large bowel obstruction

You are asked to give your opinion on an abdominal plain film radiograph of a patient with bowel obstruction. The film shows distended loops of large bowel which form a 'U' shape, giving the appearance of a big coffee bean. Select the most likely reason for the large bowel obstruction.

A.   Faecal impaction
B.   Sigmoid volvulus
C.   Obstructing carcinoma
D.   Foreign body
E.   None of the above

29. Lower gastrointestinal infection

You see a 50-year-old woman, admitted with colicky central abdominal pain, and passing blood-stained diarrhoea and mucus per rectum. She has a marked fever and tachycardia. Abdominal plain film radiography appears normal. The white cell count is raised and stool analysis reports reveal the presence of *Clostridium difficile* cytotoxins. What is the most likely diagnosis?

A.   Ulcerative colitis
B.   Crohn's colitis
C.   Ischaemic colitis
D.   Pseudomembranous colitis
E.   None of the above

30. Investigation of a diverticular abscess

A 75-year-old man, with a history of diverticular disease, is experiencing swinging fevers and left-sided abdominal pain. You suspect the patient has a diverticular abscess. Which one of the following investigations is the most appropriate to confirm your suspicion?

A.   Barium enema studies
B.   Abdominal plain film radiography
C.   Computed tomography scan of the abdomen
D.   Colonoscopy
E.   Flexible sigmoidoscopy

ANSWERS

Haematemesis

1 E **Perforated peptic ulcer**

Free air under the diaphragm, visualised on chest radiograph, suggests that there has been perforation of a hollow viscus. In this case, the history of dyspepsia, coupled with the onset of acute sudden epigastric pain, fits in more with acute peptic ulceration rather than perforated appendicitis. Acute cholecystitis typically presents with right upper quadrant or epigastric pain. Patients are usually pyrexial and nausea/vomiting may be present. Acute pancreatitis also presents with severe epigastric or upper abdominal pain which may radiate to the back. Approximately 10% of perforated peptic ulcer cases do not reveal free air under the diaphragm on chest radiograph, making it difficult to differentiate from acute pancreatitis (CT scan of an abdomen or explorative laparotomy addresses this). Patients suffering from a myocardial infarction can present with symptoms similar to an acute abdomen and should never be excluded in the differential diagnosis of abdominal pain.

Management of abdominal pain (1)

2 A **Send the patient to the emergency operating theatre for an appendicectomy**

A very important rule to remember is that a female of childbearing age is assumed pregnant until proven otherwise. In this scenario, the results of the beta-hCG test confirm that the patient is not pregnant, also ruling out ectopic pregnancy. This patient is showing clear signs and symptoms of appendicitis and needs to have an emergency appendicectomy. Delaying surgery may lead to severe complications such as perforation resulting in generalized peritonitis and sepsis. Ultrasound can be diagnosed in the hands of the experienced but should not delay surgical intervention due to the severity of the patient's symptoms. Ultrasound of the pelvis may be done to rule out pelvic pathology if in doubt after history taking and physical examination. A plain film abdominal radiograph has been rarely shown to be useful as a diagnostic aid in appendicitis. In the hands of experienced surgeons, laparoscopy can be used as a diagnostic and therapeutic tool. Therefore, making sure that this patient is sent to the theatre in the presence of a good history is the priority.

Testicular pain

3 B **Send the patient immediately for emergency surgical exploration of the scrotum**

This patient has testicular torsion which is common between the ages of 12 and 25; it is uncommon after this age but does sometimes occur in older adults. The pain is usually of sudden onset and may occur following mild trauma to the testis, straining and weight-bearing exercises. Lower abdominal pain is experienced because the testis retains its embryological nerve supply which, primarily, is from the T10 sympathetic pathway. Testicular torsion is a surgical emergency and when suspected, surgical exploration of the scrotum should not be delayed as the testes can infarct within hours. Although Doppler ultrasound can effectively show the integrity of the arterial blood flow to the testis, it should not delay surgical exploration.

Investigation of abdominal pain (1)

4 D Plain film radiograph of the abdomen
This patient has symptoms and signs consistent with small bowel obstruction. The four cardinal features of small bowel obstruction are:

- Vomiting (occurs early in small bowel obstruction)
- Colicky pain (in small bowel obstruction the pain is periumbilical)
- Absolute constipation (not passing faeces or flatus)
- Abdominal distension

Absolute constipation may not always be a feature if the site of obstruction is high up and is usually a late sign of small bowel obstruction.

The abdominal plain film radiograph is a valuable tool and should be the first line imaging investigation in confirming the diagnosis of small bowel obstruction. Barium follow-through, colonoscopy (if mechanical obstruction is suspected, but it carries the risk of perforation) and CT scan are all helpful investigations and can be performed after the initial plain abdominal film is obtained. Upper gastrointestinal endoscopy is not usually helpful in diagnosing small bowel obstruction.

Management of abdominal pain and vomiting

5 A Keep nil by mouth, administer parenteral analgesia and systemic antibiotics
Acute cholecystitis can sometimes be confused with biliary colic. Unlike biliary colic (where patients writhe around in pain), patients prefer to remain still and take shallow breaths which indicate local peritonitis. Impaction of the gallbladder outlet by a stone causes the accumulation of bile, which can initiate a chemical inflammatory process within the gallbladder. Secondary bacterial infection can arise due to this inflammation and the condition may progress to acute bacterial cholecystitis. The most important next step in managing this patient is to provide pain relief and systemic antibiotics (for example, IV cefuroxime and metronidazole) to cover any superimposed infection. As the patient has been vomiting, IV fluid resuscitation would

also be of benefit, but for the purpose of this question, answer A is the most appropriate option in the list. The next thing to do would be to order an ultrasound scan to confirm the diagnosis. Under conservative management, the cholecystitis will usually settle down within 24–48 hours. If this is the case, patients are discharged and asked to return after 6–8 weeks to have an elective laparoscopic cholecystectomy. Recent literature has shown that cholecystectomy within the first 72 hours from onset of attack has the same complication rate as elective cholecystectomy (done after 6 to 8 weeks) after the inflammation has subsided. If after 72 hours from admission the patient has still not improved, then always remember the possibility of an empyema of the gallbladder, which may require percutaneous drainage.

Diagnosis of epigastric pain

6 D   Acute pancreatitis

Symptoms of pancreatitis can easily be confused with other acute abdominal conditions such as acute cholecystitis and perforated peptic ulcer. Acute abdominal pain that is relieved by leaning forward is usu-ally associated with pancreatitis. The head and neck of the pancreas are retroperitoneal. Thus, by leaning forward, this relieves the pressure on the retroperitoneal components of the pancreas, which in turn allevi-ates the pain. Patients usually have fever and tachycardia. The abdomen is usually soft, but in severe and later stages of pancreatitis the patient may be lying still and the abdomen may show signs of guarding and rigidity which resemble peritonism. All options can cause serum amy-lase to be raised. However, the clinical symptoms and signs coupled with the raised amylase six times the upper limit of normal suggests acute pancreatitis.

Diagnosis of rectal bleeding

7 C   Acute mesenteric ischaemia

Acute mesenteric ischaemia presents with a triad of symptoms: acute colicky abdominal pain, rectal bleeding and symptoms of shock which are associated with the blood loss. This condition almost always occurs in the small bowel, involving embolism or thrombosis of the mesen-teric vessels. Arterial causes (e.g. emboli due to atrial fibrillation, mural thrombus after myocardial infarction, detached atheromatous plaques and reduced arterial flow due to low cardiac output owing to either heart failure or hypotension) are more common than venous (e.g. venous stasis due to portal hypertension or portal venous system thrombosis; sepsis; coagulopathies; occasionally it may be caused by a paradoxical embolus). Arterial thrombosis is more common than arterial embolism. Venous causes tend to occur in younger patients. Haemoglobin may be raised (owing to the loss of plasma volume), and the white cell count is also usually raised coupled with serum amylase. An early abdominal plain film radiograph may show a 'gasless abdomen'. CT angiography or mesenteric angiography can be performed if the patient is stable, but this is time consuming. If the patient is unstable, the patient will usually be sent for emergency laparoscopy or laparotomy, which will reveal areas of necrotic bowel. Diverticulitis usually presents with pain and tenderness in the left iliac fossa accompanied by fever and local signs of peritonitis. The patient usually has a history of chronic constipation. (For more information regarding perforated peptic ulcers and intestinal obstruction, please refer to the answer to Questions 1 and 4.)

Murphy's sign

8   B   Acute cholecystitis

Murphy's sign may be a useful tool when attempting to diagnose cholecystitis. Confirmation of diagnosis depends on the combination of physical and laboratory findings, coupled with imaging studies. The patient is instructed to lie flat. Locate the right upper quadrant of the abdomen and put two fingers lightly over that area, and at the same time ask the patient to take a deep breath. If the patient experiences pain on inspiration and catches their breath, the sign is positive. As the patient breathes in, the inflamed gallbladder impacts on the examining hand, causing pain and consequently cessation of inspiration. The sensitivity of Murphy's sign has been recorded at 97.2% and the specificity at 48.3%. The positive predictive value of this test has been recorded at 70% and negative predicted value at 93.3%. In summary, these results indicate that if a positive Murphy's sign is present, this is highly suggestive of cholecystitis; and if the sign is absent, then it is highly unlikely that the patient has cholecystitis.

Management of an abdominal aortic aneurysm

9   A   Establish intravenous access and begin fluid resuscitation with a colloid

This patient has a ruptured abdominal aortic aneurysm and is showing signs and symptoms of shock. The most important initial aspect of management is to establish venous access and begin fluid resuscitation. By giving IV colloid therapy, and aiming to keep systolic blood pressure less or equal to 100 mmHg, this will decrease the rate of blood volume depletion and 'buy' some time for the patient to be sent to theatre and have the aneurysm repaired. Although all the other answers (B–E) form part of management, they do not take priority over the initial fluid resuscitation, which, if not managed promptly, may be fatal. Performing a CT scan is usually helpful and should only be done if the patient is stable. An abdominal plain film radiograph will not change the course of management and will add further delay to the patient being sent to theatre. Amylase and haemoglobin are important, but should, again, be performed once the patient is stable.

Surgery for ruptured AAAs involves immediate laparotomy, clamping the aorta above the site of rupture and inserting a synthetic Dacron graft (e.g. 'tube graft' or 'trouser graft' for aneurysms extending to the common iliac arteries). A treated ruptured AAA carries a mortality rate of approximately 41% as opposed to 100% if left untreated.

Antibiotic prophylaxis

10 B   One hour before surgery
Surgical site infections account for approximately 15% of nosocomial infections and are associated with a prolonged hospital stay and increased costs. A prospective randomized control trial has shown that administering prophylactic antibiotics, and starting the initial dose one hour before surgery, decreases the incidence of postoperative surgical site infections. It is also worth noting that for a majority of surgical procedures, prophylaxis should not exceed 24 hours.

Diagnosis of left iliac fossa pain

11 B   Diverticulitis
In general, diverticula can be described as outpouchings of serosa-covered mucosa alone through gaps in the muscularis layer where terminal blood vessels are transmitted (the weakest point where diverticula protrude). Diverticula are commonly found in the descending and sigmoid colon. Patients who have diverticula and do not experience any symptoms are said to have diverticulosis. If colonic diverticula cause symptoms (either left-sided or central colicky abdominal pain, as well as bloating coupled with constipation), the patient is said to have diverticular disease.

Diverticulitis occurs when a colonic diverticulum becomes inflamed due to infection or when faeces impact within it. Classically, it presents with lower central abdominal pain which moves to the left iliac fossa, usually referred to as 'left-sided appendicitis' due to the similar symptoms experienced in appendicitis. Accompanying symptoms include fever, vomiting, local tenderness and guarding (local peritonitis). When the inflamed diverticulum perforates (perforated diverticulitis), signs of general peritonitis develop, characterized by general abdominal rigidity and guarding. Patients may show signs of shock, and on an erect chest radiograph free air may be visible under the diaphragm.

Management of left iliac fossa pain

12 D **Keep nil by mouth, administer intravenous fluids and analgesia**
The treatment of diverticulitis focuses on conservative management. This consists of resting the bowel by keeping the patient nil
by mouth, giving maintenance intravenous fluids and administering
antibiotics (e.g. cefuroxime and metronidazole or the recommended
combination of choice at the local hospital), which will resolve the
underlying infection. Diverticulitis is extremely painful and administering analgesia is imperative in providing pain relief to the patient.
This combined method of treatment will allow the inflammation to
resolve.

Right upper quadrant pain

13 C **Cholangitis**
In the context of acute abdominal conditions, the Charcot's triad is a
set of clinical signs relating to ascending cholangitis. The combination
of right upper quadrant abdominal pain, jaundice and rigours (involuntary shaking, which occurs during high fevers) are the clinical manifestations of ascending cholangitis. If a patient presents with Charcot's
triad coupled with hypotension and an altered mental state, this collection of clinical signs is called Reynold's pentad and suggests a diagnosis
of septic ascending cholangitis. A patient suspected of having ascending cholangitis requires prompt treatment with intravenous fluids and
antibiotics.

Management of an inguinal hernia

14 A **Alert theatre and send the patient for emergency surgery**
This patient is suffering from a strangulated hernia, which requires
prompt surgical intervention. The signs of bowel obstruction coupled
with the tense, irreducible, inguinal hernia and the overlying skin
being erythematous and warm suggests that this hernia is strangulated
rather than obstructed. The blood supply to the contents of the hernia
is cut off by pressure at the neck of the hernia. This causes ischaemic
necrosis/gangrene of the hernial contents (i.e. either bowel or omentum). Symptoms of intestinal obstruction are present if the bowel is
present within the hernial sac. If on the other hand, only omentum
is present, bowel obstruction is not a feature with the accompanying
strangulation.
In this case, the patient requires immediate surgical intervention.
Delaying surgery can be fatal and emergency surgery is a priority in a
patient in whom a strangulated hernia is suspected.

Constipation and abdominal pain

15 D   Large bowel obstruction

The most likely answer here is large bowel obstruction. Pain is usually colicky in nature and is felt commonly in the suprapubic area rather than the central area of the abdomen, which is experienced in small bowel obstruction. Vomiting is usually a late sign in large bowel obstruction, but an early sign in small bowel obstruction. Absolute constipation (not passing faeces or flatus) is an early feature of large bowel obstruction, due to the lower site of obstruction, and a late feature of small bowel obstruction. Abdominal distension is marked in large bowel obstruction and may be absent or slight in small bowel obstruction depending on the level of obstruction in the small bowel. For information on appendicitis, pancreatitis and diverticular disease, please refer to answers to Questions 2, 6 and 11, respectively. Irritable bowel syndrome is a chronic disorder of intestinal motility and presents as central/lower abdominal pain which is relieved by defaecation. It is accompanied by bloating, altered bowel habits (constipation alternating with diarrhoea), tenesmus (the feeling of incomplete faecal evacuation) and usually mucus production rectally.

Acute pancreatitis

16 C   (3)

The modified Glasgow criteria (sensitivity 68% and specificity 84%) are commonly used in the United Kingdom to assess the severity of an episode of pancreatitis within 48 hours of onset. Other systems used are Ranson's criteria, and the acute physiological and chronic health evaluation (APACHE) scores. The modified Glasgow criteria can be used for pancreatitis caused by gallstones and alcohol whereas Ranson's criteria have been validated for alcohol-induced pancreatitis and can only be fully put to use after 48 hours of onset. The modified Glasgow criteria are:

- paO_2 <8 kPa
- Age >55 years
- White cell count >15 × 10^9/L
- Calcium <2 mmol/L
- Urea >16 mmol/L
- LDH >600 IU/L
- AST/ALT >200 IU/L
- Albumin <32 g/L
- Blood glucose >10 mmol/L

If three or more criteria are positive and detected within 48 hours of onset, this suggests that the pancreatitis is severe.

Diarrhoea and abdominal pain

17 B   Toxic megacolon

This patient is suffering from an acute complication of ulcerative colitis called toxic megacolon. Severe inflammation rendered by the ongoing ulcerative colitis leads to dilatation of the colon, especially the transverse colon. Clinical features include toxaemia (leading to pyrexia, tachycardia and hypotension), anaemia from bleeding, acute loss of water and electrolytes and progressive abdominal distension. Along with clinical features, toxic megacolon can be diagnosed on a plain film abdominal radiograph by assessing the extent of dilatation of the transverse colon. Usually if the transverse colon is dilated more than 6 cm, this is diagnostic of toxic megacolon. For information on perforated diverticulitis and large bowel obstruction, please refer to the answers to Questions 11 and 15, respectively. Toxic megacolon can also be a complication of Crohn's colitis, but in this scenario we are told that the patient already has a 10-year history of ulcerative colitis, making Crohn's colitis unlikely.

Treatment involves initial fluid resuscitation, correcting electrolyte imbalances and administering high-dose steroids. Repeated abdominal plain film radiographs are conducted as part of ongoing assessment of the size of the colon. If the size of the colon is increasing despite medical therapy, surgery is indicated before perforation ensues. Surgery is usually indicated if the patient fails to improve within 24–48 hours of medical treatment or if the risks of perforation are high.

Bowel obstruction

18 C   Paralytic ileus

Intestinal obstruction can be broadly divided into mechanical and paralytic obstruction (also known as paralytic ileus). A paralytic ileus occurs when the intestines are in a complete state of atony. Clinical features include abdominal distension, absolute constipation, vomiting and the absence of intestinal motility (thus bowel sounds are absent). Due to the lack of intestinal movement, colicky abdominal pain is not a feature, unlike what is seen in mechanical obstruction. Postoperative abdominal surgery, peritonitis, trauma, acute pancreatitis, potassium deficiency, uraemia, anticholinergic and antidiarrhoeal drugs are some of the frequent causes of a paralytic ileus. Causes of mechanical obstruction can be divided into:

- Luminal (e.g. faecal impaction, foreign body, intussusceptions, large polyps)
- Intramural (e.g. congential intestinal atresia, Crohn's colitis, tumours, strictures)

- Extraluminal (e.g. volvulus, adhesions, strangulated hernia, extrinsic compression also known as a 'mass effect')

A gallstone ileus can be classified as a form of luminal intestinal obstruction. This occurs when a large gallstone (usually >2.5 cm) erodes through the gallbladder wall and passes into the duodenum, through a cholecysto-duodenal fistula, which is formed due to the chronic inflammatory environment of the eroding gallstone. The stone may then go on to obstruct the terminal ileum at the ileocaecal junction.

Investigation of right upper quadrant pain

19 A Ultrasound
Right upper quadrant pain coupled with a positive Murphy's sign suggests acute cholecystitis. From the list, upper gastrointestinal endoscopy, colonoscopy and barium follow-through are inappropriate and will not positively add to the management of this patient. Serum amylase, although an important test used to rule out acute pancreatitis, would not be the most useful test in this scenario. Conducting an ultrasound scan of the abdomen can confirm the presence of gallstones, identify areas of the gallbladder where oedema and wall thickening are present and know the status of the CBD.

Acute urinary retention

20 B Bladder outflow obstruction due to benign prostatic hypertrophy
The findings of the DRE suggest that this man has bladder outflow obstruction due to prostatic enlargement rather than the other causes mentioned in options C–E. From the findings of the DRE, it seems evident that the prostate enlargement is most likely due to benign prostatic hypertrophy rather than prostatic carcinoma, which usually feels 'craggy and nodular' on DRE coupled with systemic symptoms such as back pain and weight loss, which may occur as a result of metastatic spread of the primary prostate carcinoma.

Urethral strictures are uncommon in men and rare in women. They may arise due to recurrent infections of the urinary tract, trauma or cancer, and can be congenital. Symptoms include dysuria, decreased stream, terminal dribbling and 'double stream' when voiding. In addition, acute urinary retention may be caused by a spinal cord lesion which would have produced severe neurological complications such as paraesthesia and paralysis depending on the level of the spinal cord lesion; a history of trauma would also be present.

Management of acute urinary retention

21 D Urinary catheterisation
Prompt urinary catheterization is the most appropriate course of action here. This will relieve the discomfort and prevent the risk of acute renal

failure. Urethral catheterization is attempted first; if unsuccessful, supra-pubic catheterization is carried out. At some centres, administering par-enteral antibiotics (e.g. intramuscular gentamicin) 15–20 minutes before catheterization is encouraged (in elderly patients with acute urinary retention) to decrease the risk of the patient developing a urinary tract infection. An abdominal plain film radiograph would not be informative in this case and obtaining blood for urea and electrolytes is important (to check renal function) but should be done once the patient is catheterized.

Vomiting and left upper quadrant pain

22 C   **Gastro-oesophageal obstruction secondary to a gastric volvulus**
The clinical triad of vomiting (after which non-productive retching occurs), pain and failed attempts to pass a nasogastric tube are clas-sic signs of gastro-oesophageal obstruction. Gastric dilatation and a prominent fluid level seen on the plain film chest radiograph suggest that the obstruction is due to a volvulus. The pathology has been clini-cally narrowed down to the stomach, making a sigmoid volvulus an unlikely possibility in this question. The causes of a gastric volvu-lus can be divided into congenital (e.g. paraoesophageal hernia, con-genital bands, bowel malformations, pyloric stenosis) and acquired (e.g. previous gastric/oesophageal surgery, adhesion from previous abdominal surgery). If a gastric volvulus is suspected, emergency laparotomy should not be delayed so as to avoid perforation. At some centres, endoscopic manipulation is done first and if this is not suc-cessful, surgery is warranted. Perforation usually occurs secondary to ischaemia and necrosis of the stomach (caused by the twisting of the stomach). This surgical emergency is more common in adults than in children and carries a 42%–56% mortality rate.

Management of abdominal pain (2)

23 D   **Send for emergency explorative laparotomy**
Mesenteric adenitis refers to inflammation of the mesenteric lymph nodes and is regarded as the main differential diagnosis of acute appen-dicitis. It is more commonly a childhood illness, though occasionally seen in adults. It is often preceded by a viral upper respiratory tract infection. Enlargement of the mesenteric lymph nodes, due to the effects of the viral infection, causes right iliac fossa pain (can be diffused) and tenderness as well as an accompanying fever. Symptoms of nausea, vomiting, anorexia and diarrhoea may also be experienced. A white cell count may show lymphocytosis rather than a raised neutrophil count as seen with acute appendicitis.

Since the ultrasound was inconclusive, coupled with symptoms and signs paralleling acute appendicitis, the most appropriate step to take is to send the patient for an explorative laparotomy. Acute appendicitis may be mistaken for mesenteric adenitis which can lead to complications of perforation, general peritonitis and septicaemia. Usually during explorative laparotomy, the appendix will be removed (even if it is normal) so that subsequent attacks of abdominal pain of this nature are not confused with appendicitis. Treatment of mesenteric adenitis involves analgesia and observing the patient for 24 hours; symptoms usually settle down within 24 hours of onset. In severe cases, intravenous antibiotics may be given and anti-emetics for the nausea and vomiting.

Management of intussusception

24 B **Barium enema per rectum and abdominal plain film radiography**
Intussusception can be defined as the invagination of a portion of bowel into its own lumen. The invaginated portion of the bowel is called the intussusceptum. Common types of intussusception are ileo-ileal, ileo-caecal and colocolic. This condition is common in children (the cause is idiopathic enlarged Peyer's patch) and rare in adults. After the age of 3 years certain factors can predispose to the condition such as intestinal polyps, carcinoma, intestinal lymphoma, foreign bodies or an inverted Meckel's diverticulum. It presents as intermittent abdominal colic (screaming and pallor are seen in children), vomiting, and the passage of mucus and bloody stools per rectum (sometimes referred to as red-currant jelly). On examination the child will appear pale and anxious and will be irritable. On palpation of the abdomen, a sausage-shaped mass may be felt. Plain film abdominal radiography may be normal in early stages or there may be signs consistent with bowel obstruction. Ultrasound scanning has been used in some centres, but with variable success in diagnosing intussusception. The initial steps of treatment involve the use of barium enemas per rectum and plain abdominal film radiographs (which highlight the site of intussusception). The pressure at which the barium flows through the bowel can reduce the intussusception and this can be confirmed by conducting another plain abdominal film radiograph. If this fails, surgical reduction can be carried out. If the bowel is gangrenous, resection will be carried out. The chances of bowel ischaemia and gangrene are reduced if the intussusception is reduced within 24 hours of diagnosis.

Diagnosis of abdominal pain

25 C Renal colic
The most likely diagnosis here is renal colic caused by obstruction of the urinary tract. Commonly the obstruction is caused by calculi impacting the pelvi-ureteric junction or anywhere along the course of the ureters.

Stones within the renal parenchyma of the kidney rarely produce pain but if they do, dull loin pain may be experienced. The pain is caused by dilatation, stretching and spasm of the ureters. This is an extremely painful condition and clinically presents with colicky pain which radiates from 'loin to groin'. The pain is usually so intense that patients are classically described as 'writhing around in pain'. Associated symptoms include vomiting and sweating. In small bowel obstruction, the pain is centrally positioned and bowel sounds are usually raised (please refer to the answer to Question 4). Acute diverticulitis presents with left iliac fossa pain and tenderness with local guarding, usually with accompanying fever (please refer to the answer to Question 11). A ruptured ectopic pregnancy would produce signs of left or right iliac fossae pain, generalized peritonitis (generalized guarding and abdominal rigidity), fever, hypotension and tachycardia; serum b-hCG is raised. In this case the patient is postmenopausal making a ruptured ectopic pregnancy unlikely. For information on ruptured aortic aneurysms please refer to the answer to Question 9.

Investigation of abdominal pain (2)

26 A Computed tomography scan of the abdomen

Urine dipstick shows blood but is not diagnostic. Intravenous urogram and CT scanning (more specifically, CT-KUB) are investigations of diagnostic value for renal stones. CT scans are able to detect 99% of renal stones and, therefore, have now been classed as the gold standard diagnostic investigation for renal calculi. In addition, the CT scan is able to exclude other causes of an acute abdomen and contrast media is not needed unlike IVU which may be nephrotoxic. A KUB film, although not the investigation of choice, should always be performed when the patient is admitted with symptoms of renal colic. It should be noted that a KUB film alone will detect 80% of renal stones. Ultrasound scanning, when combined with a KUB film, has been shown to be sensitive in detecting renal calculi, but not as sensitive as CT-KUB scanning. An abdominal plain film radiograph would not be of value in this condition; KUB is a larger abdominal plain film radiograph which incorporates visualization of the kidneys, ureters and bladder.

Causes of acute pancreatitis

27 C Gallstones

The causes of pancreatitis can be remembered by the pneumonic 'GET SMASHED' (see the answer to Question 33 in Section 6). The most common causes are gallstones followed by alcohol (especially binge drinking).

Causes of large bowel obstruction

28 B Sigmoid volvulus

Sigmoid volvulus is the most common type of volvulus in its category. It is common in elderly and mentally retarded patients who have a chronic history of constipation and who have redundant loops of sigmoid colon on a long mesentery, making the chances of 'twisting' more likely. The patient usually presents with severe acute colicky abdominal pain, abdominal distension and absolute constipation. Abdominal plain film radiography may reveal, first, distended loops of the sigmoid colon in an inverted 'U' shape orientation, which extend from the pelvis under the diaphragm. The classical 'coffee bean sign' is seen as a result of compression of two medial walls of the distended sigmoid colon. Second, free air may be present under the hemi-diaphragms as a result of bowel perforation (secondary to ischaemia and necrosis of the bowel).

Lower gastrointestinal infection

29 D Pseudomembranous colitis

Pseudomembranous colitis is an infection of the colon caused by the Gram-positive anaerobic bacteria *Clostridium difficile*. The signs and symptoms of this condition are similar to those experienced in ulcerative, Crohn's and ischaemic colitis: watery diarrhoea (with or without blood), passing of mucus per rectum, cramping abdominal pain and fever. Toxin A, a proinflammatory enterotoxin released by *C. difficile*, acts as an intestinal receptor causing loosening of junctions between intestinal epithelia. Toxin B, which is also produced by this organism, is then able to pass through the loosened epithelial cell junctions and initiates an inflammatory cascade. This process ultimately leads to fluid secretion, mucosal cell injury, oedema and inflammation. The development of *C. difficile* infection has been associated with a history of recent or prolonged antibiotic use, increasing age and prolonged hospital stay.

Diagnosis is by stool analysis; the stool cytotoxin test is highly sensitive and specific and considered to be the first line diagnostic investigation. A highly effective, but expensive, PCR testing method is also available, but due to the costs involved, stool cytotoxin testing is favoured. Colonoscopy or sigmoidoscopy may show pseudomembrane plaque appearance (present in 50% of patients). In some cases, histological examination may be performed for confirmation. First line treatment is usually with metronidazole, or vancomycin, if the *C. difficile* is resistant to metronidazole. *C. difficile* colitis can cause toxic megacolon (see the answer to Question 17). This cannot be treated with antibiotics and therefore warrants emergency surgery.

Investigation of a diverticular abscess

30 C Computed tomography scan of abdomen
The most appropriate investigation here is an abdominal CT scan. Barium enema evaluation was the diagnostic investigation of choice before CT scanning was introduced. The plain film abdominal radiograph, although a quick and simple imaging investigation, is not useful in diagnosing diverticular abscesses. Colonoscopy and flexible sigmoidoscopy carry a risk of perforation and may not be able to visualize the abscess and are therefore not used. Diverticular abscess could be treated with antibiotics and CT guided drainage.

SECTION 9:
BREAST SURGERY AND ENDOCRINE DISEASE

Questions

1.	Breast lumps (1)	184
2.	Breast pain (1)	184
3.	Breast infection	184
4.	Breast lumps (2)	185
5.	Breast pain (2)	185
6.	Nipple discharge	185
7.	Management of breast pathology (1)	185
8.	Pathological breast enlargement	186
9.	Rash	186
10.	Breast pain (3)	186
11.	Breast lump assessment	187
12.	Management of fat necrosis of the breast	187
13.	Management of breast cysts	187
14.	Management of breast infection	187
15.	Management of fibroadenoma	188
16.	Mammary duct ectasia	188
17.	Management of breast pathology (2)	188
18.	Ductal carcinoma *in situ*	189
19.	Management of breast cancer	189
20.	Ductal carcinoma	189
21.	Management of breast pathology (3)	190
22.	Complications of breast surgery	190
23.	Management of endocrine disease (1)	190
24.	Management of endocrine disease (2)	190
25.	Management of breast pathology (4)	191
Answers		192

QUESTIONS

1. Breast lumps (1)

A worried 23-year-old woman, who started taking the combined contraceptive pill 3 months ago, presents with a 1-day history of discovering a painless lump in the right breast. The patient states that the lump was not there a month ago. On examination, a slightly mobile, discrete, well-defined, non-tender, firm 1 cm diameter lump is found. There is no lymphadenopathy. The most likely diagnosis here is

- A. Breast cyst
- B. Lipoma
- C. Fibroadenoma
- D. Sebaceous cyst
- E. Carcinoma of the breast

2. Breast pain (1)

A 36-year-old nulliparous woman attends your clinic with a 7-day history of left breast pain after being involved in a car accident. On examining her breast, you notice a hard, irregular 3 cm, immobile, tender lump. You also notice some skin tethering and overlying bruising in the region of the lump. Ultrasound features suggest a benign pathology. The most likely diagnosis at this point is

- A. Fat necrosis
- B. Breast cyst
- C. Mammary duct ectasia
- D. Breast abscess
- E. Fibroadenosis

3. Breast infection

A 33-year-old, non-smoking, breastfeeding woman is 10 days postpartum. She has a 4-day history of a slight crack on the surface of her left nipple. She presents with a 2-day history of severe continuous pain in the left breast, spiking pyrexia up to 38.8 with rigours which has prevented her from sleeping. On examination, you find the outer quadrants of the left breast to be red, warm and tender with a hard 3 cm lump at the edge of the left nipple. The most likely diagnosis is

- A. Acute mastitis
- B. Breast cyst → findings not in line
- C. Fat necrosis no hx of local trauma
- D. Breast abscess → spiking fever
- E. Periductal mastitis
  → in non lactating brest

4. Breast lumps (2)

A 65-year-old nulliparous woman presents to your clinic with a lump in her left breast, which was discovered 7 months ago. On examination you find a hard, ill-defined, non-tender, 3.5 cm lump behind the left nipple. The patient has also had bloody, non-purulent discharge from a single duct on the left nipple for over 3 months. The most likely diagnosis here is

A. Mammary duct ectasia → green discharge
B. Breast carcinoma
C. Duct papilloma → young
D. Periductal mastitis → no fever
E. Acute mastitis

5. Breast pain (2)

A 43-year-old woman presents to your clinic with a 2-month history of local-ized dull pain in the right breast. The pain intensifies just before her period. On examination, you find a discrete 2.5 cm mobile, tense, tender, fluctuant lump in the lower inner quadrant of the right breast. The most likely diagnosis here is

A. Fibroadenosis
B. Periductal mastitis
C. Breast cyst
D. Fat necrosis
E. Fibroadenoma

6. Nipple discharge

A 47-year-old perimenopausal woman presents with a 3-week history of green discharge from the right nipple. On examination, the right nipple is non-tender, has a 'slit-like' appearance and is retracted. The most likely diagnosis is

A. Galactorrhoea
B. Duct papilloma
C. Breast carcinoma
D. Mammary duct ectasia
E. Fibroadenoma

7. Management of breast pathology (1)

A 25-year-old woman presents to your clinic after discovering, for the first time, two lumps in the inner lower quadrant of her left breast. On examination you find these lumps to be 2 cm in size, solid, discrete, mobile and non-tender. The right breast is normal and there is no lymphadenopathy. The most appropriate course of management is

A. Request a mammogram
B. Reassure the patient and discharge her

All lumps should be investigated!

C. Request an ultrasound of the left breast
D. Request fine needle aspiration
E. Request a core biopsy

8. Pathological breast enlargement

A 67-year-old woman, with a 25-year smoking history, on hormone replacement therapy, presents to clinic expressing concerns regarding an increase in the size of her right breast over the last 4 months. On examination, you find a non-tender, mobile, lobulated 10 cm mass with relatively smooth edges in the right breast. The right breast is significantly larger than the left and has a 'teardrop' appearance and the skin looks normal. The most likely diagnosis here is

A. Paget's disease of the nipple *→ non-itchy unilateral usually*
B. Inflammatory breast carcinoma *— pain erythema lump*
C. Breast abscess *→ no fever*
D. Malignant phylloides tumour
E. Fibroadenoma *— benign*

eczema of nipple → bilateral → itchy and itchy

9. Rash

A worried 59-year-old city worker arrives at your clinic with a 1-month history of having noticed a non-itchy, persistent, burning rash in the region of her right breast. On examination, you find the right nipple and the skin overlying the areola to be red and eczematous. The most likely cause is

A. Breast abscess *→ no spiking fever*
B. Malignant phyllodes tumour *→ no ↑ in size*
C. Paget's disease of the nipple
D. Basal cell carcinoma *→ Pearly edge, Rodent ulcer*
E. Mastitis *→ no pain*

10. Breast pain (3)

A 21-year-old nulliparous woman presents to your clinic with a 1-month history of bilateral breast pain. The pain, which is dull and achy in nature, is poorly localized and widespread across both breasts. The pain gradually increases in severity and is worse just before her menses. The pain usually starts to get better once her menses start. On examination, both breasts are tender. There are no lumps, skin changes or obvious swellings. The most likely diagnosis here is

A. Non-cyclical mastalgia
B. Tietze's syndrome
C. Cyclical mastalgia
D. Acute bacterial mastitis
E. Traumatic fat necrosis

11. Breast lump assessment

You are attending a breast multidisciplinary team (MDT) meeting where the core biopsy histology results of a suspicious breast lesion are being discussed in a 55-year-old woman presenting with a right sided breast lump. The histopathologist states that the breast lesion possesses 'B5b' histology features. What is the most likely diagnosis?

    A. Fibroadenoma
    B. Benign breast cyst   ??
    C. Ductal carcinoma *in-situ*
    D. Invasive breast carcinoma
    E. No breast abnormality

12. Management of fat necrosis of the breast

A 25-year-old woman is diagnosed with a 1.5 cm palpable area of fat necrosis of the left breast by core biopsy following a traumatic injury 14 days earlier. She has slight bruising of the lower outer quadrant of the left breast with moderate tenderness. What would be the most appropriate course of management?

    A. Reassurance and discharge
    B. Follow-up appointment for ultrasound in 3 months
    C. Wide local excision
    D. Left mastectomy
    E. Follow-up appointment for ultrasound in 6 months

13. Management of breast cysts

A 38-year-old woman, and mother of two healthy children, is diagnosed with a fluid-filled simple cyst after triple assessment. On ultrasound the inner surface of the cyst looks entirely smooth. The woman does not have any significant family history of carcinoma and the cyst is located in the outer-lower quadrant of the right breast. What would be the most appropriate course of action?

    A. Wide local excision
    B. Follow-up appointment in 3 months
    C. Annual follow-up
    D. Reassure and discharge
    E. Core biopsy

- Usually collapse after fluid is aspirated.
- If not → Investigate with triple test.

14. Management of breast infection

A 30-year-old woman who is 12 days postpartum and breastfeeding is diagnosed with acute mastitis of the left breast. Four days earlier, she discovered a painful crack in the region of the left nipple and noticed that the surrounding skin was tender, warm and red in colour. The patient is not allergic to penicillin and you decide to prescribe a course of antibiotics. What would be the most appropriate antibiotic for treating this condition?

    A. Erythromycin
    B. Amoxicillin
    C. Ciprofloxacin
    D. Flucloxacillin
    E. Cephalexin

15. Management of fibroadenoma

if small <2.5 cm ↓ no need to do anything.

After a triple assessment, including core biopsy, a 28-year-old woman is diagnosed with a fibroadenoma of the left breast. The patient has a significant family history of breast carcinoma. The non-tender lump is situated in the inner lower quadrant of the left breast. The lump is approximately 1.5 cm × 1.5 cm. What is the most appropriate course of management?

    A. Excision of the lump *→ because of hx of Ca., reassures patient*
    B. Reassure and follow-up after 3 months
    C. The patient should be given the choice of excision or not and if not she could be discharged
    D. Fine needle aspiration
    E. Perform triple assessment again in 6 weeks

16. Mammary duct ectasia

for small amt of discharge

A 45-year-old perimenopausal woman is diagnosed with mammary duct ectasia of the right breast after having had small and infrequent amounts of milky green discharge from multiple ducts of the right nipple for over 2 months. The patient has no significant family history and mammography findings are normal. What is the most appropriate course of management?

    A. Reassure and discharge
    B. Surgical resection of the duct system of the right breast (Hadfield's operation) *if discharge excessive*
    C. Commence antibiotic therapy
    D. Perform mammography of the right breast in 3 months
    E. Mastectomy of the right breast

17. Management of breast pathology (2)

1) hx and exam
2) Imaging
3) Cytology

A 48-year-old perimenopausal woman presents with a 2-month history of a painful lump in her right breast. On examination you find a 2.5 cm tense, fluctuant, mobile lump in the outer lower quadrant of the right breast. The most appropriate next course of action is

    A. Computed tomography scan
    B. Mammography and ultrasound

C. Fine needle aspiration
D. Core biopsy
E. Mammography and core biopsy

18. Ductal carcinoma *in situ*

A 60-year-old woman was found to have one focal area of microcalcification (approximately 20 mm in diameter) in the left breast. A stereotactic core biopsy of this area was taken for histological assessment, which revealed low-grade ductal carcinoma *in situ*. In light of this, what would be the most appropriate treatment modality for this patient?

A. Mastectomy → if multiple foci, tumor > 40mm, aggressive type
B. Mastectomy + postoperative radiotherapy
C. Wide local excision + postoperative radiotherapy → preserves normal breast tissue
D. Mastectomy + axillary clearance + postoperative radiotherapy
E. Wide local excision + axillary clearance + postoperative radiotherapy

19. Management of breast cancer

Invasive → invaded BM. → axillary nodes likely to be affected

A 47-year-old woman is diagnosed with an unofficial 2.5 cm Grade 3 invasive ductal carcinoma of the right breast. Following MDT discussion the consultant sees the patient in clinic to convey management options. Which of the following would be the most appropriate management plan for this patient?

A. Wide local excision
B. Wide local excision and axillary clearance
C. Mastectomy and sentinel node biopsy
D. Wide local excision and sentinel node biopsy —because
E. Mastectomy and axillary clearance

Sentinel node biopsy → to see if LN involved → to plan for axillary clearance if needed.

tumor < 40 mm

20. Ductal carcinoma

, Surgery for Stage 1 and 2 only.

A 46-year-old man is diagnosed with an oestrogen receptor positive invasive ductal carcinoma of the right breast after having discovered a lump 3 months before. The patient is found to have multiple involved axillary lymph nodes and the tumour is of an aggressive phenotype. The most appropriate treatment option for this patient is

← for Stage 3 and 4.

A. Cytotoxic chemotherapy and Tamoxifen but no surgery
B. Mastectomy + axillary clearance + systemic chemotherapy + radiotherapy and tamoxifen
C. Wide local excision and Tamoxifen only → cannot determine clear margins
D. Mastectomy + postoperative radiotherapy only
E. Palliative care programme → Stage 4

21. Management of breast pathology (3)

A 34-year-old premenopausal woman presents to your clinic with a lump in her right breast. On examination you find a 2.5 cm fluctuant, mobile, tender lump in the inner lower quadrant of the right breast. The ultrasound report suggests a benign fluid-filled cyst. The most appropriate course of action is

    A. Breast magnetic resonance imaging
    B. Ultrasound guided fine needle aspiration
    C. Ultrasound guided core biopsy
    D. Reassure and discharge
    E. Mammography

22. Complications of breast surgery

In which one of the following scenarios is the complication of lymphoedema of the arm more likely to occur after resection of a breast tumour and axillary clearance?

    A. Mastectomy + axillary clearance + postoperative radiotherapy to the chest wall
    B. Mastectomy + axillary clearance + systemic chemotherapy
    C. Mastectomy + axillary clearance + postoperative radiotherapy to the axilla
    D. Mastectomy + axillary clearance
    E. Mastectomy + postoperative radiotherapy

23. Management of endocrine disease (1)

A 28-year-old woman, who was hospitalized 2 months ago following a head injury, attends the outpatient clinic with a 6-week history of polyuria and polydipsia and no other symptoms. Her blood pressure is 117/83 mmHg and her heart rate is 68 beats/min. From the list below, select the most appropriate management option.

ADH = reabsorption of water

ADH insufficiency

    A. Carbimazole
    B. Desmopressin
    C. Spironolactone
    D. Thyroxine
    E. Octreotide

24. Management of endocrine disease (2)

↑ Catecholamines

During a ward round, you are asked by your surgical registrar about the management of a phaeochromocytoma. Select from the list below the most appropriate management plan for a phaeochromocytoma.

    A. Surgical resection, followed by β blockade, followed by α blockade
    B. Lifelong β and α blockade

C. Surgical resection

D. β blockade, followed by α blockade, followed by surgical resection

E. α blockade, followed by β blockade followed by surgical resection

25. Management of breast pathology (4)

A 58-year-old postmenopausal woman has been seen in clinic following discovery of a 3 cm, non-tender, irregular, firm lump in the upper outer quadrant of the left breast. Mammography and ultrasound imaging respectively reveal that the lump has areas of calcification and is a solid mass. The most appropriate course of action is

⤷ features suggestive of malignancy

A. Repeat mammography and ultrasound scans in 6 months

B. Reassure and discharge

C. Repeat mammography and ultrasound scans in 3 months

D. Fine needle aspiration to ensure that the lump is not really fluid filled

E. Core biopsy

Management of Pheochromocytoma

α-blockade given 7-10 days before surgery

β-blockade

ANSWERS

Breast lumps (1)

1 C Fibroadenoma

Fibroadenomas classically present in females below the age of 35 and are infrequent after the age of 35–40. They are described as painless, rubbery to firm, non-fluctuant, discrete mobile breast lumps commonly referred to as 'breast mice'. Breast cysts occur more frequently after the age of 35 and may present with breast pain. They can be fluctuant if fluid filled and characteristically are tense, discrete, mobile lumps. Carcinoma of the breast is rare under the age of 35, and usually presents as a solitary, painless, ill-defined lump of varying size which may show signs of skin tethering. Lipomas, although very common, are usually soft, fluctuant, irregularly defined lumps. Sebaceous cysts are typically round, soft lumps attached to the skin and have a central punctum.

Breast pain (1)

2 A Fat necrosis

The most likely answer here is fat necrosis. Although the irregularity and hardness of the breast lump with overlying skin tethering suggests breast carcinoma, the history of recent trauma coupled with overlying breast lump tenderness and bruising indicates fat necrosis rather than breast cyst, fibroadenosis and breast abscess. Breast cyst, fibroadenosis and breast abscess are all unlikely here because of the history.

Breast infection

3 D Breast abscess

Lactational breast abscesses are caused by the skin's commensal microorganisms, nearly always staphylococci, infiltrating cracks in the nipple during breastfeeding. Segmental breast inflammation occurs, leading to cellulitis which, if not treated promptly, results in breast tissue necrosis, pus build up and abscess formation within the breast segment. Continuous pain and sleepless nights coupled with the hard 3 cm painful lump suggest an abscess rather than acute mastitis. Fat necrosis is unlikely here with no history of previous minor local trauma. Periductal mastitis is possible, but classically occurs in non-lactating women of reproductive age and is associated with smoking. From the nature of the history and physical examination findings, it is unlikely to be a breast cyst.

Breast lumps (2)

4   B   Breast carcinoma

The most likely diagnosis here is breast carcinoma. The patient is in her sixth decade with a nulliparous history. Furthermore, blood-stained nipple discharge coupled with the non-tender breast lump place her at high risk of breast cancer. Milky to dirty-green nipple discharge is usually seen with mammary duct ectasia (common in postmenopausal women) and often, but not always, occurs bilaterally. Acute and periductal mastitis are unlikely here due to the absence of mastalgia. Although duct papillomas are relatively common causes of blood-stained discharge, they do not classically present with a breast lump and other symptoms are rarely present. Owing to the similar presentation of breast carcinoma, it is difficult to distinguish it from a duct papilloma by clinical examination alone.

Breast pain (2)

5   C   Breast cyst

Breast cysts usually occur in women over the age of 40 years through to the menopause. The aetiology in unclear, but it is thought that they occur due to hormonal imbalances around the menopause. Not all breast cysts manifest as pre-menstrual tenderness. The lump is mobile and fluctuant, suggesting that it is a fluid-filled cyst. Fibroadenomas classically present in females below the age of 35 and are infrequent after the age of 35–40. Fibroadenosis presents at a similar age, however the lump is fluctuant, making it more likely to be a cyst. Fat necrosis is unlikely here in the absence of previous minor local trauma (which is not stated in the history). Periductal mastitis is commonly seen in non-lactating women in their thirties (with a history of smoking) with pain usually developing in the areolar area.

Nipple discharge

6   D   Mammary duct ectasia

This presentation is typical of mammary duct ectasia, which is common in the decade around the menopause. The nipple discharge can vary, ranging from milky, brown to a dirty green colour. The nipple discharge can be bilateral and occasionally it is associated with cyclical mastalgia. The history of nipple retraction can cause confusion, leading the clinician to suspect breast carcinoma. However, the presence of the slit in the nipple, coupled with the colour of the nipple discharge and the perimenopausal age of the patient, make it more likely to be duct ectasia. Galactorrhoea is unlikely here as nipple discharge is usually bilateral and milky in appearance and this usually follows lactation. Duct papillomas usually present with blood-stained nipple discharge. Fibroadenoma does not usually present with nipple discharge and is common in women under the age of 35.

Management of breast pathology (1)

7　C　Request an ultrasound of the left breast

US if <35

mammogram >35

All breast lumps are investigated using 'triple assessment' which involves clinical examination, ultrasound breast scans for women younger than 35 (due to relatively denser breast tissue) or mammograms for women older than 35, followed by fine needle aspiration cytology and/or core biopsy for cytological and histological assessment, respectively. Women over the age of 35 tend to have less dense breast tissue, which increases the sensitivity and specificity of mammography.

This patient is 25, which coupled with the discovery of two new lumps, indicates that the next line investigation, following clinical examination, would be an ultrasound of the left breast. Mammography would not be suitable as this patient is under the age of 35. Reassurance and discharge is clearly wrong as all breast lumps should undergo triple assessment before the patient is discharged. Fine needle aspiration and core biopsy, although they will be carried out, are not considered until radiological assessment has been performed.

Pathological breast enlargement

8　D　Phyllodes tumour

The most likely answer here is a malignant phyllodes tumour which accounts for 0.5% of all breast tumours. The recent increase in size of the right breast coupled with the discovery of a non-tender, mobile lump, giving the right breast a 'tear drop' appearance, is suggestive of a malignant phyllodes tumour. Phyllodes tumours have many of the clinical and histological features of fibroadenomas (which are common in women in their early to late twenties). Inflammatory breast carcinoma, as its name suggests, is associated with pain (unlike other breast cancers), breast erythema, *peau d'orange* (the skin overlying the breast resembles that of red-coloured orange peel) and skin ridging with or without a palpable mass. Paget's disease of the nipple presents as a unilateral, non-itchy, irregular eczematoid eruption of the nipple. It can be easily confused with eczema of the nipple, which usually occurs bilaterally, with pruritus, and can be nipple sparing. Breast abscess is unlikely here, and for more information, please refer to the answer to Question 2.

Rash

9　C　Paget's disease of the nipple

The most likely answer here is Paget's disease of the nipple. The non-itchy, eczematoid changes in the overlying skin of the right nipple and accompanying lymphadenopathy suggests underlying breast malignancy rather than eczema. Paget's disease of the nipple is almost always associated with an underlying intraductal or invasive carcinoma. Early BCC lesions consist of raised pearly pink papules with fine overlying areas of telangiectasia. Late BCC lesions gradually ulcerate and are often referred to as 'rodent ulcers'. A malignant phyllodes tumour is unlikely here due to the absence of a lump and increase in size of the breast. Mastitis and breast abscess are also unlikely due to the presenting history and clinical findings (please refer to the answer to Question 2).

Breast pain (3)

10 C Cyclical mastalgia

The history of bilateral cyclical breast pain, which gradually intensifies before the start of the menses, and which is relieved once the menses start, is highly suggestive of cyclical mastalgia. The absolute cause of this condition is not yet clear, although it is thought to arise due to the sensitivity and responsiveness of breast tissue to hormones. Non-cyclical mastalgia does not fit the history as it is not usually associated with the menstrual cycle. Tietze's syndrome is characterized by tenderness usually over the second, third or fourth costochondral junctions because of chondritis of the costal cartilages. Acute bacterial mastitis is possible, but usually does not present bilaterally and is not associated with the menstrual cycle. The affected breast is usually erythematous, swollen and extremely tender. Traumatic fat necrosis is clearly wrong as there is no history of recent trauma to the breasts.

Breast lump assessment

11 D Invasive breast carcinoma

Triple assessment is adopted when investigating all breast lumps. Clinical history and examination is followed by imaging and then by cytological or histological analysis.

On palpation of a breast lump, a grade of 1-5 is given based on its clinical characteristics. These are:

- P1 – Normal breast tissue
- P2 – Benign breast tissue
- P3 – Suspicious but probably benign
- P4 – Suspicious but probably malignant
- P5 – Malignant

The same 1-5 grading is used for imaging, but an 'M' is used for mammography and 'U' for ultrasound.

Cytological grades are given as follows:

- C1 – Normal cell architecture or inadequate sample
- C2 – Benign cytology
- C3 – Suspicious but probably benign

- C4 – Suspicious but probably malignant
- C5 – Malignant

Histology grades for needle core biopsy are

- B1 – Normal breast tissue or inadequate sample
- B2 – Benign breast tissue
- B3 – Suspious but probably benign
- B4 – Suspicious but probably malignant
- B5a – Carcinoma *in-situ* (e.g. ductal/lobular carcinoma *in situ*)
- B5b – Invasive carcinoma (e.g. invasive ductal/lobular carcinoma)

With regard to the question, the breast lesion was given a 'B5b' histology grade from the needle core biopsy sample. This histology result implies invasive malignancy.

Management of fat necrosis of the breast

12 A   Reassurance and discharge

Traumatic fat necrosis of the breast, in most cases, does not warrant any treatment or follow-up and will usually resolve with time. In some cases, fat necrosis can leave a hard, irregular lump (with some overlying skin tethering) which can be mistaken for carcinoma. History of recent trauma to the breast(s) makes carcinoma unlikely. Core biopsy can be performed to confirm the diagnosis. Therefore, follow-up appointment in 3 months, wide local excision, left mastectomy, and follow-up appointment in 6 months are all incorrect.

Management of breast cysts

13 C   Annual follow-up

Once a breast cyst is diagnosed and imaging features are benign, there is usually a follow-up with the patient in 1 year. Wide local excision, follow-up appointment in 3 months, reassure and discharge and core biopsy are incorrect. Benign breast cysts usually produce a straw-coloured aspirate. Once drained, fluid-filled benign cysts usually collapse and the lump disappears. If the aspirate is blood stained or the lump fails to resolve, re-evaluation with triple assessment is done within a few weeks.

Management of breast infection

14 D   Flucloxacillin

Flucloxacillin is the antibiotic of choice for treating lactational acute mastitis. The crack in the left nipple allows invasion by skin commensal *Staphylococcus aureus*, the most common cause of breast infection. Flucloxacillin is a penicillinase-resistant antibiotic that is very effective against *S. aureus* infections. Breastfeeding or milk expression is still encouraged during treatment and has shown to quicken recovery. Amoxicillin (from the penicillin family), and ciprofloxacin (from the quinolone family) are ineffective against *S. aureus*. Erythromycin (from the macrolide family) is usually administered to patients who are allergic to penicillin formulas. It is not as effective as penicillinase-resistant antibiotics against *S. aureus*. Cephalexin (from the cephalosporin family), a moderate-spectrum antibiotic, can be used for *S. aureus* infections. However, cephalosporins are not considered a first line antibiotic therapy for the treatment of breast abscesses due to moderate-spectrum activity. In this case, the patient is not allergic to penicillin and thus flucloxacillin is the more appropriate choice of treatment.

Management of fibroadenoma

15 A Excision of the lump

After a diagnosis of fibroadenoma is made, small lesions (i.e. <2.5 cm) do not warrant excision. In most cases, patients are reassured and discharged from clinic, but due to the patient's significant family history of breast carcinoma, it is essential, and reassuring to her, for the lump to be excised. Therefore, excision of the lump is the most appropriate answer in this clinical vignette.

Mammary duct ectasia

16 A Reassure and discharge

Mammary duct ectasia does not warrant treatment providing investigations are normal. Duct excision is only performed if the discharge is frequent and excessive. Antibiotic therapy is not usually a treatment option for this condition and will not provide a cure. Performing a mammography in 3 months is unlikely to be beneficial. Mastectomy of the right breast is not a recommended treatment modality.

Management of breast pathology (2)

17 B Mammography and ultrasound

After clinical examination of a breast lump, the next step is radiological assessment. This patient is over 35 and should therefore be offered mammography and ultrasound. CT scanning does not indicate in the triple assessment protocol. Fine needle aspiration and core biopsy are not considered until radiological assessment is performed. A combination of mammography and core biopsy is incorrect for reasons explained in the answer to Question 7.

Ductal carcinoma *in situ*

18 **C**   Wide local excision + postoperative radiotherapy

Although mastectomy and mastectomy + postoperative radiotherapy are accepted treatment options for DCIS, wide local excision + postoperative radiotherapy is now frequently offered to women with tumours less than 40 mm in diameter of not an aggressive grade. Wide local excision attempts to conserve the unaffected breast tissue, thus avoiding the need for complete mastectomy, which carries greater psychological trauma to the patient. Mastectomy + postoperative radiotherapy is offered when DCIS is found in multiple areas of the breast, the tumour grade is aggressive, the size of the tumour is greater than 40 mm and if the oestrogen receptor status is negative. Ductal carcinoma *in situ* implies that the tumour is still confined to the basement membrane and has not broken through the latter. Thus axillary lymph nodes are at a greater chance of being affected once the tumour has broken through the basement membrane. With some exceptions, axillary staging and clearance is performed when multiple foci of extensive and aggressive DCIS are found.

Management of breast cancer

19 **D**   Wide local excision and sentinel node biopsy

The patient has a unifocal 2.5 cm malignant tumour in the right breast. The most appropriate management would be to perform a wide local excision of the breast tumour and it is essential to establish whether axillary disease is present or not. To assess disease positivity/negativity in the axilla, sentinel node biopsy should be performed. If the axillary sentinel lymph node is involved with metastatic tumour deposits originating from the primary breast tumour (e.g. macrometastases; tumour deposits. 2 mm), depending on the level of involvement of the axilla, the patient will undergo axillary clearance. This involves removing level 1–3 axillary lymph nodes to remove residual malignancy.

It is not common practice for a patient diagnosed with breast cancer to undergo axillary clearance if the axilla has not been assessed. In some cases, an axillary lymph node FNA cytology assessment may be performed if there is palpable axillary disease. If the result confirms malignant disease, then the patient will undergo axillary clearance. Otherwise, sentinel node biopsy is usually performed to plan, whether the patient requires axillary clearance.

The main indications for mastectomy are patients who have large tumours (>5 cm) that are unresponsive to chemotherapy, multifocal breast tumours, diffuse DCIS, and a large tumour relative to the patient's breast tissue.

Ductal carcinoma

20 B   Mastectomy + axillary clearance + systemic chemotherapy + radiotherapy and Tamoxifen

The treatment options for male breast cancer are similar to those for
female breast cancer. The most common form of breast cancer in males
is invasive ductal carcinoma, which is also the most common type in
women. There are four clinical stages of ductal carcinoma and determining the clinical stage allows for the selection of initial treatment.
Patients who have stage 1 or 2 (early breast cancer) are more suitable for
surgery whereas surgery should be avoided in patients who have stage 3
and 4 breast cancer, that is locally advanced cancer or metastatic spread
at presentation, respectively, and they should be treated with chemotherapy. In this case, the patient has stage 2 breast cancer, implying that
he is suitable for surgery. In addition, this tumour is oestrogen receptor
positive; 90% of male breast cancers are oestrogen receptor positive.

Mastectomy + axillary clearance, followed by systemic chemotherapy,
radiotherapy and Tamoxifen, is the most suitable answer out of the
five options. Chest wall radiotherapy coupled with systemic chemotherapy carries a better prognosis for the patient. Mastectomy alone
would ensure tumour removal, but would not ensure the clearance of
micrometastases, and the risk of recurrence/metastases would be higher
without chemo/radiotherapy. Wide local excision would be difficult due
to the invasive nature of the tumour and ensuring tumour clear margins of tissue. Mastectomy + radiotherapy is possible, but the addition
of chemotherapy and hormonal therapy with Tamoxifen carries a better
prognosis because of the higher likelihood of removal of micrometastases. Patients who have stage 4 breast cancer (metastases at presentation)
are usually offered palliative care.

Management of breast pathology (3)

21 B   Ultrasound guided fine needle aspiration

Ultrasound assessment of this patient's breast lump confirms that it is
a fluid-filled cyst with benign features. The next best course of action
is therefore to offer the patient fine needle aspiration of the cyst. The
extracted fluid is usually discarded. In some cases, if the Radiologist
suspects that the cyst has indeterminate features, the aspirated cystic
fluid may be sent off for cytological analysis (if but in some cases the
fluid may be blood). Breast MRI is used in the assessment of multifocal/
bilateral disease and also in patients with cosmetic implants who are at
a predisposed risk of breast cancer. Core biopsy, reassure and discharge
and mammography are thus incorrect answers. For further clarifica-
tion, please refer to the answer to Question 7.

Complications of breast surgery

22 C Mastectomy + axillary clearance + postoperative radiotherapy to the axilla

Observation?

Lymphoedema of the arm usually occurs following the combination of surgical axillary clearance and postoperative radiotherapy to the axilla. This therapeutic combination is therefore not offered to patients as it is associated with an unacceptably high incidence of lymphoedema. Mastectomy + axillary clearance + postoperative radiotherapy to the chest wall, mastectomy + axillary clearance + systemic chemotherapy, mastectomy + axillary clearance and mastectomy + postoperative radiotherapy are incorrect options where the incidence of lymphoedema is relatively lower compared with mastectomy + axillary clearance + postoperative radiotherapy to the axilla.

Management of endocrine disease (1)

23 B Desmopressin

Hyper : Carbimazole

Hypo : Thyroxine

GH ↑ : Octreotide

Conn's : Spironolactone

Symptoms of polyuria and polydipsia are common in many conditions. From the patient's history, she had suffered a head injury (the triggering factor for her symptoms) and after 2 weeks her symptoms started. The fact that she has no other symptoms makes it likely that this patient is suffering from diabetes insipidus, where vast amounts of dilute urine are secreted. Two forms exist: cranial diabetes insipidus (causes include head injury, cranial surgery, sarcoidosis), where there is a lack of ADH secretion from the posterior pituitary gland; and nephrogenic diabetes insipidus (causes include hypokalaemia, hypercalcaemia, drugs such as lithium and demecycline, genetic defects and heavy metal poisoning), where there is a lack of response of the kidneys to ADH. Diagnosis can be confirmed using the water deprivation test.

This patient has cranial diabetes insipidus. From the list of options, the most likely answer is treatment with desmopressin (a synthetic analogue of ADH). Carbimazole is given to patients with hyperthyroidism. Spironolactone, in the context of endocrine medicine, is given to patients with Conn's syndrome. Thyroxine is given to hypothyroid patients and octreotide (a somatostatin analogue) can be used in patients with excessive growth hormone production (e.g. acromegaly) and patients with carcinoid syndrome.

Management of endocrine disease (2)

24 E α-blockade, followed by β-blockade followed by surgical resection

Definitive treatment of a phaeochromocytoma is surgical resection, but before this is performed, pharmacological therapy is required to antagonize the effects of serum circulating catecholamines. α blockade with phenoxybenzamine is usually commenced 7–10 days before surgery, which allows blood volume expansion. Once this is achieved, β blockade therapy is started. β blockade cannot be initiated too early as unopposed a receptor stimulation may precipitate a hypertensive crisis. Once the patient has been established on adequate α and β blockade, surgical resection of the tumour is carried out.

Management of breast pathology (4)

25 E   Core biopsy

After confirmation with mammography and ultrasound imaging, a core biopsy of the lump is warranted for histological analysis. Ultrasound confirmation of the lump being solid is sufficient. This lump is highly suggestive of underlying malignancy and requires urgent assessment. Repeat mammography and ultrasound scans in 6 months, reassure and discharge and repeat mammography and ultrasound scans in 3 months are therefore all incorrect.

SECTION 10:
VASCULAR SURGERY

Questions

1.	Diabetic foot ulceration	204
2.	Ankle–brachial pressure index	204
3.	Lower limb pain	204
4.	Intermittent claudication	204
5.	Critical limb ischaemia	205
6.	Severe limb ischaemia	205
7.	Leg ulcers	205
8.	Diagnosis of acute lower limb pain	206
9.	Management of acute lower limb pain	206
10.	Acute upper limb pain	206
11.	Popliteal aneurysms	207
12.	Abdominal aortic aneurysm	207
13.	Elective abdominal aortic aneurysm repair	207
14.	Varicose veins	208
15.	Venous embolism prophylaxis	208
16.	Deep vein thrombosis	208
17.	Trendelenburg's tourniquet test	209
18.	Amaurosis fugax	209
19.	Investigation of amaurosis fugax	209
20.	Carotid endarterectomy	209
21.	Postoperative complications of carotid endarterectomy	210
22.	Investigation of an aortic dissection	210
23.	Raynaud's syndrome	210
24.	Lymphoedema	210
25.	Acute mesenteric ischaemia	210
Answers		212

QUESTIONS

1. Diabetic foot ulceration

You assess a patient with a plantar ulcer who has poorly controlled diabetes. From the list of options below, select the most likely management plan.

    A. Optimise glycaemic control
    B. Reduce plantar pressure by ensuring good footwear
    C. Ensure podiatry input
    D. Assess vascularity of the limb
    (E.) All of the above

2. Ankle–brachial pressure index

As part of the peripheral vascular examination, you are asked to record the ankle–brachial pressure index of the patient. Which one of the following values reflects a normal ankle–brachial pressure index?

    A. Between 0.9 and 0.6
    B. Greater than 1.3
    C. Between 0.6 and 0.3
    (D.) Greater than or equal to 1.0
    E. Less than or equal to 0.3

3. Lower limb pain

A 55-year-old man, with a positive smoking history, presents to you in the out-patient clinic with pain in the lower leg which is brought on by walking. The pain is cramping in nature, well localized to the left calf only, and is relieved by rest. The patient has noticed that his walking distance has progressively decreased because of the cramps in the left calf. There are no abnormal findings on physical examination. What is the most appropriate way to investigate the patient's symptoms?

    (A.) Measure the ankle–brachial pressure index
    B. Angiography
    C. Radiograph of the lower limbs
    D. Duplex ultrasound
    E. None of the above

4. Intermittent claudication

A 60-year-old woman has been diagnosed as having claudication of the lower limbs which does not impair her lifestyle. The patient is a smoker and has hyper-lipidaemia for which she is taking a 'statin'. You are asked to discuss with the patient the treatment options available to her. From the list below, choose the recommended treatment option for this patient.

    A. Angioplasty
    B. Amputation
    C. Lower limb bypass
    D. Start an antiplatelet, increase exercise and quit smoking
    E. Continue with the cholesterol-lowering medication and follow up in outpatients in 3 months

5. Critical limb ischaemia

You see a 60-year-old man with a history of coronary heart disease, diabetes and hyperlipidaemia in your clinic. The patient has found it increasingly hard to walk due to the gradual increase in intensity of the cramping pain he experiences in his right leg on walking, which is relieved by resting a few minutes. In addition, he tells you that cramps have started to occur at night when he is sleeping. On examination of the right leg, you notice that there is a 'punched out' ulcer on the right heel. The right posterior tibial and dorsalis pedis pulses are weak. You suspect that this patient has critical limb ischaemia. What is the most appropriate next line investigation that would support your diagnosis?

    A. Computed tomography angiography
    B. Ankle–brachial pressure index
    C. Radiograph the lower limbs
    D. Magnetic resonance angiography
    E. None of the above

6. Severe limb ischaemia

You are asked to see a 67-year-old woman admitted with severe limb ischaemia. Your senior colleague asks you to examine the patient and report your findings. What are the two most likely clinical features that suggest the patient has severe limb ischaemia?

    A. Pulselessness and pain
    B. Paraesthesia and paralysis — usually late sign → impending limb loss
    C. Perishingly cold limb and pallor
    D. Pallor and pain
    E. Paraesthesia and pallor

7. Leg ulcers

A 65-year-old man presents for the first time to your clinic with a painless wound in his right leg, which has been present for over 2 months. On examination you notice a 3 cm × 4 cm leg ulcer in the gaiter area of the right leg, covering the medial malleolus. The shallow bed of the ulcer is covered with granulation tissue, which is surrounded by sloping edges. There is no history of trauma. From the list below, choose the most likely diagnosis.

    A. Arterial leg ulcer
    B. Neuropathic ulcer
    C. Venous ulcer
    D. Traumatic ulcer
    E. Neoplastic ulcer

8. Diagnosis of acute lower limb pain

You are asked to see a 56-year-old homeless man who presented to the emergency department with a severe pain in his right leg, which started over 12 hours ago. On examination, the right leg is pale in colour in comparison with the left leg from below the knee to the toes and has fixed mottling. The right leg is cold and the popliteal, posterior tibial and dorsalis pedis pulses are absent. There is no sensation in the right leg and the patient is unable to flex the knee or move the toes due to fixed flexion deformities. In addition, the patient is apyrexial and heart rate is 85 beats per minute and regular. What is the most likely diagnosis?

    A. Critical limb ischaemia
    B. Acute limb ischaemia
    C. Intermittent claudication
    D. Necrotizing fasciitis
    E. Spinal claudication

9. Management of acute lower limb pain

From the list below, select the most appropriate treatment option for the patient in Question 8.

    A. Percutaneous transluminal angioplasty
    B. Revascularization through endarterectomy
    C. Revascularization through bypass grafting
    D. Endoluminal stent grafting
    E. Amputation

10. Acute upper limb pain

You see a 50-year-old woman with a history of atrial fibrillation, who presents to the emergency department with a sudden onset of pain in the left forearm. The pain started 3 hours ago, and has been increasing in intensity since. On examination, the left forearm is cold and pale. The left axillary pulse is present, *acute limb = surgical emergency.*

but distal pulses are absent. Movement and sensation are intact in the left hand. There is no history of trauma. What is the most appropriate next step in this patient's management?

A. Commence a heparin infusion and send the patient to theatre for vascular intervention
B. Give analgesia and manage the patient in the emergency department
C. Administer oral aspirin and send the patient to theatre for vascular intervention
D. Request an angiogram
E. Request anteroposterior and lateral plain radiographs of the left forearm

11. Popliteal aneurysms

In association with a diagnosed popliteal aneurysm, a patient is more likely to have

A. A berry aneurysm
B. A femoral aneurysm
C. An aortic aneurysm
D. A carotid artery aneurysm
E. None of the above

12. Abdominal aortic aneurysm

You see a 65-year-old man in your clinic who is under surveillance for an abdominal aortic aneurysm. The patient smokes 20 cigarettes a day and has a 25-year history of poorly controlled hypertension. From the list below, select the most appropriate investigation that can be used to monitor the progression of this patient's condition.

A. Computed tomography scan of the abdomen
B. Angiography
C. Abdominal plain film radiography
D. Magnetic resonance imaging
E. Ultrasound

13. Elective abdominal aortic aneurysm repair

During a ward round you are asked about the conditions that must be met in order to qualify a patient for elective abdominal aortic aneurysm repair. From the list below, select the most likely abdominal aortic aneurysm size that warrants elective repair providing the patient is fit for surgery.

A. Greater than 5.0 cm
B. Greater than 5.5 cm

C. Less than 5.0 cm
D. Greater than 4.5 cm
E. Less than 5.5 cm

14. Varicose veins

A 41-year-old woman, diagnosed with varicose veins in the left leg, presents to your clinic with a 2-month history of severe pain in the left leg on prolonged standing. The patient is obese and the pain has affected her working and social lifestyle and she asks you about the most effective treatment option. From the list below, choose the most effective treatment option that you would discuss with this patient.

tortuous dilatation of superficial veins

A. Use of compression stockings → conservative Mx.
B. Injection sclerotherapy → for Smaller varicosities
C. Surgery
D. Weight loss
E. None of the above

15. Venous embolism prophylaxis

A 55-year-old woman, who is obese and has a positive smoking history, is to have varicose vein surgery in the next 12 hours. Your senior colleague asks you to ensure that deep vein thrombosis prophylaxis is commenced. From the list below, choose the most appropriate form of deep vein thrombosis prophylaxis that you would use.

A. Low-molecular-weight heparin
B. Warfarin
C. Aspirin
D. Clopidogrel
E. None of the above

16. Deep vein thrombosis

You are told by your colleague that a 44-year-old woman, who underwent elective right hip replacement, is suspected of having deep vein thrombosis of the left calf. You are asked to carry out a pretest clinical probability score (Wells score) and a D-dimer test. Which is the most likely scenario where deep vein thrombosis can be excluded from your list of differential diagnoses?

A. Wells score of 2 and a positive D-dimer result
B. Wells score of 1 and a positive D-dimer result
C. Wells score of 0 and a negative D-dimer result
D. Wells score of 3 and a positive D-dimer result
E. None of the above

17. Trendelenburg's tourniquet test

You are told that a 45-year-old woman, who presented to the vascular surgery clinic, has a positive tourniquet test in the left leg. On the basis of the information conveyed to you, choose the most likely diagnosis that is associated with a positive tourniquet test.

A. Varicose veins
B. Chronic leg ischaemia
C. Deep vein thrombosis
D. Arterial ulcer
E. Acute leg ischaemia

18. Amaurosis fugax

Your colleague consults you with regard to a 56-year-old patient who has suffered an episode of amaurosis fugax. From the list below, choose the most likely site of pathology which may give rise to amaurosis fugax.

A. Vertebrobasilar artery territory
B. Carotid artery territory
C. Posterior communicating artery territory
D. Spinal artery territory
E. Anterior communicating artery territory

19. Investigation of amaurosis fugax

You have decided to investigate the symptom experienced by the patient in Question 18. From the list below, select the most appropriate investigation that you would order first to investigate the site of pathology.

A. Magnetic resonance angiography
B. Digital subtraction angiography
C. Computed tomography scan of the head and neck
D. Duplex ultrasound scanning
E. None of the above

20. Carotid endarterectomy

You are in the vascular surgery outpatient clinic explaining the indications for undergoing carotid endarterectomy to a patient. From the list below, select the most likely scenario where carotid endarterectomy is likely to be indicated.

A. Symptomatic carotid artery stenosis of greater than 50%
B. Asymptomatic carotid artery stenosis of between 70% and 80%
C. Asymptomatic carotid artery stenosis of between 50% and 60%
D. Symptomatic carotid artery stenosis of less than 50% → optimal medical management
E. None of the above

21. Postoperative complications of carotid endarterectomy

The most common postoperative complication associated with carotid endarterectomy is

    A. Surgical site infection
    B. Cranial nerve injury
    C. Stroke
    D. Hypertension
    E. Patch rupture

22. Investigation of an aortic dissection

From the list below, select the most appropriate investigation for the prompt diagnosis of an aortic dissection.

    A. Electrocardiogram
    B. Echocardiogram
    C. Computed tomography scan
    D. Chest radiograph
    E. Magnetic resonance imaging

23. Raynaud's syndrome

Raynaud's syndrome can be caused by which one of the following antihypertensives?

    A. α-blockers
    B. Angiotensin-converting enzyme inhibitors
    C. β-blockers
    D. Calcium channel blockers
    E. Angiotensin receptor blockers

24. Lymphoedema

You see a 26-year-old woman in clinic presenting with lower limb lymphoedema. Which of the following conditions is associated with lymphoedema?

    A. Post lymph node dissection
    B. Radiotherapy
    C. Filarisis
    D. Post trauma
    E. All of the above

25. Acute mesenteric ischaemia

A 45-year-old man presents to A&E with acute onset of abdominal pain. Following clinical assessment, he is found to have acute mesenteric ischaemia.

Which of the following is the diagnosis of acute mesenteric ischaemia based on?

    A. An elevated lactate

    B. A high white cell count

    C. A metabolic acidosis

    D. Pain out of keeping with the clinical signs

    E. Any of the above and a high index of suspicion

ANSWERS

Diabetic foot ulceration

1 E All of the above

Diabetic foot ulceration occurs in 15% of diabetics and is a common cause for major and minor amputations. Many ulcers are preventable if there is good communication between the patient, podiatrist and multidisciplinary foot team. Patients are screened on a yearly basis and are risk assessed as high, medium or low. These patients need to be signposted to the appropriate foot care providers and educated that if ulceration does occur, then help should be sought within 24 hours. Optimisation of glycaemic control, reducing pressure at ulcer sites by offloading devices, ensuring podiatry input and assessing the neurovascular status of the foot is essential. Common causes of ulceration are poor vascularity, incomplete sensation and abnormal bone structure or gait of the patient.

Ankle–brachial pressure index

2 D Greater than or equal to 1.0

The ABPI is measured by dividing the highest systolic blood pressure measured in any ankle artery (either the dorsalis pedis or posterior tibial artery) by the systolic pressure at the brachial artery. This test is performed using a Doppler and blood pressure cuff (sphygmomanometer). The cuff is inflated above the artery while the Doppler probe, connected to a pulse volume recorder, is placed just below or at the site of the artery. The cuff is gently deflated and the pressure, at which the first pulse sound is heard, is noted.

An ABPI greater than or equal to 1.0 is usually normal. ABPI values between 0.9 and 0.6 usually suggest peripheral vascular occlusive disease such as intermittent claudication. This is progressive symptomatic arterial occlusion of the lower limbs due to atherosclerosis, resulting in pain on movement which is relieved by rest. Values between 0.6 and 0.3 usually suggest critical limb ischaemia and these patients usually have limb pain at rest. An ABPI less than or equal to 0.3 implies impending gangrene of the affected limb.

Patients with diabetes or renal disease may have ABPI of greater than 1.3 which implies that the lower limb arterial walls may be calcified and are incompressible.

Lower limb pain

3 A Measure the ankle-brachial pressure index

The iliac and lower limb arteries are commonly affected in PVD. The main effect of PVD, of which the commonest cause is atherosclerosis, is to restrict blood flow to the limbs due to stenotic narrowing or occlusion of the arterial lumen. An increase in metabolic demand from muscles due to an increase in physical activity cannot be met due to the reduced blood flow and results in ischaemia. Patients are usually asymptomatic until a critical arterial stenosis is attained (75% of the cross-sectional area or 50% of the vessel diameter is reached).

Intermittent claudication can be clinically described as cramp-like pain experienced in the muscles of the leg on walking, which is alleviated in minutes of resting. Cramp-like pain of intermittent claudication can be experienced in the calf, thigh or buttock muscles depending on the level at which the arterial occlusion is present.

The ABPI may be used as a first line diagnostic investigation for PVD in patients presenting with lower limb symptoms. This test is non-invasive, quick and cheap and is usually performed in an outpatient clinic setting. Duplex ultrasound scanning enables assessment of the distribution and extent of the disease and allows the risks and benefits of intervention to be discussed with the patient. A plain film radiograph of the lower limbs may not reveal any abnormalities. Angiography is not used as a first line investigation in the initial stages of forming a diagnosis of PVD. It is used for surgical planning in patients who are to undergo surgical or radiological interventional revascularization.

Intermittent claudication

4 D Start an antiplatelet, increase exercise and quit smoking
A majority of patients who are initially diagnosed with vascular claudication will usually be counselled about their condition, and in most cases, no further treatment is required providing the claudication is not severe. Risk factors (e.g. hyperlipidaemia, smoking, poor exercise, and obesity) are usually identified and the patient is asked to correct these as part of managing their condition. Exercise and smoking cessation are factors which, if taken up by the patient, will most likely improve symptoms of claudication as well as decreasing overall cardiovascular risk.

Structured exercise programmes are relatively cheap and safer than endovascular intervention (e.g. percutaneous transluminal angioplasty) and surgery, and have shown to be beneficial if followed for at least 6 months. Patients are asked to walk to near maximum pain tolerance as well as increasing their maximum walking distance; compliance is usually a confounding factor.

Where claudication is concerned, percutaneous transluminal angioplasty and surgery are usually offered to patients after careful assessment of long-term efficacy of intervention, balanced by procedural risks and costs. These are patients who have severe claudication that has major implications on their social and working lifestyle (e.g. if the patient is unable to work or unable to look after themselves without help).

Critical limb ischaemia

5   B   Ankle-brachial pressure index
This patient is showing signs of critical limb ischaemia which is characterized by gradual worsening of claudication progressing to rest pain, ulceration and ultimately gangrene. Nocturnal limb pain, which occurs when the patient is asleep, results from a decrease in cardiac output, which in turn decreases systemic blood pressure, leading to a reduction of perfusion pressure on the foot; hence ischaemic pain ensues. The ABPI would be the most appropriate next line investigation in this scenario. An ABPI between 0.6 and 0.3, coupled with a clinical history of rest pain, is highly suggestive of critical limb ischaemia.

Doppler ultrasound, which was not an option in the question, is also another non-invasive investigation that can be performed to locate the stenosed area and confirm diagnosis. A plain film radiograph of the lower limbs would not be informative. Magnetic resonance imaging and CT angiography are possible investigations, but would not classically be the next line in this situation.

Severe limb ischaemia

6   B   Paresthesia and paralysis
The clinical signs and symptoms associated with acute limb ischaemia can be remembered using the list of '6 Ps':

- Pain
- Pallor
- Pulselessness
- Perishingly cold
- Paresthesia
- Paralysis

Paraesthesia and paralysis are late signs of severe limb ischaemia and urgent surgical intervention is required as these features threaten loss of the limb. Acute limb ischaemia results either from a thrombus *in situ* (~40% of cases), an embolus (~38%) or graft/angioplasty occlusion (~15%) or trauma.

Leg ulcers

7   C   Venous ulcers
Venous ulcers: These account for 80% of all skin ulcers, the majority being painless. They occur due to venous hypertension, which develops as a result of either increased hydrostatic pressure due to valve failure

and weight of blood pressing distally, or due to the transmission of blood from the deep venous system to the superficial system (subcutaneous veins and dermal capillaries) through incompetent valves. It is thought that white cells become trapped, leading to an increase in peripheral resistance and tissue ischaemia. Another school of thought postulates that tissue ischaemia develops due to the formation of fibrin plugs. Patients with venous ulcers usually have varicose veins, and 95% of venous ulcers occur in the gaiter area and characteristically around the medial malleoli. Venous ulcers may be discrete or circumferential, shallow, with irregular sloping edges and prominent granulation tissue in the bases. Prolonged ulceration with lipodermatosclerosis gives the leg a look of an inverted champagne bottle.

- *Arterial ulcers:* These can be painful, have deep bases and bear a 'punched out' appearance. They are well demarcated and usually occur on the toes, heels and bony prominences of the foot. The base of the arterial ulcer may be pale, non-granulating and necrotic. The surrounding skin may be cool to touch, hairless, thin, brittle, and erythematous and have a shiny texture. There are usually associated stigmata with peripheral arterial disease.

- *Neuropathic ulcers (cross-over with patients with peripheral arterial disease and diabetes):* Patients with diabetes are more likely to get neuropathic ulcers. These occur at high pressure sites (i.e. the heel and metatarsal heads) and usually appear cleanly punched out of the surrounding callous. The patient may be suffering from neuropathic pain in the leg and the foot may be numb. Neuropathic ulcers are often painless and the patient may not have noticed them.

- *Traumatic ulcers:* The patient will usually present with symmetrical damage, i.e. across the toes and margins of the feet due to wearing tight shoes. Other causes include burns, injections, sclerosants and cortisone.

- *Malignant ulcers:* This can either be due to a primary or a secondary malignant lesion or may be caused by a malignant change in a pre-existing ulcer (e.g. Marjolin's ulcer). Some examples of malignant ulcers are epithelioma, basal cell carcinoma, squamous cell carcinoma and lymphoma.

Diagnosis of acute lower limb pain

8 B Acute limb ischaemia

This patient has classic clinical signs of an acute ischaemic limb. The patient has the '6 Ps' (pain, pallor, pulselessness, paraesthesia, paralysis and perishingly cold) which indicate that the limb is unsalvageable.

- Necrotizing fasciitis is an infection of the deep layers of the skin and subcutaneous tissues which spreads within the fascial plane of the subcutaneous tissue. Of the many organisms that cause this condition (group A streptococcus, *Vibrio vulnificus*, *Clostridium perfringens*, *Bacteroides fragilis*), group A streptococcus is the most common. The infection usually starts at the site of local trauma and clinical features may include severe pain in the affected area and evidence of cellulitis, followed by swelling, erythema, vesicle and bullae formation on the skin surface; these may be absent if the bacteria are deep within the tissue. Patients are usually very ill with fever and, sometimes, diarrhoea and vomiting. Blood cultures and aspiration of pus at the site of the infected tissue can confirm the diagnosis. Prompt antibiotic therapy is required and the patient should be sent for emergency surgical debridement.
- Spinal stenosis/claudication occurs as a result of nerve root compression (a history of recent trauma may be evident) at the level of the lumbosacral vertebra and usually affects patients in a dermatomal distribution. Weakness and paraesthesia of the limb supplied by the compressed nerve may be present. The pain is of rapid onset and made worse by movement and may be relieved when the patient sits down. Peripheral vascular examination is usually normal and diagnosis is made using MRI, although a plain film radiograph may show signs of vertebral disk space narrowing.

Management of acute lower limb pain

9 E Amputation

In addition to having pain, pallor, absent pulses and cold right leg, there is loss of sensation coupled with complete paralysis which indicates that the right limb (below the knee) is completely gangrenous, warranting an amputation procedure.

Indications for amputation are

- Useless limb (i.e. fixed flexion deformities, vestigial fingers)
- Dead limb (i.e. extensive tissue loss due to trauma or widespread necrosis or peripheral vascular disease that cannot be treated with reconstructive surgery)
- Lethal limb (i.e. malignancy or ischaemia)

Types of amputations include:

- Hind quarter (the entire lower limb is removed from the sacroiliac joint – Not commonly performed)

- Above knee amputation
- Through knee amputation
- Below knee amputation (knee joint left intact)
- Foot amputation
- Forefoot amputation (transmetatarsal amputation)
- Metatarsal amputation – A ray amputation may be used if necrosis is present in the digits and the muscles of the foot. The incision is made from either side of the affected digit(s) to the base of the metatarsal. This creates a 'V shape' and narrows the foot.
- Toe amputation – Removal of the head of the metatarsal (requires revascularization in order to be successful)

Acute upper limb pain

10 A Commence a heparin infusion and send the patient to theatre for vascular intervention
Emboli are the commonest cause of acute upper limb ischaemia. Occlusive disease leading to *in situ* thrombosis is rare in the upper limbs. Acute limb ischaemia is a surgical emergency and needs prompt surgical intervention. The classic clinical picture of severe pain, pallor, coldness with absent pulses, loss of sensation and paralysis points to acute limb ischaemia (the '6 Ps': pain, pallor, pulselessness, perishingly cold, paraesthesia and paralysis). The patient has a history of atrial fibrillation, which most likely points to the origin of the embolus.

Movement and sensation of the left upper limb are preserved, indicating that the limb is salvageable. The fact that the left axillary pulse is present and distal pulses absent suggests that the level of the occlusion is in the brachial artery. Although collateral blood supply to the left arm will keep the limb viable, revascularization of the brachial artery will need to be initiated in order to alleviate symptoms and prevent claudication. Therefore, definitive management includes commencing a heparin infusion and sending the patient immediately to theatre for surgical exploration and embolectomy using a Fogarty catheter.

The anticoagulant effects of aspirin are not as effective as heparin. Aspirin therefore is not commonly used in the setting of intervention of acute limb ischaemia. Requesting an angiogram will delay the definitive management of this patient and should not take priority over surgical intervention. There is no history of trauma, making an underlying fracture unlikely; and being a surgical emergency, managing the patient in A&E with analgesia is wrong.

Popliteal aneurysms

11 C   An aortic aneurysm

Popliteal aneurysms account for 80% of all peripheral aneurysms and patients diagnosed with popliteal aneurysms (of which 50% are bilateral) are more likely to have an associated aortic aneurysm (approximately 40% of cases) compared with other types of aneurysms. Reasons for operative intervention are size, distal embolisation, or occlusion.

Abdominal aortic aneurysm

12 E   Ultrasound

An aneurysm can be defined as an abnormal permanent widening of a portion of a weakened or diseased blood vessel. It can occur in the aorta (most common), popliteal vessels (arterial and venous), circle of Willis, mesenteric arteries (rare) and splenic arteries (rare). The exact aetiology of aneurysms is unclear, although they are associated with hypertension, atherosclerosis, connective tissue disorders and trauma. Abdominal aortic aneurysms are common in the elderly (over 60 years old) with men more commonly affected than women. A patient with an AAA usually presents with a pulsatile and expansile mass visible in the abdomen. Most AAAs are asymptomatic and discovered on either routine abdominal examination or by ultrasonography.

Ultrasound scanning is usually used to screen for, and monitor the growth of, AAAs. CT imaging is regarded as the investigation of choice in terms of diagnostic confirmation, defining aortic size, aneurismal position, that is, assessing the extension of the aneurysm into the suprarenal aorta. It has a sensitivity of nearly 100% where AAAs are concerned. Once an AAA is diagnosed, and is found to be less than 5.5 cm, the patient is routinely monitored. Ultrasound scanning (safe, non-invasive and usually requiring no patient preparation) is preferred for screening and monitoring patients with abdominal aortic aneurysms. Abdominal plain film radiography may show calcification of the abdominal aortic walls (this may suggest an AAA) but will be of no use in terms of screening and diagnosis. The role of angiography is uncertain in the assessment of patients with AAAs; it is invasive, and carries potential renal and embolic complications.

Elective abdominal aortic aneurysm repair

13 B   Greater than 5.5 cm

Patients diagnosed with an AAA greater than or equal to 5.5 cm, who are otherwise fit for surgery, qualify for elective repair of the AAA. Abdominal aortic aneurysms greater than 5.5 cm carry a significant risk of rupture and mortality. Therefore, prompt surgical intervention is required. The risk of mortality secondary to surgical intervention is lower when compared with mortality resulting from a ruptured aneurysm of greater than 5.5 cm in diameter.

Abdominal aortic aneurysms which are less than 5.5 cm are usually monitored with yearly ultrasound scanning. Abdominal aortic aneurysms up to 5 cm in size grow at an average rate of 1–4 mm per year, whereas those greater than 5.0 cm grow at a rate of 4–6 mm per year. Other indications for surgical repair year and the rate of the AAA of greater than 1 cm per year and the aneurysm becoming symptomatic (e.g. back pain, distal embolisation of one or both legs causing acute ischaemia) or tender. In addition, if a patient suddenly experiences an acute onset of back pain associated with hypotension, tachycardia and hypovolaemic shock, this indicates rupture of the AAA and emergency surgery is warranted, which has a mortality rate between 50% and 75%.

Elective surgical repair of an AAA can be performed either via the traditional laparotomy route, whereby a Dacron artificial graft is used to replace the aneurysmal aorta, or via the minimally invasive route known as endovascular aneurysm repair. EVAR is increasingly being practised for the elective repair of AAAs. EVAR involves accessing the femoral artery and, under radiological guidance, and endoluminal stent-graft is placed at the site of the aneurysm. Successful EVAR leads to a shorter hospital stay and decreased frequency of blood transfusions. In addition, EVAR can be performed in patients who are unfit for surgery, such as the elderly or those with other significant co-morbidities.

Varicose veins

14 C **Surgery**

Patients with asymptomatic varicose veins can either be treated conservatively (i.e. patient education: avoiding long periods of standing; use of compression stockings; losing weight; frequent periods of walking – this helps to aid superficial to deep venous return in the legs) or by injection sclerotherapy, which is particularly effective in below-the-knee varicosities. Sclerosants, such as ethanolamine and sodium tetradecyl, work by increasing the amount of intravascular granulation tissue, resulting in the occlusion of the vein lumen. Sclerosant is injected into the superficial varicosities at various sites, after which compression bandaging is applied for a few weeks to prevent the formation of thrombi. Other techniques include the injection of sclerosant foam into the superficial venous system. The injection is placed in a superficial varicose vein (at one single site) and the distribution of foam is monitored using ultrasound. Sclerosant therapy may cause long-term hypo/hyperpigmentation and ulceration at the injection site. If the sclerosant is passed into the femoral vein, anaphylaxis may ensue.

If quality of life is severely affected by varicose veins (i.e. severe impact on working and social lifestyle due to leg pain, venous ulceration, thrombophlebitis) surgery can be offered. Surgery is the most effective treatment for large varicose veins, and aims to correct the deep to superficial reflux and to remove varicosities. Various forms of surgery for varicose veins are now available, for example:

- Ligation of either the saphenofemoral (tributaries of long saphenous vein are also ligated) or saphenopopliteal (ligation of short saphenous vein deep in the popliteal fossa) junctions
- Multiple avulsions of the varicosities and endoluminal radiofrequency ablation of the long saphenous vein followed by multiple avulsions of superficial varicosities
- Multiple avulsions of the varicosities and laser ablation of the long saphenous vein followed by multiple avulsions of superficial varicosities

Postoperatively, compression stockings are worn for several weeks and exercise is encouraged. Patients are able to resume normal daily activities considerably quicker compared with the conventional methods of varicose vein surgery. In this question the patient's quality of life is being affected by the varicose veins in her left lower limb. Surgery is therefore the most appropriate treatment modality, although recurrence rates are approximately 50%.

Venous embolism prophylaxis

15 A   Low-molecular-weight heparin
Low-molecular-weight heparin has been shown to be effective for the use of DVT prophylaxis in those undergoing surgery. It is given subcutaneously and does not require laboratory monitoring. It should be used with caution in patients with renal dysfunction.

Warfarin has a prothrombotic effect within the first 48 hours of administration and usually takes up to 72 hours to exert its antithrombotic effect. It is usually given along with LMWH (where high-risk DVT patients are concerned) and is monitored using the INR (the ratio of a patient's prothrombin time to a normal control sample). When the INR reaches 2–3, LMWH can be stopped and warfarin can be continued for 3–6 months postoperatively, depending on the patient's clotting risk. Aspirin and clopidogrel are not as effective as LMWH and warfarin at preventing venous thrombus. They are preferred in anti-arterial thrombus prophylaxis.

Deep vein thrombosis

16 C   A Wells score of 0 and a negative D-dimer result
Venous stasis, potential injury to the vessel wall, and/or a hypercoagulable state are the three classic causes of venous thrombus formation

described by Virchow (also known as Virchow's triad). The legs are common sites for the development of DVT.

There are two main types of DVT: below knee and above knee. Below knee DVTs occur most frequently in the calf veins, with those in the soleal plexus being commonly affected. Above knee DVTs are considered relatively more dangerous than below knee DVTs as there is a higher risk of developing pulmonary emboli.

There are numerous risk factors for developing DVTs. The major risk factors include age over 40; pregnancy; obesity; contraceptive pill; clotting abnormalities; malignancy; recent pelvic or orthopaedic surgery; trauma; immobility; long-haul flights; and failure to provide DVT prophylaxis for high-risk patients postoperatively. The majority of patients who have DVT are asymptomatic. If symptoms are present, pain is the commonest followed by swelling of the affected limb. In some cases, distension of the superficial veins with erythema may be present.

D-dimers are small protein fragments of fibrin (fibrin degradation product) which are formed when a thrombus is degraded by fibrinolysis. D-dimer blood tests are sensitive but not specific for DVT.

The pretest clinical probability (Wells) score (based on a series of questions) is used to assess the probability of a patient having a DVT.

A score above or equal to 2 is regarded as a 'likely DVT' and the patient is treated as suspected DVT. A proximal leg vein ultrasound scan should be carried out within 4 hours of being requested and if the result is negative, a D-dimer test should be carried out. If a proximal leg vein ultrasound scan cannot be obtained within 4 hours, a D-dimer test should be carried out and an interim 24-hour dose of parenteral anticoagulant should be given; however, the proximal leg vein ultrasound should be performed within 24 hours of being requested. A repeat proximal leg vein ultrasound scan should be performed 6–8 days later for all patients with a positive D-dimer test (and Wells score of 2 or above) and a negative proximal leg vein ultrasound scan.

A score less than or equal to 1 is regarded as an 'unlikely DVT' and with this a D-dimer test is performed. If this is positive, the patient should undergo a proximal leg vein ultrasound scan within 4 hours of being requested. If a proximal leg vein ultrasound cannot be performed within 4 hours, the patient is commenced on an interim 24-hour dose of parenteral anticoagulant whilst waiting for an ultrasound scan which should be performed within 24 hours of being requested.

A DVT can be excluded if the D-dimer result is negative.

Trendelenburg's tourniquet test

17 A Varicose veins

The tourniquet test, a modification of Trendelenburg's test, where the SFJ is occluded using a tourniquet rather than the fingers, is used to assess the level at which venous insufficiency occurs – commonly at the SFJ. This test is used as part of the vascular examination of varicose veins. Varicose are long, tortuous and dilated veins of the superficial venous system and can either be primary, due to congenital abnormality or even absence of valves in the perforator system, or secondary, due to thrombosis of deep or superficial veins, pregnancy, abdominal and pelvic masses and obesity. Although this test is not commonly performed, it is worth knowing the principles for the purposes of exams.

[handwritten margin note: Trendelenburg's test.]

The patient is asked to lie down on the examination couch and the affected leg is elevated and the varicosities are milked and emptied. After sufficient drainage of the veins, with the patient's leg still elevated, a tourniquet is placed as high on the thigh as possible. The patient is then asked to stand up and the rate of filling of the varicosities is assessed. If the varicosities do not fill, it implies that the defect lies above the tourniquet. On the other hand, if the veins refill rapidly, this means that the defect lies below the tourniquet. This has largely been replaced by a venous duplex which is now the gold standard.

Amaurosis fugax

18 B Carotid artery territory

Amaurosis fugax, a Greek derived word which means 'fleeting blindness', can be described as transient monocular loss of vision. The description usually given by patients is of a 'black curtain descending vertically and obscuring vision in one eye'. It usually occurs as a result of atherogenic emboli arising from the carotid artery territory (therefore, option B is the most likely from the list), which unilaterally obstruct the lumen of the retinal arterial circulation. This leads to decreased blood flow to the retina, resulting in ischaemia.

Other less common causes of amaurosis fugax are cardiac emboli and temporary vasospasm of the retinal artery (usually occurs in young people during exercise) and atherosclerosis of the ophthalmic artery. Giant cell arteritis causes chronic granulomatous inflammation of the central retinal artery, which can occlude and produce symptoms similar to that of amaurosis fugax.

Investigation of amaurosis fugax

19 D Duplex ultrasound scanning

Amaurosis fugax is highly suggestive of carotid artery disease (i.e. atherosclerosis of the carotid arteries) and patients will usually undergo duplex ultrasound scanning of the carotid arteries for further assessment. In comparison with DSA, the duplex ultrasound scan is cheap, time efficient and non-invasive. Therefore, the duplex scan is considered the mainstay of an initial assessment. MRI angiography is used, but is usually performed after screening with duplex ultrasound scanning. Plain CT scanning of the head (and neck) is not usually recommended for the initial assessment of carotid artery disease.

Carotid endarterectomy

20 A   Symptomatic carotid artery stenosis of greater than 50%

Studies have shown that patients who are otherwise well, but have symptomatic carotid artery stenosis (i.e. transient ischaemic attacks and amaurosis fugax) greater than 50% are good candidates for carotid endarterectomy; the procedure carries a morbidity and mortality rate of approximately 3%. If this patient group is given optimal medical therapy (i.e. lipid-lowering medication and anti-hypertensives coupled with stopping smoking and an increase in physical activity) after the carotid endarterectomy, this reduces the risk of stroke by 6- to 10-fold. On the other hand, if patients who fall into this category are treated medically, rather than surgically, they have a significant increased chance of developing a stroke.

Patients with a symptomatic carotid stenosis of 50%–70% are usually given optimal medical therapy first. If symptoms continue, carotid endarterectomy is warranted within 48 hours. Patients with symptomatic carotid stenosis of less than 50% are usually given optimal medical therapy, and if symptoms persist they are usually referred for investigations.

Asymptomatic patients with carotid stenosis greater than 80% are candidates for carotid endarterectomy, although this is a controversial topic.

Postoperative complications of carotid endarterectomy

21 D   Hypertension

Approximately 66% of patients who undergo carotid endarterectomy suffer from postoperative hypertension (aetiology unclear). Therefore, close control of blood pressure is warranted within usually the first 72 hours of postoperative care. The risk of stroke ranges from 3% to 8%, of which two-thirds are due to postoperative carotid stenosis and one-third are because of intracranial haemorrhage. Cranial nerve injury occurs in approximately 5% of patients. Wound infection and patch rupture occur in approximately 1% of procedures.

Investigation of an aortic dissection

22 C Computer tomography scan

Providing the patient is stable, the CT scan is used for *rapid* diagnosis of an aortic dissection although MRI has a greater sensitivity.

An aortic dissection, a surgical emergency, can be defined as a split in the intimal lining and internal portion of the tunica media of the aorta. Blood then passes into the media and extends either proximally or distally leading to the formation of a double lumen (occluding important branches of the aorta: coronary, carotid or renal arteries) or rupture into the pericardium (leading to cardiac tamponade) or mediastinum (resulting in a fatal haemorrhage) or affecting the attachments of the aortic valve (leading to aortic incompetence). The most common site for an aortic dissection is in the arch of the aorta.

Seventy per cent of aortic dissections affect the ascending aorta (type A) while 30% affect the descending aorta (type B). Congenital causes include associations with Marfan's disease and Ehlers–Danlos syndrome. Acquired causes include hypertension and atherosclerosis. Patients usually present with sudden onset of severe tearing chest pain that radiates to the back between the scapulae. The pain may radiate to the neck, shoulder or abdomen. Associated symptoms include shortness of breath, dizziness, hemiplegia (carotid involvement) and haematuria (renal involvement). The patient may be pale, sweaty (signs of shock) and there may be differing blood pressure measurements in each arm with the disappearance and reappearance of distal pulses. Fundamental aspects of management include fluid resuscitation while maintaining systolic blood pressure below 100 mmHg (to prevent excessive blood loss), cross-matching 10 units of blood, blood tests (full blood count, urea and electrolytes and coagulation screen) and call for senior help. Usually type A dissections are treated surgically due to high risk of tamponade. Type B dissections tend to be managed conservatively, but secondary symptoms may necessitate an endovascular approach.

Raynaud's syndrome

23 C β-blockers

Raynaud's disease (primary Raynaud's – idiopathic cause) can be described as a syndrome of unknown aetiology that causes digital ischaemia by reflex vasospasm of normal arterioles. It occurs predominantly in women and clinically presents as digital pallor due to vasoconstriction, followed by cyanosis (relaxation of arterioles, but not venules) and reactive hyperaemia (a complete reversal of vasospasm).

[handwritten margin notes: pallor / cyanosis / reactive hyperaemia]

Raynaud's syndrome (secondary Raynaud's), which presents as the same clinical features as Raynaud's disease, can occur as a result of scleroderma, systemic lupus erythematosus, polyarteritis nodosa, rheumatoid arthritis, cervical rib, cryoglobulinaemia, polycythaemia and drugs such as β-blockers and ergot alkaloids. Raynaud's syndrome can be unilateral whereas Raynaud's disease is systemic and occurs bilaterally.

Raynaud's disease is diagnosed by exclusion of the other causes which may be due to Raynaud's syndrome. Blood tests (such as full blood count, thyroid function tests, liver function tests, cryoglobulins, antinuclear antibodies and rheumatoid factor), cold provocation tests and upper limb and digital pressures can be performed to search for an underlying cause. Treatment may be conservative (i.e. remove underlying cause, avoid cold, stop smoking), medical (i.e. calcium antagonists, 5-HT antagonists or admission as inpatient and treatment with prostacyclin) and surgical (i.e. sympathectomy – although symptoms may return).   ↳ not effective

Lymphoedema

24 E   All of the above
Lymphoedema is classified as primary and secondary. Primary lymphoedema has a genetic cause and therefore there is a hereditary component seen in families and is seen more commonly in females. There are many causes of secondary lymphoedema including post lymph node dissection for cancer clearance, post radiotherapy due to infections such as filarisis as well as post trauma. Other recurrent bacterial infections leading to cellulitis can also trigger lymphoedema. Venous disease can lead to swelling secondary to superficial or deep venous incompetence or thrombosis.

Acute mesenteric ischaemia

25 E   Any of the above with a high index of suspicion
This may occur due to an arterial or venous occlusion to the bowel mesentery which, if untreated, leads to bowel infarction and a high risk of mortality. The clinical condition can be diagnosed with a high index of suspicion in an arteriopath, a patient with previous abdominal surgery and documented atrial fibrillation who presents with sudden severe abdominal pain. This is out of keeping with the clinical signs and is associated with a metabolic acidosis, very high white cell count and an elevated lactate. Early diagnosis allows treatment prior to the development of irreversible bowel ischaemia.

SECTION 11:
UROLOGY

Questions

1.	Covering layers of the kidney	229
2.	Anatomy of the kidney	229
3.	Anatomy of the renal tract	229
4.	Vascular supply of the kidney (1)	229
5.	Vascular supply of the kidney (2)	229
6.	Anatomy of the reproductive system	230
7.	The male urethra	230
8.	Renal stone disease (1)	230
9.	Investigation of urinary calculi	230
10.	Renal stone disease (2)	231
11.	Renal stone disease (3)	231
12.	Urological infection (1)	231
13.	Urological infection (2)	232
14.	Urethral discharge	232
15.	Urological disease	232
16.	Rhabdomyolysis	233
17.	Inherited urological disease	233
18.	Paediatric urology (1)	233
19.	Paediatric urology (2)	234
20.	Preoperative assessment	234
21.	Renal cell carcinoma	234
22.	Bladder malignancy (1)	235
23.	Bladder malignancy (2)	235
24.	Testicular malignancy (1)	235
25.	Testicular malignancy (2)	235

26. Carcinoma of the penis 236
27. Peyronie's disease 236
28. Anatomy of the prostate gland 236
29. Prostatic disease 236
30. Prostate cancer 237

Answers 238

QUESTIONS

1. Covering layers of the kidney

All of the following form a covering layer over the kidney, except

    A. Gerota's fascia (peri-renal fascia)
    B. Peri-renal fat
    C. Liver
    D. Para-renal fat
    E. Fibrous capsule

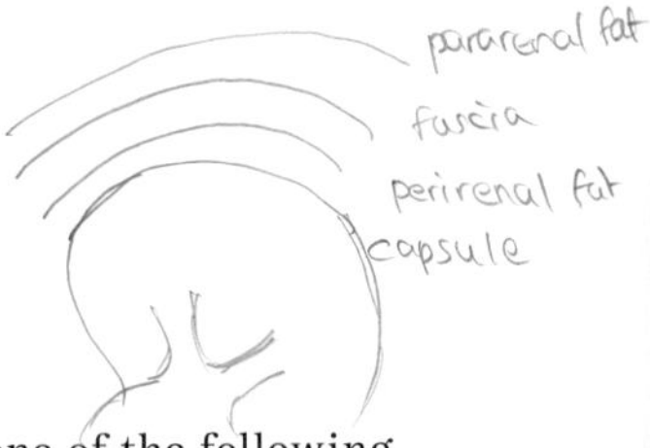

[handwritten annotations: pararenal fat, fascia, perirenal fat, capsule]

2. Anatomy of the kidney

The posteromedial aspect of the kidneys is related to which one of the following structures?

    A. Psoas muscle
    B. Ilio-inguinal nerve
    C. Diaphragm
    D. Pancreas
    E. 12th rib

3. Anatomy of the renal tract

In its course from the kidney to the bladder, the ureter runs on the top of which muscle?

    A. Quadratus lumborum
    B. Transversus abdominis
    C. Psoas
    D. Iliacus
    E. Latissimus dorsi

4. Vascular supply of the kidney (1)

[handwritten: below S. Mesenteric artery]

The renal arteries arise at intervertebral level

    A. T11/T12
    B. T12/L1
    C. L1/L2
    D. L2/L3
    E. L3/L4

5. Vascular supply of the kidney (2)

In a non-exercising individual, the proportion of cardiac output supplied to the kidneys is approximately

A. 5%
B. 10%
C. 15%
D. 20%
E. 25%

6. Anatomy of the reproductive system

A 34-year-old father of five children attends the family planning clinic for advice on birth control. After discussing the various options available, he requests a vasectomy. Which of the following structures lies most proximal to the vas deferens (ductus deferens)?

A. Superficial scrotal fascia (Dartos fascia)
B. Internal spermatic fascia
C. Tunica vaginalis
D. External spermatic fascia
E. Preperitoneal fat

7. The male urethra

With regard to the male urethra, which one of the following segments is the narrowest?

A. Pre-prostatic
B. Prostatic
C. Membranous
D. Bulbar
E. Penile

8. Renal stone disease (1) renal colic

A 40-year-old office executive presents with a 4-hour history of excruciating left loin pain radiating to the groin. The pain has been constant with short spells of more severe pain every 30–40 minutes. He informs you that his father has gout and has had similar pains in the past. A KUB and IVU confirm the presence of a radio-opaque stone in the left ureter, measuring approximately 4 mm in diameter. What type of stone is more likely to be present in this patient?

A. Xanthine
B. Uric acid   rare
C. (Triple) phosphate
D. Calcium oxalate
E. Cysteine

9. Investigation of urinary calculi

A 30-year-old PhD student presents with acute-onset colicky left loin pain and describes a history suggestive of urinary calculi. Which one of the following would be the initial investigation of choice to determine the presence of a calculus in the renal tract?

(handwritten: for calcium oxalate and triple phosphate stones)

A. Dimercaptosuccinic acid (DMSA) scan
B. Kidney ureter bladder (KUB) radiograph
C. Intravenous urogram/pyelogram
D. Flexible cystoscopy
E. Diethylene triamine pentaacetic acid (DTPA) scan

10. Renal stone disease (2)

A 35-year-old housewife presents to her GP with a week-long history of dysuria, frequency and extremely strong smelling urine. A urine dipstick test confirms the presence of leucocytes and nitrites. She has previously suffered from multiple urinary tract infections, which have resolved with a short course of antibiotics. To rule out further complications of the urinary tract, an ultrasound scan is performed, which suggests the presence of a large calculus within the left pelvicalyceal system. Which one of the following microorganisms is *not* associated with the formation of such stones?

(handwritten: Staghorn calculus → UTI)

A. *Proteus*
B. *Klebsiella*
C. *Pseudomonas*
D. *Mycoplasma*
E. Mycobacteria

11. Renal stone disease (3)

A 75-year-old man presents to the surgical unit with a 24-hour history of acute-onset left loin pain, which seems to worsen intermittently and has not settled with regular simple analgesia. He suffers from mild dementia and is unable to recall the details of his past medical history. The foundation year 2 doctor on call suspects that a urinary calculus is the cause of this man's pain and spots an old pathology report in the patient's notes showing the presence of negatively birefringent crystals in a synovial fluid aspirate. Which one of the following substances is likely to make up the majority of this man's calculus?

(handwritten: radiolucent — Xanthine, Cysteine, uric acid)

A. Xanthine
B. Uric acid
C. (Triple) phosphate
D. Calcium oxalate
E. Cysteine

12. Urological infection (1)

A 24-year-old sexually active medical student is diagnosed as having a urinary tract infection by her GP. Which one of the following organisms is most commonly associated with community acquired urinary tract infection?

A. *Escherichia coli*   90% community   50% hospitalized UTIs.
B. *Pseudomonas* → associated with foreign body (catheter) and stones.
C. *Staphylococcus saprophyticus*   2nd most common. In sexually active women.
D. *Staphylococcus aureus*   recent surgery
E. *Streptococcus faecalis* → un common cause of uncomplicated UTI.

13. Urological infection (2)

A 40-year-old female lawyer is referred to the urology outpatient clinic with a history of multiple urinary tract infections over the preceding 10 years, which have required increasingly longer courses of antibiotics to treat. She also reports feeling more lethargic of late, despite leading a relatively active lifestyle. An ultrasound scan of this patient's renal tract indicates chronic pyelonephritis. Which of the following sonographic features would be diagnostic of her condition?

A. Absent kidney
B. Hydronephrotic kidney
C. Multiple renal stones
D. Atrophic kidney
E. Poor urinary concentration

14. Urethral discharge

A 28-year-old student presents with a 2-day history of dysuria and mucopurulent urethral discharge. He reports recently having had unprotected sex while on holiday in the Mediterranean. A urethral discharge smear inoculated into Thayer–Martin medium confirms infection with *Neisseria gonorrhoeae* and appropriate antibiotics are started. What type of organism is *N. gonorrhoeae*?

A. Lactose-fermenting Gram-negative rod → E. coli → Klebsiella → Enterobacter.
B. Maltose-fermenting Gram-negative coccus → N. meningitides
C. Coagulase-positive Gram-positive coccus → S. aureus
D. Glucose-fermenting Gram-negative coccus
E. Lactose-non-fermenting Gram-negative rod → Shigella, Salmonella → Proteus (oxidase neg)

oxidase +ve → pseudomonas.

15. Urological disease

A 69-year-old diabetic man presents to the acute surgery unit with a 5-day history of mild dysuria, frequency and feeling generally unwell. On examination, he is found to be pyrexial and tachycardic. A genital examination reveals both the penis and the scrotum to be swollen, red and tender to touch, with erythema also extending into the groin bilaterally. Of note, the examining surgeon believes that there is palpable crepitus in the perineum. Routine bloods and cultures are taken (which later grow both aerobic and anaerobic organisms), and fluid resuscitation and broad-spectrum antibiotics are commenced. Following further discussion with a urologist, he is taken promptly into the operating theatre for definitive management. The most likely diagnosis in this patient is

A. Fournier's gangrene → perineal crepitus = diagnostic
B. Epididymo-orchitis
C. Testicular tumour
D. Testicular torsion
E. Prostatitis

16. Rhabdomyolysis

A 45-year-old railway worker is admitted following a crush injury to his left leg. He is talking in full sentences and complaining of pain in his leg. Further examination reveals a blood pressure of 90/58 mmHg, pulse of 99 beats/min, and a swollen and bruised left leg. Intravenous access is gained, routine blood samples are taken and fluid resuscitation is commenced. In addition, the patient is catheterized for monitoring purposes but passes only a small volume of red-brown urine, which, on microscopy, is confirmed to contain myoglobin. The admitting physician makes a working diagnosis of rhabdomyolysis. Which one of the following metabolic abnormalities is *not* associated with this condition?

A. Hypocalcaemia
B. Hyperkalaemia
C. Hypernatraemia
D. Hyperphosphataemia
E. Hyperuricaemia

17. Inherited urological disease

A 41-year-old man presents to the emergency department with a severe headache that started suddenly following a weight-training session. He is treated appropriately and further examination some days later reveals a palpable lump in the left loin. An ultrasound scan confirms multiple kidney cysts and hepatomegaly, suggestive of adult polycystic kidney disease. On further questioning, he reports that his father died of a brain haemorrhage at the age of 35. Adult polycystic kidney disease is most commonly inherited by which one of the following modalities?

A. Autosomal recessive gene chromosome 16
B. Autosomal dominant gene chromosome 16
C. Autosomal dominant gene chromosome 8
D. Autosomal recessive gene chromosome 4
E. Autosomal dominant gene chromosome 4

18. Paediatric urology (1)

A 6-week-old boy presents with his parents to the specialist paediatric urology outpatients department. The family is Jewish and at the time of the boy's circumcision were told by their rabbi that the urethral meatus was not in the normal position. On examination, the meatus is on the ventral surface just below the glans penis. What is the most likely diagnosis?

A. Hypospadias
B. Epispadias *urethral meatus on dorsum*
C. Phimosis — *in small children physiological*
D. Chordee → *head of b   curves down in ventral position*
E. Perineal urethra

adesion of prepuce to glans penis.
Congenital disorder

19. Paediatric urology (2)

A young girl presents to her GP with a 2-day history of fever and swelling on the left side of her abdomen. Examination confirms a raised temperature and left loin swelling extending into the mid-line. In addition, microscopic haematuria is found on a urine dipstick test. She is referred to the local hospital where an ultrasound scan of the abdomen and biopsy confirm Wilm's tumour (nephro-blastoma). Which one of the following statements regarding Wilm's tumour is true?

A. The tumour may be associated with anophthalmia
B. 5-year survival in stage IV disease is approximately 65%
C. Children most commonly present at the age of 8–10 years
D. Some cases are associated with a gene mutation on chromosome 13
E. It commonly metastasizes to the brain

20. Preoperative assessment

A 65-year-old hypertensive man attends the preoperative assessment clinic 7 days before he is due to undergo a transurethral resection of the prostate for benign prostatic hypertrophy. He is currently taking furosemide for blood pressure control but no other regular medication. A routine set of bloods is taken, the results of which show a potassium level of 2.7 mmol/L. On the basis of this an electrocardiogram is requested. All of the following electrocardiographic changes are characteristic of hypokalaemia, except

A. Left bundle branch block
B. Flattened T waves
C. U waves
D. ST segment depression
E. Prolonged QT interval

21. Renal cell carcinoma

Which one of the following statements regarding renal cell carcinoma is true?

A. It is an incidental finding in approximately 30% of patients
B. Women are more commonly affected than men
C. Approximately 5% of cases are familial
D. Renal cell carcinoma accounts for around 3% of adult cancers
E. Metastases are poorly visualized by standard imaging techniques

22. Bladder malignancy (1)

With regard to carcinoma of the bladder, which one of the following statements is *not* correct?

A. Epithelial tumours account for the majority of bladder tumours
B. It accounts for 1 in every 5000 new cases of cancer in the United Kingdom
C. Males are more commonly affected than females
D. There is a strong correlation with exposure to industrial dyes
E. It frequently presents with painful haematuria

23. Bladder malignancy (2)

A 69-year-old retired canal engineer who has previously worked in North Africa presents to the urology outpatients department with a 2-month history of intermittent painless haematuria. A cystoscopy is performed showing a sessile mass on the posterior bladder wall. A biopsy is taken of this mass, which confirms transitional cell carcinoma invading the bladder muscle, but no local nodes are involved. A further staging computed tomography scan shows no distant metastases. According to the TNM classification, the tumour stage in this individual is

A. Tis Nx Mx
B. T2 N0 M0
C. T2 N1 M0
D. T3 N1 M1
E. T3 N0 M1

24. Testicular malignancy (1)

Which one of the following statements regarding testicular tumours is true?

A. They account for 5%–10% of male malignancy in the United Kingdom
B. Seminomas are more common than non-seminomatous germ cell tumours
C. Teratomas commonly present between the ages of 30 and 50 years
D. Seminomas secrete α-fetoprotein and ß-human chorionic gonadotrophin
E. 5-year survival for seminomas is approximately 90%

25. Testicular malignancy (2)

A 36-year-old carpenter is diagnosed with a seminoma. To which lymph nodes do a seminoma most commonly spread first?

A. Para-aortic lymph nodes
B. Superficial inguinal lymph nodes
C. Anterior cervical chain

D. Posterior cervical chain
E. Deep inguinal lymph nodes

26. Carcinoma of the penis

All of the following statements regarding carcinoma of the penis are true, except

A. It is a squamous cell carcinoma
B. Incidence is lower in men infected with the human papilloma virus
C. Incidence is lower in men circumcised at birth
D. Staging of disease is by the tumour node metastasis (TNM) system
E. 5-year survival in patients with localized disease is around 80%

27. Peyronie's disease

A 55-year-old solicitor presents to the urology outpatients department with a 6-month history of abnormal angulated penis on erection. This has made sexual intercourse particularly difficult and painful and has been affecting his relationship with his wife. After further questioning, a diagnosis of Peyronie's disease is offered. All of the following statements regarding Peyronie's disease are true, except

A. It is a connective tissue disorder of unknown origin
B. Around 1% of men are affected
C. It is the result of a gene mutation on chromosome 5
D. Surgical treatment is considered only 1 year after initial presentation
E. There is an association with Dupuytren's contracture

28. Anatomy of the prostate gland

Which of the following vessels contributes to the blood supply of the prostate gland?

A. Coeliac plexus
B. Superior mesenteric artery
C. Inferior mesenteric artery
D. Internal iliac artery
E. External iliac artery

29. Prostatic disease

An 80-year-old man presents to his GP with a 6-month history of increasing urinary frequency. He passes urine approximately eight times during the day and six times each night, but feels that he has not completely voided. In addition, he reports that his stream is very slow and finds it hard to stop, with micturition prolonged due to terminal dribbling. He is otherwise fit and healthy with no other symptoms reported. On rectal examination, the prostate is found to be smoothly enlarged with no other significant findings on systemic examination. Which of the following layers of the prostate gland is likely to be enlarged in this man?

- (A) Transition zone
- B. Central zone
- C. Peripheral zone
- D. Anterior fibromuscular stroma
- E. All of the above

30. Prostate cancer

A 75-year-old man presents to the urology outpatient clinic with a 6-month history of urinary frequency associated with difficulty initiating micturition, dribbling on reaching the end of his stream and nocturia. A digital rectal examination reveals a hard prostate gland. Core biopsy is performed on the gland and the pathology report indicates the presence of a tumour involving most of the right lobe. According to the TNM classification, the tumour stage is

- A. T2 N1 M0
- B. T3 Nx Mx
- C. T3 N1 M0
- (D) T2 Nx Mx
- E. T1 N1 M0

ANSWERS

Covering layers of the kidney

1   C   Liver

The kidneys are a pair of retroperitoneal organs lying on the posterior abdominal wall. The right kidney lies lower in the body in comparison with the left as a result of the liver, which due to its large size pushes the kidney down during development. Meanwhile, the renal hila of the left and right kidney lie above and below the transpyloric plane respectively, approximately 5 cm from the midline.

Left – above
right – below

The kidneys have four covering layers, which are as follows (from most proximal, i.e. in contact with the kidney substance to distal):

out Inside

- Fibrous capsule
- Peri-renal fat
- Peri-renal/Gerota's fascia – a layer of connective tissue that surrounds the kidneys and adrenal glands. It is continuous with the fascia transversalis laterally.
- Para-renal fat – the outermost covering layer of the kidney, forming part of the retroperitoneal fat.

Outside

The liver (more specifically the right lobe of the liver) forms the superior border/relation of the right kidney. It does not however form a covering layer of the kidney itself.

Anatomy of the kidney

2   A   Psoas muscle

Anatomical relations are shown in Table 11.1.

Table 11.1 Anatomical relations of the kidneys

Anterior	Left kidney	Right kidney
Superior	Stomach	Adrenal gland
	Spleen	Right lobe of liver
Medial	Pancreas	Second part of duodenum (D2)
Inferior	Left colon	Right colon; small bowel

Posterior	Left and right kidney
Superior	Diaphragm; costo-diaphragmatic recess
Inferior	12th rib; ilio-hypogastric nerve; ilio-inguinal nerve
Medial	Psoas muscle
Lateral	Quadratus lumborum; transversus abdominis muscle

*Ureters
= retroperitoneal*

Anatomy of the renal tract

3   C   Psoas

The ureters are a pair of muscular tubes that emerge from the hilum of each kidney and run vertically downwards behind the parietal peritoneum on the psoas muscle. The psoas muscle separates the ureter from the tips of the lumbar vertebrae transverse processes. Each ureter is approximately 25 cm in length and has three natural constrictions at the renal pelvis (pelvi-ureteric junction or PUJ), the pelvic brim and on joining the bladder itself (vesico-ureteric junction or VUJ). Within the pelvis, the ureter runs down the lateral wall in the region of the ischial spine, where it turns forward and enters at the lateral angle of the bladder.

Quadratus lumborum is an intra-abdominal muscle that arises from aponeurotic fibres of the iliolumbar ligament and the iliac crest. It is involved in lateral flexion and extension of the vertebral column and fixes the ribs in forced expiration. In addition, it forms the posterolateral border of the kidney. Transversus abdominis is a muscle of the abdominal wall that also forms the posterolateral border of the kidney. Iliacus is a muscle of thigh flexion and lateral rotation found in the iliac fossa, lateral to the psoas muscle. Latissimus dorsi is a large muscle of the back that is involved in pulling the arm dorsally and caudally (backwards and downwards).

Vascular supply of the kidney (1)

4   C   L1/L2

The renal arteries are branches of the abdominal aorta, arising at the level of L1/L2, immediately below the origin of the superior mesenteric artery (vertebral level L1).

Vascular supply of the kidney (2)

5   D   20%

While an individual is at rest, the kidneys receive around 20% of the cardiac output via the renal arteries. The right renal artery lies posterior to the inferior vena cava and is longer than the left renal artery.

The renal artery divides into five segmental branches, each independently supplying a parenchymal zone unrelated to the anatomical arrangement of the pyramid and calyx (the base unit of the kidney). The areas supplied are the apical, upper, middle, lower and posterior zones. The segmental arteries are further divided into arcuate branches that run in the boundary between the kidney cortex and medulla. Finally, the arcuate arteries branch into smaller vessels that run up and down, parallel with the collecting tubules, and form the afferent artery to each glomerulus.

The renal veins are anterior to the artery and communicate freely with each other, necessitating multiple ligations at the time of operation.

Anatomy of the reproductive system

6　C　Tunica vaginalis

The vas deferens (or ductus deferens) is one of a pair of ducts that connect to the testis via the epididymis. It functions to transmit sperm to the urethra. It is supplied by the artery of the vas deferens, which arises from the superior vesical artery, a branch of the internal iliac artery.

Vasectomy is a method of contraception in which the vasa deferentia are (usually surgically) ligated or injected to prevent the flow of sperm. Active sperm can remain in the seminal vesicles for up to 12 weeks after and the patient must be informed of this when the procedure is undertaken. Several layers must be cut through in order to reach the vas. From superficial to deep, these are:

superficial
- Skin
- Superficial scrotal fascia (Dartos fascia)
- External spermatic fascia
- Cremasteric fascia and muscle
- Internal spermatic fascia
- Preperitoneal fat
deep - Tunica vaginalis

vas deferens

The male urethra

7　C　Membranous

The urethra is a tubular structure that connects the bladder to the external environment in males and females alike. Although its main function is to excrete urine, in males, it has the added function of acting as a conduit for semen.

In females, the urethra is a short perineal structure approximately 3–5 cm in length, opening in the vulva between the clitoris and vagina. Given its short length and location in the perineum, females are especially prone to ascending urinary tract infections (UTIs).

In comparison, the male urethra is around 20 cm long and has five components. These are

- Pre-prostatic or intramural urethra – Approximately 0.5–1.5 cm in length (varies according to bladder fullness).
- Prostatic urethra – Approximately 3 cm in length and the widest/most dilatable part of the urethra. The vas deferens and prostatic ducts (contributing sperm and seminal fluid) open into this portion.

- Membranous urethra – Approximately 2 cm long portion of the urethra piercing the urogenital diaphragm. It is also the narrowest part of the urethra.
- Bulbar urethra.
- Penile urethra – Runs along the ventral surface of the penis and is the longest portion, comprising most of the urethral length.

Renal stone disease (1)

8 D Calcium oxalate

Renal tract stones (calculi) are common, affecting approximately 1%–2% of the adult population. They are more prevalent in young and middle-aged men and caused mainly by factors that increase urine solute concentration, e.g. calcium salts, urine concentration and urinary stasis. They can arise in any part of the urinary tract and present with intense colicky loin to groin pain, and are associated with nausea, vomiting and lower urinary tract symptoms. *(freq, dys, urgency)*

Most stones (approximately 90%) are formed of calcium oxalate and magnesium/calcium/ammonium phosphate (so-called triple phosphate stones). These substances are radio-opaque and as a result mostly seen on a plain KUB scan. Xanthine, uric acid and cysteine stones are rarer and usually the result of an acquired or genetic biochemical abnormality. These types of stones are generally radiolucent and therefore not seen on a KUB scan. *struvite*

Initial treatment consists of adequate analgesia, fluid rehydration (oral ± intravenous) and correcting any underlying abnormality that could predispose to stone formation. Further treatment depends on the size of the stone. Most calculi (95%) <5 mm in diameter will tend to pass spontaneously (although this can be painful). Patients can therefore be treated conservatively with fluid rehydration and analgesia. For calculi >5 mm in diameter or in individuals in whom pain is not resolving, further investigation may be needed, with treatment dependent on calculus size and location.

Approximate frequency of stone types is

- Xanthine – <1% *⎫ radiolucent*
- Cysteine – <2% *⎬*
- Uric acid – 5% *⎭*
- (Triple) phosphate (Mg^{2+}, Ca^{2+}, PO_4^{3-}) – 33% *⎫ radio-opaque* → staghorn calculus.
- Calcium oxalate – 60% *⎭*

Investigation of urinary calculi

9 B Kidney ureter bladder (KUB) radiograph

Renal colic is the result of ureter spasm and hyper-peristalsis secondary to stone impaction in the urinary tract. Calculi impact at sites of narrowing in the ureter, which can be pathological in origin (e.g. strictures) or naturally occurring (e.g. the pelvi–ureteric junction, crossing of the ureter at the SIJ and at the vesico-ureteric junction).

Several methods of imaging are available to visualize the renal tract and urinary calculi. Traditionally, the most frequently used technique has been an x-ray KUB (also called the control film) which visualizes the kidneys, ureters and bladder. It relies on the fact that more than 90% of urinary calculi are radio-opaque and will therefore appear on a plain radiograph. This is the correct answer here.

Intravenous urography/pyelography is an X-ray technique consisting of a control film, i.e. taking a KUB and giving a contrast solution. Following contrast injection, another film is immediately taken followed by more radiographs at 20 and 60 minutes. An IVU will indicate the level of an obstruction, whether there is prevention of flow of contrast (seen as filling defect), or tumours in the bladder. Although an excellent technique, it is contraindicated in those with contrast allergy, poor renal function and diabetic patients taking metformin. It is incorrect in this scenario as there is no indication of a KUB having been taken already.

DMSA and DTPA scans are used for cortical imaging and can give an estimate of renal function. They are not commonly used as first line imaging tools in cases of suspected renal tract stones. Ultrasound KUB is also a commonly used technique to determine acute obstruction and can detect some stones, but is generally unreliable for detecting ureteric calculi. More recently, many units have begun to use CT-KUB as a first line investigative tool, however this is not yet universal practice. Flexible cystoscopy is used to directly visualize the urethra, bladder and ureters. It is more commonly used as a minimally invasive method of stone removal in the presence of large renal tract stones or if conservative management of small stones is unsuccessful.

Renal stone disease (2)

10 E   Mycobacteria

Repeated UTI predisposes individuals to so-called infection stones that account for approximately 10% of renal tract stones. They are the result of repeated infection with organisms such as *Proteus*, *Pseudomonas*, *Staphylococcus*, *Mycoplasma* and *Klebsiella*. These are referred to as urea-splitting organisms as they hydrolyse urea to ammonium with a resulting alkalinization of urine. The alkalinization process results in deposition of various ions and formation of struvite stones (magnesium ammonium phosphate) especially in the pelvicalyceal system. The stones can appear to have the shape of deer antlers and are therefore also referred to as staghorn calculi.

Mycobacteria species include the organisms *Mycobacterium tuberculosis* (TB) and *Mycobacterium leprae* (leprosy), which are not usually involved in the formation of struvite stones.

Renal stone disease (3)

11 B Uric acid

Gout is a disorder of purine metabolism exacerbated by dehydration, resulting in hyperuricaemia and acute recurrent attacks of synovitis due to urate crystal deposition in the (predominantly) large joints of the body.

Aspiration of joint fluid and examination under polarized light shows negatively birefringent crystals, which are characteristic of the condition and suggested in this individual. Hyperuricaemia also predisposes individuals to urate and calcium oxalate stones. Treatment is as for other urinary tract stones, but also includes allopurinol and diet modification in order to lower levels of serum uric acid.

Given the age of this man, it is important to exclude other important differentials (as for any patient), particularly a ruptured AAA, which can present with similar symptoms and is occasionally missed in such individuals resulting in a catastrophic outcome. The aetiology of other types of urinary calculi is discussed in the answer to Question 8.

Urological infection (1)

12 A *Escherichia coli*

Many factors contribute to the impairment of urinary tract defence mechanisms, thereby predisposing an individual to developing a UTI. These include:

- Female sex – Women have shorter a urethra than men, which can allow the transfer of faecal flora. Vaginal flora can be transferred during sexual intercourse and hormonal changes during pregnancy/menopause alter the acidity and composition of urine.
- Diabetes – Causes immunosuppression and glycosuria, which provides a sugar-rich environment in which bacteria can flourish.
- Urinary stasis secondary to obstruction.
- Foreign bodies, e.g. catheterization.

E. coli is a Gram-negative organism that accounts for some 90% of UTIs in the community and approximately 50% of infections in hospitalized patients. *Pseudomonas* infection is associated with the presence of a foreign body, such as an indwelling urinary catheter or urinary tract calculus. *Staph. saprophyticus* infection occurs most commonly in sexually active women and is the second commonest cause of community-acquired UTI. *Staph. aureus* infection is associated with recent surgery or presence of surgical instruments within the urinary tract. *Strep. faecalis* is an Enterobacter (this group also includes *Proteus* and *Klebsiella* species), which are urea-splitting organisms that predispose to the formation of struvite stones in affected individuals. They are uncommon causes of uncomplicated UTI.

Urological infection (2)

13 D Atrophic kidney

Pyelonephritis is an infection of the renal pelvis and the substance of the kidney itself. It is divided into acute and chronic. Acute pyelonephritis occurs as a result of ascending infection of the urinary tract or septicaemia, leading to fever, rigours and loin pain as the classic triad of presentation. A variety of methods are used to investigate acute pyelonephritis including a urine dipstick test, as well as urine and blood cultures (to exclude a possible bacterial cause and direct treatment). Radiological investigations such as CT-KUB and ultrasound may demonstrate obstructing points indicative of renal stone disease, while an IVU can indicate kidney enlargement and poor urinary concentration.

Chronic pyelonephritis is the result of recurrent UTI and vesico-ureteric reflux. It is diagnosed by the radiological finding of a small, contracted, scarred and atrophic kidney. Occasionally, patients may present later with signs and features of chronic renal failure. Treatment is by addressing the underlying cause, correcting metabolic and renal abnormalities, antibiotics and occasionally nephrectomy in the presence of severely diseased kidneys.

Urethral discharge

14 D Glucose-fermenting Gram-negative coccus

N. gonorrhoeae, a glucose-fermenting Gram-negative diplococcus, is the causative organism in gonorrhoea, which is a common sexually transmitted illness. It can involve many parts of the body, including the throat, joints and urogenital organs in men, women and also children. In addition, it can cause conjunctivitis in newborn infants. It can present with dysuria and profuse, purulent urethral discharge, particularly in affected males. In addition to urethral smear showing Gram-negative diplococci, inoculation of discharge into Thayer–Martin medium is also used to confirm the disease. Treatment is with broad-spectrum antibiotics (which also cover *Chlamydia*) and encouraging the use of condoms as a preventive measure.

Lactose-fermenting Gram-negative rods include *Klebsiella* species, *E. coli*, *Enterobacter* species, *Citrobacter* species and *Serratia* species.

Neisseria meningitides is a maltose, sucrose and glucose-fermenting, Gram-negative coccus. *Staphylococcus aureus* is a cluster-forming, coagulase-positive, Gram-positive coccus. Lactose non-fermenting, Gram-negative rods comprise the oxidase-negative *Shigella*, *Salmonella* and *Proteus* species and oxidase-positive *Pseudomonas* species.

Urological disease

15 A Fournier's gangrene

Fournier's gangrene is a relatively rare necrotizing fascitis of the perineal, perianal and genital areas (secondary to infection by aerobic and anaerobic bacteria), affecting predominantly middle-aged and elderly men with pre-existing co-morbidities (it is seen more frequently in diabetic patients). It is a urological emergency that often presents with swelling, pain and erythema of the genital region accompanied by systemic features such as fever and rigour. This is commonly preceded by a several-day history of pruritus and discomfort of the external genitalia. External necrotic areas may or may not be evident. The presence of perineal crepitus is virtually diagnostic. Given the potential for rapid spread and tissue destruction, early diagnosis and debridement is an essential component of management, along with broad-spectrum antibiotic cover. Mortality is high and related to the level of existing co-morbidity.

Prostatitis is an inflammation of the prostate gland related to bladder outflow obstruction that presents with frequency, urgency, dysuria and occasional haematuria (i.e. symptoms of a UTI) as well as fever, haemospermia and occasionally a tender prostate and pain on ejaculation. Treatment is with antibiotics and further investigations such as a trans-rectal ultrasound may be employed to rule out (and if necessary, drain) any abscess that has formed as a result of the inflammatory process. Testicular tumours, torsion and epididymo-orchitis are discussed elsewhere in this chapter.

Rhabdomyolysis

16 C Hypernatraemia

Rhabdomyolysis is the destruction of striated muscle due to injury, which may be physical, chemical or biological in origin. Causative factors for rhabdomyolysis include:

- **Common causes** – e.g. crush injury, ischaemia, prolonged epileptic fits, heavy physical exercise (especially if dehydrated) and alcohol withdrawal.
- **Rare causes** – e.g. infection (viral necrotizing myositis), inflammatory myopathy (polymyositis), drugs (statins), hypothyroidism, snake bites, malignant hyperthermia and electric shock.

The presentation will be dependent on the cause, but may include pain, swelling and weakness of an obviously affected muscle in crush injury. Occasionally, this can cause compartment syndrome as surrounding tissues are compressed by swelling, requiring urgent fasciotomy. Patients may also present with nausea, confusion, disorientation, coma, hypotension and physiological shock due to volume depletion and metabolic disturbance.

Classically, expected metabolic abnormalities are hyperkalaemia, hyperuricaemia and raised creatinine (indicative of acute renal failure), hypocalcaemia (from calcium binding to necrotic muscle), hyperphosphataemia (as a reaction to hypocalcaemia), raised creatine kinase (from muscle breakdown) and occasionally, deranged liver function tests. Furthermore, a urine dipstick test may reveal blood, which is confirmed as myoglobin on microscopy. Myoglobin can accumulate to form casts in renal tubules, leading to obstruction of urine flow and acute tubular necrosis. Myoglobinuria is also suggested by the presence of red-brown urine.

[handwritten margin notes: hyperical, hyperuric, hyperphos, hypo cal, ↑ Creat, ↑CK, myoglobinuria]

Initial management consists of stabilizing the patient, followed by fluid resuscitation (for rehydration and prevention of myoglobin deposition and tubular necrosis) and catheterization (to monitor urine output and guide rehydration). Urine alkalization with isotonic sodium bicarbonate can be used to make myoglobin more soluble, but evidence for its overall benefit is limited. Electrolyte abnormalities, particularly hyperkalaemia, will need correction, given its potential to cause fatal arrhythmias. Dialysis can be used in severe cases.

Inherited urological disease

17 B   Autosomal dominant gene chromosome 16

Adult polycystic kidney disease is an autosomal dominant disease caused by a defect on chromosome 16 affecting the *PKD1* gene (in 85% of patients, while the majority of remaining cases is due to a gene defect on chromosome 4). The condition is characterized by the formation of multiple kidney cysts (which are present at birth), with progressive enlargement and reduced renal function in affected adults.

Patients may present with features of renal dysfunction such as loin pain, haematuria (due to bleeding into a cyst), renal failure, hypertension and UTI or with systemic features of the disease such as

- Intracranial haemorrhage – Especially subarachnoid haemorrhage due to rupture of berry aneurysms of the circle of Willis
- Liver, breast and pancreatic cysts
- Mitral valve prolapse   *click murmur.*
- Aortic root dilatation

- Thoracic aorta dissection
- Abdominal wall hernias

There may also be a family history of unexplained intracranial bleed or renal failure, with most patients developing end-stage renal failure by age 60. Treatment is with dialysis and renal transplantation. Affected families can also be offered genetic counselling and testing.

Paediatric urology (1)

18 A   Hypospadias

Hypospadias is the name for the abnormal ventral opening of the urethral meatus along the urethral groove between the glans penis and the scrotum or perineum, occurring in around 1:125 births. The meatus opens on the glans penis in the majority of cases (so-called first-degree hypospadias) and usually causes little functional problem. Opening of the urethra on the shaft and scrotum/perineum (second- and third-degree hypospadias) can result in difficulty urinating, along with psychosexual and fertility problems, necessitating repair at a young age (usually between 9 and 18 months). Common methods of repair include:

- Meatal advancement and glanuloplasty – Involving the creation of a new meatus and closure of the existing opening.
- Mathieu flap – Used for proximal shaft hypospadias, creating a flap based on the ectopic meatus, which is folded over, and the remaining lateral flaps closed over the new urethra.

Epispadias is a condition in which the urethral meatus opens on the dorsum of the penis. It results from failure of mid-line structures below the umbilicus to fuse and is associated with the split symphysis pubis, low umbilicus, bifid clitoris (in girls), undescended testes, bladder exstrophy and cloacal exstrophy (in rare cases). Phimosis is a contraction of the foreskin, preventing its retraction from the head of the penis. In infants, it is usually a physiological process due to adhesion of the prepuce to the glans penis. Pathological phimosis occurs usually in older children and adults as a result of a disease process or infection. Treatment depends on the extent of functional disability and the commonest surgical intervention is circumcision. Paraphimosis occurs when retracted foreskin is not fully replaced, resulting in a tight and irreducible band around the penis, e.g. after insertion of a urinary catheter. Chordee is a congenital abnormality in which the head of the penis curves down in a ventral direction. It is usually corrected surgically during infancy. Perineal urethra refers to a urethral opening in the perineum. It is most common in women.

Paediatric urology (2)

19 B   5-year survival in stage IV disease is approximately 65%

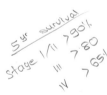

Wilm's tumour (nephroblastoma) is a malignant tumour of embryonic origin, most commonly affecting children aged 3–4 years. It is associated with a gene mutation on chromosome 11 that leads to the loss of the tumour suppressor gene *WT-1*. Occasionally, Wilm's tumour may be associated with other systemic abnormalities such as WAGR syndrome (Wilm's tumour, aniridia (absence of the iris), genito-urinary abnormalities and mental retardation) or Denys–Drash syndrome (associated with hemi-hypertrophy), but most patients are otherwise healthy and present acutely with fever, abdominal swelling and haematuria.

The tumour is classified into four stages, depending on the extent of tumour spread:

- Stage I – Disease is limited to the kidney and can be completely excised. It does not breach the renal capsule.
- Stage II – Disease extends beyond the kidney but can be excised with no residual beyond the excision margin.
- Stage III – There is an unresectable primary tumour with lymph node metastasis.
- Stage IV – Distant metastases are present, especially in the lungs.

Treatment is by surgical resection, which may be delayed to allow pre-resection chemotherapy. After resection, further chemotherapy may be required depending on the tumour stage. Disseminated disease, particularly lung secondaries, can be treated with radiotherapy. Five-year survival is dependent on tumour stage, but overall prognosis is excellent. Individuals with stage I/II disease (the most common presentation) have a >90% 5-year survival, those with stage III disease have a >80% 5-year survival, and finally patients with disseminated stage IV disease have an approximately 65% 5-year survival.

Preoperative assessment

20 A   Left bundle branch block

Hypokalaemia is the presence of a low serum potassium level. The normal range of serum potassium varies from laboratory to laboratory, but is approximately 3.5–5.0 mmol/L. The serum potassium level is usually strictly controlled, but may be altered as a result of disease, physiological response or medication. Causes of low serum potassium include:

- Diuretics, e.g. furosemide, bumetanide and ethacrynic acid, which are all loop diuretics that inhibit the $Na^+/K^+/2Cl^-$ symporter in the thick ascending limb of the loop of Henle, resulting in reduced serum potassium levels

- Vomiting and diarrhoea
- Pyloric stenosis
- Villous adenoma of the rectum
- Intestinal fistula
- Steroids/Cushing's syndrome (excess steroid production)
- Conn's syndrome 1ry hyperald.
- Alkalosis

Hypokalaemia may present asymptomatically or with muscle weakness, hypotonia, cramp, tetany and potentially fatal cardiac arrhythmias (this is in common with hyperkalaemia).

ECG changes in *hypokalaemia* are small or inverted T waves, prominent U waves, prolonged PR interval, ST segment depression and a prolonged QT interval. Although left bundle branch block may occur in hypertension, it is not classically associated with hypokalaemia. ECG changes in *hyperkalaemia* include tall (tented) T waves, small P waves and wide QRS complexes.

Treatment of hypokalaemia involves removing any causative agents and treating underlying conditions. For acute cases, oral or intravenous potassium supplementation is indicated with slow correction in order to prevent possible overload and arrhythmias.

Renal cell carcinoma

21 D Renal cell carcinoma accounts for around 3% of adult cancers
Renal cell (adeno)carcinoma is a malignant cancer of proximal renal tubule cells accounting for around 3% of all adult cancers. It is a highly vascular malignancy with a slightly higher incidence in men than women. Risk factors for renal cell carcinoma include:

- Acquired renal cystic disease (affects 90% of patients on dialysis)
- Smoking
- Exposure to lead
- Asbestos
- Polycarbons

Triad
· pain
· palpable mass
· hematuria

Although the majority of cases are sporadic, a small proportion (~2%) are familial and associated with Von Hippel–Lindau disease, haemangioblastomas of the cerebellum and spine, retinal haemangiomas, phaeochromocytoma and islet cell tumours.

A significant number of patients will present with pain, palpable loin mass and haematuria, a triad of symptoms considered classical for the disease. In the majority of patients, however, the disease is an incidental finding (~50%) or associated with signs of systemic illness, e.g. weight loss, anaemia. Some patients may present with paraneoplastic syndromes indicative of disseminated disease. This will include release of renin, erythropoietin, ACTH or parathyroid-like hormone and will cause, among other symptoms, hypercalcaemia, polycythaemia, hypertension and night sweats. Metastatic spread of the disease is by direct extension into the paranephric fat, fascia and into the renal vein/inferior vena cava; or haematogenous, presenting as cannonball metastases in the lung, brain and bone.

Treatment is dependent on stage and spread of disease. Localized disease is treated mainly with radical nephrectomy. This involves removal of the kidney and surrounding Gerota's fascia via either an extra-peritoneal lateral loin approach or trans-abdominal approach. A partial nephrectomy may be performed in certain cases, e.g. poor renal function. Treatment for metastatic disease (which affects around 30% of patients on initial presentation) includes palliative nephrectomy, embolization, chemo/radiotherapy and immunotherapy.

Five-year survival is dependent on tumour stage and grade. In cases of localized disease, there is approximately 90% 5-year survival, but in patients with distant metastases, this drops to around 20%.

Bladder malignancy (1)

22 E   **It frequently presents with painful haematuria**
Carcinoma of the bladder is a malignancy that arises more commonly in middle-aged and elderly individuals, particularly men. It accounts for approximately 1 in 5000 cancers in the UK. There are several predisposing factors, including cigarette smoking, exposure to industrial chemicals (historically aromatic amines and aniline dyes used in the dying industry, but also those involved in printing, processing and rubber industries), drugs such as phenacetin and cyclophosphamide, and chronic inflammation (e.g. secondary to schistosomiasis/Bilharzia).

Malignant bladder cancers are predominantly (<90%) transitional cell carcinomas, arising from transitional cells found in the kidneys, ureters and bladder. Rarer bladder malignancies include squamous cell carcinoma, adenocarcinoma and sarcoma, which account for around 10% of bladder cancers. Squamous cell carcinomas arise typically in an area of metaplasia and can follow chronic inflammation, e.g. post schistosomiasis. They form large, bulky masses in the bladder. Adenocarcinomas arise from urachal remnants on the bladder dome.

Bladder cancers usually present with painless haematuria and occasionally symptoms of renal failure due to ureteric obstruction. In more advanced disease, patients can present with dysuria, frequency, urgency, clot formation and urinary retention.

Treatment depends on the level of differentiation as determined by biopsy, staging and presence of metastatic spread. Modalities of treatment typically consist of chemotherapy, radiotherapy and surgical resection. Five-year survival is variable, depending on the stage and grade of the tumour.

Bladder malignancy (2)

23 B   T2 N0 M0

The TNM classification of bladder cancer is shown in the table below.

Tis	Carcinoma *in situ*
Ta	Papillary non I–IV carcinoma
T1	Tumour extends through lamina propria
T2	Tumour invades muscle
T2a	Tumour invades superficial muscle
T2b	Tumour invades deep muscle
T3	Tumour invades peri-vesical tissue
T3a	Microscopic invasion
T3b	Macroscopic invasion
T4	Tumour invades adjacent structures
T4a	Invades prostate, uterus or vagina
T4b	Pelvic/abdominal wall invasion
Nx	Level of nodal involvement unknown
N0	No nodes involved
N1	Single lymph node metastasis <2 cm
N2	Single node 2–5 cm or multiple nodes >5 cm
N3	Metastasis >5 cm
Mx	Degree of metastatic spread unknown
M0	No distant metastasis
M1	Distant metastasis present

Treatment of bladder carcinoma depends on tumour stage:

- Superficial disease (i.e. Tis, Ta and T1) is treated with trans-urethral resection of bladder tumour (TURBT) ± intravesical therapy. Patients are followed up with regular cystoscopy as there is a risk of developing invasive disease.
- Intravesical therapy consists of mitomycin C or BCG for 6 weeks.
- Radical therapy is reserved for patients with extensive disease and those who fail to respond to intravesical treatment.

Intervention includes radical cystectomy (with bladder reconstruction surgery) and radiotherapy.
- Metastatic disease can be treated with platinum-based chemotherapy.

Testicular malignancy (1)

24 E 5-year survival for seminomas is approximately 90%

Testicular malignancy is the commonest solid tumour in young men, but accounts for approximately 1%–2% of all male cancers in the United Kingdom. Individuals with undescended testicles, infertile parents and a previous contralateral malignancy are at an increased risk.

Testicular tumours are divided into three broad groups: stromal tumours, lymphomas and germ cell tumours. Stromal tumours are those arising from Leydig's cells (which secrete androgens and can cause infantile Hercules' syndrome) and Sertoli's cells (these secrete androgens and individuals can present with testicular feminization). Approximately 10% are malignant. Lymphomas account for <10% of testicular tumours, occurring predominantly in elderly men, and have a poor prognosis.

Germ cell tumours comprise the majority of testicular tumours (80%–90%) and are subdivided into two main types: seminomas and non-seminomatous germ cell tumours. Seminomas arise from germinal cells in the testes and are solid and slow growing. They comprise approximately 42% of germ cell tumours and are extremely radiosensitive, giving an excellent prognosis with a 5-year survival rate of around 90%. NSGCTs account for almost 60% of germ cell tumours and also have many subtypes of which teratomas are the most common. Teratomas usually affect individuals aged 15–35 years and are believed to originate from totipotent cells. They can be solid or cystic in nature.

Most patients will present with a painless lump in the testicle although a small proportion may present with testicular pain. Occasionally, patients will complain of haematospermia and gynaecomastia (as a result of ß-hCG production). Infrequently, patients will present with signs of disseminated disease such as shortness of breath, bone pain and a palpable abdominal mass (due to enlarged para-aortic lymph nodes). These malignancies can also produce tumour markers including AFP and ß-hCG. Both markers are produced by teratomas whereas seminomas may produce AFP alone. Treatment is dependent on the type, grade and stage of the malignancy, and includes radical orchidectomy, chemotherapy and radiotherapy.

Testicular malignancy (2)

25 A **Para-aortic lymph nodes**

Seminoma is a type of germ cell tumour of the testicle, predominantly affecting individuals aged 20–40 years. Vascular supply to the testicles is from the testicular artery, a branch of the abdominal aorta that travels through the inguinal canal to reach the testicles. Lymphatic drainage of the testicles follows the arterial supply back to the aorta and as a result initial dissemination of testicular malignancies is in the para-aortic lymph nodes.

The anterior cervical chain of nodes lies above and below the sternocleidomastoid muscle in the neck and drains the throat, posterior pharynx, tonsils and thyroid gland. Meanwhile, the posterior cervical chain lies posterior to the sternocleidomastoid muscle (and anterior to the trapezius) and can become enlarged during upper respiratory tract infections. The superficial inguinal lymph nodes drain lymph from the scrotum, while the deep nodes can become enlarged as a result of spread from anal and vulval malignancies. The deep nodes drain to the external iliac, pelvic and finally para-aortic lymph nodes.

Carcinoma of the penis

26 B **Incidence is lower in men infected with the human papilloma virus**

Carcinoma of the penis is a rare squamous cell carcinoma originating predominantly in the glans penis or foreskin and accounting for around 1% of male malignancy. It is extremely rare in individuals circumcised at a young age and thought to result from chronic irritation due to balanitis and smegma. Incidence is also higher in individuals with HPV infection (particularly serotypes 16, 18 and 31).

Patients usually present with a painless lesion (an erythematous indurated area, ulcer or wart) on the glans, prepuce or foreskin. Patients will often delay consulting a medical practitioner, and as a result may have palpable inguinal lymph nodes at the time of initial presentation.

The disease is staged by the TNM classification, with treatment being dependent on staging. Local disease may be treated simply with local biopsy or circumcision, while more advanced disease may require topical chemotherapy (e.g. with 5-fluorouracil) or even partial or total amputation of the penis if there is poorly differentiated or locally advanced disease. Patients with palpable inguinal lymph nodes may or may not have disseminated disease. Antibiotic therapy is used to treat the underlying infection that could be confounding an individual's presentation. If lymph nodes remain palpable despite treatment, then bilateral inguinal lymphadenectomy with *en bloc* dissection may be needed to clear the disease.

The 80% 5-year survival is dependent on tumour stage and the presence of metastatic disease. Overall survival is approximately 50%, but can be as low as 20% in patients with iliac node involvement or as high as 90% in those with only local disease without metastatic spread.

Peyronie's disease

27 C **It is the result of a gene mutation on chromosome 5**

Peyronie's disease is an eponymously named connective tissue disorder of unknown origin, resulting in growth of fibrous plaques in the tunica albuginea and the corpus cavernosum. The disease affects approximately 1% of mainly middle-aged men, causing the penis to curve abnormally on erection (at the point at which fibrous plaques are present), and resulting in pain. The presence of pain and abnormal penile curvature can make sexual intercourse difficult and lead to erectile dysfunction. The condition is also associated with Dupuytren's and plantar fascial contractures.

Treatment is initially conservative for 1 year to allow the disease process and pain to stabilize. ESWL can be used to soften or destroy the penile plaque, but there haven't been any long-term follow-up studies of this procedure.

Surgical management is generally considered after 1 year especially if the condition is causing sexual dysfunction. Three main procedures are used:

- Nesbit's operation – Tunica albuginea on the opposite side of the offending plaque is excised, leading to return of normal curvature but also penile shortening.
- Plaque excision and patching – Can lead to softer erections.
- Implantation of penile prosthesis – Straightens penis in men with pre-existing erectile dysfunction.

Anatomy of the prostate gland

28 D **Internal iliac artery**

The prostate gland is a conical shaped structure lying inferior to the bladder in men and surrounds the prostatic urethra. It functions to produce an alkaline fluid that builds up seminal fluid. It is supplied by branches of the inferior vesical and middle rectal arteries, which are two of the branches of the internal iliac artery. Venous drainage is via the prostatic venous plexus, which drains into the internal iliac vein and occasionally into the vertebral venous plexus. Lymphatic drainage of the gland is to the internal iliac nodes.

Prostatic disease

29 A   Transition zone

This scenario describes a case of BPH. The prostate gland is composed primarily of glandular tissue, with fibromuscular stroma contributing the rest of its mass. It is composed of three lobes (anterior, posterior and median) formed by four tissue layers:

- Transition zone – Innermost tissue layer of the prostate that surrounds the urethra proximal to the ejaculatory ducts and is enlarged in BPH, leading to the associated signs and symptoms described.
- Central zone – Surrounds the ejaculatory ducts and projects beneath the bladder to the seminal vesicles.
- Peripheral zone – Most cancers of the prostate arise here (causing the bulky and the irregular prostate to be palpable on rectal examination).
- Anterior fibromuscular stroma.

ant .fibr .

perip.

Benign prostatic hypertrophy is the benign enlargement of stromal and glandular tissue within the inner transition zone of the prostate gland. This process is thought to result from a steroid hormone imbalance causing a proportionately increased level of oestrogen as compared with testosterone within the body. As a result, the elevated levels of oestrogen inhibit the elimination of DHT from the prostate. It is more common in middle-aged and elderly individuals, affecting most men by the age of 80. Presentation can be asymptomatic, i.e. found coincidentally, with lower urinary tract symptoms (which may develop over weeks or months) or urinary retention.

Lower urinary tract symptoms include:

- Voiding symptoms, e.g. hesitancy, straining, poor stream, terminal dribbling and strangury (the sensation of incomplete voiding).
- Storage symptoms, e.g. frequency, urgency, nocturia, overflow incontinence.
- Other symptoms – UTI, bladder stones due to stasis, occasional haematuria.

Physical examination may reveal a palpable, enlarged bladder, which may also cause pain. This must be relieved by urinary or suprapubic catheterization. In addition, a digital rectal examination will reveal a smoothly enlarged prostate but this does not always correlate with the patient's symptoms. Key investigations in addition to routine blood tests are PSA level, although this is not specific for investigation of LUTS, and ultrasound scan of the renal tract, to rule out any other abnormalities.

doxazosin

Medical treatment is with α-blockers such as alfuzosin and tamsulosin, which relax prostatic and bladder neck smooth muscle to increase urine flow, or with 5-α-reductase inhibitors, e.g. finasteride or dutasteride, which prevent the formation of dihydrotestosterone and reduce prostate size.

Surgical management is reserved for those with ongoing symptoms despite medical intervention and most commonly involves TURP to reduce prostatic volume.

Prostate cancer

30 D   T2 Nx Mx

Cancer of the prostate is the most common cancer in men and the third most common cause of death (in men) due to cancer. Several different classification systems exist to stage prostate cancers, of which the TNM classification is the most widely used (see Table 11.2). In the case described, it is known that the prostate gland is mis-shapen on rectal examination and in addition the tumour remains within the capsule of the prostate gland. There is no indication in the scenario of lymph involvement or the presence of metastases. As a result the tumour stage would be T2 Nx Mx – x indicating that the involvement of lymph nodes and presence of metastases is unknown.

Table 11.2 TNM classification of prostate cancer

Tis	Carcinoma *in situ*
T1	Incidental finding
T2	Intracapsular tumour with deformation of the prostate
T3	Extra-prostatic extension
T4	Tumour fixed to the pelvis
Nx	Level of nodal involvement unknown
N0	No lymph node involvement
N1–4	One or more lymph node systems involved to varying levels
Mx	Degree of metastatic spread unknown
M0	No distant metastases
M1	Metastases to a distant site, e.g. spine

SECTION 12: ORTHOPAEDICS

Questions

1. Orthopaedic disease and management
    of fractures   259
2. Orthopaedic examination   259
3. Common musculoskeletal pathology (1)   259
4. Common musculoskeletal pathology (2)   259
5. Common musculoskeletal pathology (3)   260
6. Rheumatoid arthritis   260
7. Systemic manifestations of rheumatoid arthritis   260
8. Dupuytren's contracture   260
9. Fracture patterns   260
10. The carpal tunnel   261
11. Carpal tunnel syndrome (1)   261
12. Arthritis and the hand   261
13. Soft tissue pathology   261
14. Carpal tunnel syndrome (2)   262
15. Anatomy of the shoulder   262
16. Common shoulder pathology (1)   262
17. Common shoulder pathology (2)   262
18. Muscle lumps   263
19. Bone pathology   263
20. Disorders of bone   263
21. Paget's disease of the bone   263
22. Bone disease   264
23. Management of osteoporosis   264
24. Acute limb pain   264
25. Septic arthritis   265
26. Crystalline arthropathy   265

27. Acutely hot joint   265
28. Spinal cord injury   265
29. Spinal cord compression   266
30. Lumbar disc herniation   266

Answers   267

QUESTIONS

1. Orthopaedic disease and management of fractures

You are asked to see a patient in the outpatient clinic. The patient has weakness in her left arm following a car accident 1 month ago when she fractured her left arm. On examination, there is weakness of extension of the fingers and wrist on the left side. However, the sensation is maintained in all distributions and there is *no* wrist drop. Which one of the following fractures classically associated with nerve damage is the most likely cause of this palsy?

- Ⓐ   Fracture of head of radius
- B.   Fracture of shaft of humerus
- C.   Medial epicondyle of humerus
- D.   Fracture of shaft of ulna
- E.   Fracture of neck of femur

injury of radial.n
wrist extension
(extensor carpi radialis longus)
and sensation spared.

2. Orthopaedic examination

On assessment of a patient in the outpatients department you identify that they are Trendelenburg's test positive. This indicates a possible palsy of which nerve?

one gluteal muscle weak.

- A.   Sciatic
- B.   Femoral
- C.   Obturator
- Ⓓ   Superior gluteal → *medius and minimus (hip abductors)*
- E.   Inferior gluteal → *maximus*

3. Common musculoskeletal pathology (1)

The most common cause of an acquired valgus deformity of the knee joint is

- A.   Rheumatoid arthritis
- B.   Osteoporosis
- C.   Trauma
- Ⓓ   Osteoarthritis
- E.   Osteomalacia

Valgus   *Varus*

4. Common musculoskeletal pathology (2)

Which of the following is the most common secondary cause of haemarthrosis of the knee?

- A.   Meniscal tear   *10% if tear extends to cartilage*
- Ⓑ   Anterior cruciate ligament injury   *80%*
- C.   Osteophyte fracture *important but rare cause*
- D.   Posterior cruciate ligament injury → *less significant hemarthrosis*
- E.   Patella dislocation *(10%)*

5. Common musculoskeletal pathology (3)

Which of the following options is *not* a clinical feature common in osteoarthritis and rheumatoid arthritis of the knee?

A. Muscle wasting
B. Joint effusion
C. Baker's cyst
D. Raised C-reactive protein
E. Subcutaneous nodules

shared by both

RA has extra-articular features

OA does not

6. Rheumatoid arthritis

Rheumatoid arthritis is a multisystem connective tissue disease. Which of the following is *not* a pulmonary complication of rheumatoid arthritis?

A. Effusion
B. Obstructive lung disease *35-50%*
C. Restrictive lung disease
D. Cavitation *→ of pulmonary nodules*
E. Emphysema

7. Systemic manifestations of rheumatoid arthritis

All of the following are dermatological manifestations of rheumatoid arthritis, except

A. Palmar erythema
B. Erythema nodosum *→ IBD?*
C. Pyoderma gangrenosum
D. Livedo reticularis
E. Skin nodules

8. Dupuytren's contracture *(ABCDEFF Mnemonic)*

Dupuytren's contracture is caused by a thickening of the palmar fascia. It is associated with the following conditions, except

A. Alcoholic cirrhosis
B. Peyronie's disease *— Bent penis*
C. Acquired immune deficiency syndrome
D. Epilepsy
E. Syphilis

AIDS
Bent Penis
Cirrhosis
DM
Epilepsy
Familial
Fibromatoses

9. Fracture patterns

Your registrar tells you that his patient has a boxer's fracture. From this, you know that the bone which is fractured is

Snuffbox →
area of scaphoid

A. The fifth metacarpal
B. The fourth metacarpal
C. The fifth proximal phalanx
D. Hamate
E. Styloid process

10. The carpal tunnel

Which one of the following intrinsic muscles of the hand is *not* innervated by the median nerve?

A. First lumbrical
B. Abductor pollicis brevis
C. Opponens pollicis
D. Adductor pollicis
E. Flexor pollicis brevis

Median

thenar musc. {
Abductor poll brevis
Flexor pollicis
Opponens pollicis
}
2 lumbricals

11. Carpal tunnel syndrome (1)

All of the following are causes of carpal tunnel syndrome, except

A. Hypothyroidism
B. Amyloidosis
C. Alcoholism
D. Gout
E. Rheumatoid arthritis

12. Arthritis and the hand

Which of the following pathological changes is not a feature of rheumatoid disease of the hand?

A. Boutonnière's deformity
B. Z line thumb
C. Squaring of the thumb   → *in OA   (+ Bouchard and Heberden nodes)*
D. Ulnar deviation
E. Swan-neck deformity

13. Soft tissue pathology

A patient presents to his GP surgery complaining of a swelling on his wrist. On examination, there is a focal swelling on the dorsal aspect of the wrist. It is smooth and non-tender. The overlying skin is normal and moves freely over the mass, however it seems to be fixed to the tendon. What is the likely diagnosis?

A. Sebaceous cyst   *← usually fixed to skin*
B. Lipoma
   ↖ no fat in tendon

C. Ganglion
D. Giant cell tumour of the tendon sheath ⟩ extremely rare
E. Fibroma

14. Carpal tunnel syndrome (2)

A patient presents to the outpatients department following referral for carpal tunnel syndrome. While taking the history and examining the patient you attempt to evaluate whether any permanent nerve injury has occurred. Which sign is often the first indicator of lasting nerve injury?

A. Pins and needles
B. Thenar muscle wasting
C. Night pain
D. Reduced two-point discrimination
E. Positive Phalen's test

15. Anatomy of the shoulder

Which of the following muscles is not part of the rotator cuff?

A. Pectoralis minor
B. Subscapularis   u. and L. subscap.n
C. Supraspinous — suprascap n
D. Teres minor — axillry n
E. Infraspinous — suprascup n
    circumflex scapa
    Subscap a

16. Common shoulder pathology (1)

A patient presents with symptoms suggestive of adhesive capsulitis (frozen shoulder). Which of the following systemic conditions is most commonly associated with this?

A. Fibrotic lung disease
B. Systemic lupus erythematosus
C. Sjögren's syndrome
D. Osteoarthritis
E. Diabetes

17. Common shoulder pathology (2)

A patient with longstanding osteoarthritis presents with pain on movement of his shoulder. You perform a full shoulder exam. You note that you can re-create the pain by asking the patient to abduct his shoulder against resistance. You conclude that there is impingement of which one of the following structures?

A. Teres minor
B. Supraspinatus   abduction

C.   Infraspinatus   → *lat rotation*
D.   Subscapularis   → *medial rotation*
E.   Subacromial bursa

18. Muscle lumps

A 37-year-old patient presents to you having noticed a lump on the lateral aspect of his leg. The lump was first noticed while the patient was in the gym on a rowing machine. There is no associated pain. On examination when the patient tenses his quadriceps a smooth lump can be appreciated, which disappears when the leg is relaxed. With the leg relaxed, it is possible to identify a depression in the fascia lata. The diagnosis is

A.   Intramuscular haematoma   → *less prominent when muscle is tensed*
B.   Partial quadriceps rupture
C.   Muscle hernia
D.   Intermuscular lipomata   *— less prominent like hematoma, found on back or trunk.*
E.   Myosarcoma

19. Bone pathology

Out of the following bone pathologies, which is *not* correctly matched to the most common site at which it occurs?

A.   Enchondroma – Bones of hands and feet
B.   Osteoma – Cranial vault and skull
C.   Ewing's sarcoma – Mid-shaft femur
D.   Osteosarcoma – Femur, just above the knee
E.   Osteomyelitis – Mid-shaft long bone
     affects metaphysis → usually in childhood

20. Disorders of bone

A 19-year-old man presents having noticed a hard lump above his knee. He initially noticed the lump 3 years ago, but presents now after his girlfriend persuaded him to find out what it is. He does not complain of any associated symptoms. Radiographic investigation demonstrates a knob of bone on the surface of the distal femur, which projects away from the knee joint. The most likely diagnosis is

A.   Ossification of quadriceps tendon
B.   Exostosis *development abberant*
C.   Enchondroma   *— benign — hands and feet*
D.   Osteoma   *— forehead and vault of skull → Slow growing.*
E.   Osteosarcoma   *— long bones*

21. Paget's disease of the bone

Which one of the following statements regarding Paget's disease of the bone is *not* correct?

A. It most commonly occurs in the pelvis
B. It more commonly affects a single bone
C. It occurs in 3% of all individuals over 40 in the United Kingdom
D. Characteristic biochemical findings include raised serum alkaline phosphatase, normal calcium and normal phosphate
E. 1% of cases will develop osteosarcoma

22. Bone disease

Looser's zones (also known as pseudofractures) are a radiographic feature characterizing which one of the following bone diseases?

A. Osteomalacia Vit D deficiency in adults
B. Osteoporosis
C. Gout
D. Paget's disease
E. Osteomyelitis

23. Management of osteoporosis

According to the current National Institute for Health and Clinical Excellence guidelines all of the following are indications for the use of bisphosphonates in the treatment of osteoporosis, except

A. Any patient with a fracture over the age of 65 → 75 not 65!.
B. Any patient with a fracture aged 65–75 *and* a T score less than –2.5
C. Any patient with a fracture aged <65 *and* a T score less than –3.0
D. Any patient taking high-dose systemic steroids for more than 3 months with a T score less than –1.3
E. Any smoker with a fracture aged <65 *and* a T score less than –2.5

24. Acute limb pain

sicklecell disease?

A 10-year-old African Caribbean boy is referred to the orthopaedic team with an acutely painful arm. On examination, there is a notable swelling of the limb above and around the elbow joint. There is no reduced range of passive movement of the joint, but the boy is holding his arm very still and will not actively move the limb. Investigations include haemoglobin 8.3 g/dL, white cell count 10.5×10^9/L, and C-reactive protein 12 mg/L. The child is apyrexial with a blood pressure of 110/75 mmHg, and a pulse rate of 85 beats/min.

A. Septic arthritis } Inflammatory markers are normal
B. Osteomyelitis }
C. Bony infarct
D. Gout — rare in this age unless its syndromic
E. Juvenile arthritis
   ↓ also rare
   but poly articular.

25. Septic arthritis

Which one of the following organisms is most commonly associated with septic arthritis?

A. Gram negative bacilli → 2° to GII Infections
B. *Haemophilus influenzae* → <3y
C. ß-haemolytic streptococci
D. *Streptococcus pneumoniae* — may also have pneumonia
Ⓔ *Staphylococcus aureus* — most common

26. Crystalline arthropathy

Which of the following conditions/factors does *not* predispose to gout?

A. Lesch–Nyhan syndrome → deficient enzyme in salvage pathway?
B. Psoriasis — ↑ cell turnover
C. Aspirin — inhibits urate excretion
Ⓓ Xanthine oxidase deficiency   XO → converts xanthine
E. Alcohol   to urate

27. Acutely hot joint

A 56-year-old man is admitted with pyrexia and an acutely painful knee. On examination, the patient is holding the joint rigidly still and is extremely reluctant to let you manipulate the joint. The knee is obviously effused and erythematous. Joint aspirate is strongly positive for white cells ($75000/mm^3$) with polymorphs accounting for 90% of these. Blood tests show a raised urate level. The diagnosis is

A. Osteomyelitis → rare in adults unless other comorbidities present
Ⓑ Septic arthritis
C. Gout → high urate does not always mean gout
D. Pseudogout
E. Monoarticular acute rheumatoid arthritis

28. Spinal cord injury

A patient presents to the outpatients department following a car accident in which she has hurt her neck. Since then she has noticed some numbness in her right shoulder and neck pain. On examination you note weakness in shoulder abduction, elbow flexion, absent biceps reflex, and paraesthesia affecting the badge area over her right shoulder. The most likely diagnosis is

A. Spinal cord compression   C5
Ⓑ Radiculopathy
C. Musculocutaneous nerve injury
D. Axillary nerve injury
E. Brown–Séquard syndrome

29. Spinal cord compression

A patient is admitted from the emergency department with new and sudden-onset urinary incontinence. The patient has previously been seen in the back pain clinic by the orthopaedic team. On examination you note a large palpable bladder. Neurological examination reveals weakness of knee flexion on the right, plantar flexion of the left and reduced ankle jerks bilaterally. Plantars are down-going on both sides. You also note patchy mixed sensory loss bilaterally. The diagnosis is

A. Cauda equina syndrome
B. L3 radiculopathy
C. Conus medullaris
D. S1 level cord compression
E. Anterior cord syndrome

30. Lumbar disc herniation

A patient is being investigated for sciatica. On detailed neurological examination you elicit the following signs: sensory loss over the outer calf and dorsum of foot, weakness in dorsiflexion of toes, normal ankle reflexes, normal knee reflexes, painful straight leg raise, normal femoral nerve stretch test. At which level is the disc protrusion?

A. L2/3
B. L3/4
C. L4/5
D. L5/S1
E. S1/S2

affecting L5

femoral n stretch test will be +ve.

√ Straight leg will be painful

ANSWERS

Orthopaedic disease and management of fractures

1 A Fracture of head of radius

Candidates who are able to answer this level of question are those heading for honours. It tests candidates' knowledge of the functional anatomy of the nerve supply to the upper limb. The nerve involved is obviously the radial nerve; its course winds around the shaft of the humerus before entering the forearm laterally and running adjacent to the head of the radius. Option E is obviously wrong. Options C and D are also wrong as the radial nerve runs laterally. Medial epicondyle fractures are associated with ulnar nerve palsies, and not radial nerve injury.

Both fractured head of radius and a fractured shaft of the humerus may cause radial nerve damage. However, in the above case the sensation to the arm is maintained, as is wrist extension. This implicates a fracture of the head of the radius; proximal to the elbow, the radial nerve gives off several branches: the posterior interosseous nerve, the superficial radial nerve, which is the sensory branch, as well as a branch supplying the extensor carpi radialis longus. Head of radius fractures damage the posterior interosseous nerve only. This fracture therefore results in a palsy that spares sensation and wrist extension, while all other extensor function is lost.

Orthopaedic examination

2 D Superior gluteal

The detail of anatomy teaching varies greatly between medical schools. However, some essential points should be consistently taught. Trendelenburg's sign and gait should be correctly elicited or described by all final year candidates and candidates should expect to be able to talk about common causes and compartmental anatomy of the lower limb.

Trendelenburg's gait and test manifest secondary to hip abductor weakness. This may occur due to an abnormality in the muscle, the nerve or in the connections between the two. The most common cause is muscle wasting in patients with degenerative joint disease or chronic hip pain. Other causes include muscle damage following multiple surgeries, structural joint diseases such as developmental hip dysplasia and neuromuscular diseases such as polio and Guillian-Barré.

The nerve supply to the hip abductors (gluteus medius and minimus) is from the superior gluteal nerve; the inferior gluteal nerve supplies gluteus maximus. The superior gluteal nerve exits the greater sciatic foramen and lies in close approximation to the greater trochanter, where it may become damaged following trauma or surgery.

Common musculoskeletal pathology (1)

3 D Osteoarthritis

The concept that OA predominantly causes a varus deformity of the knee, whereas RA causes a valgus deformity, is a favoured question in exams but is of limited use in clinical practice. In reality, both diseases can cause either valgus or varus deformity, depending on the pattern of joint involvement. What is true is that OA more commonly affects the medial compartment of the knee, and therefore more commonly causes a varus deformity, and the inverse can be said of RA. However, since OA of the knee affects 40% of those over the age of 75, the most common cause of valgus deformation of the knee is OA, not RA.

If candidates are asked to differentiate between OA and RA in an exam, they should take account of the patient's age and other joint involvement, and ask for a radiograph of the joint in question. It is not possible to differentiate between OA and RA on examining an isolated knee joint alone.

Common musculoskeletal pathology (2)

4 B Anterior cruciate ligament injury

Haemarthrosis may be primary or secondary. Primary haemarthrosis indicates a spontaneous bleed into the joint, which may be because of inherited coagulopathy or may be drug (warfarin) induced. Secondary haemarthrosis is consequent to traumatic injury.

Anterior cruciate ligament injury causes rapid accumulation of blood within the joint and accounts for 80% of traumatic haemarthrosis. Posterior cruciate ligament injury is less commonly associated with significant haemarthrosis. Ten per cent of haemarthrosis is caused by patella dislocation, and an additional 10% is caused by meniscal injury where the tear extends into the peripheral third of the cartilage where it is vascularised. Osteophyte fracture is an important cause, but rarer than capsular/ligament injury.

NB: 25% of ligament/capsular injuries severe enough to cause haemarthrosis also have significant associated cartilage injury. Therefore, all such injuries will require follow-up MRI/arthroscopy.

Common musculoskeletal pathology (3)

5 E Subcutaneous nodules

Osteoarthritis and RA are both degenerative diseases affecting the joints. Osteoarthritis is commonly thought of as a disease of 'wear and tear'. However, a clinician should be aware that aetiology is multifactorial and local joint inflammation has a significant role in the progression, probably as part of a deranged repair response to cartilage injury.

Therefore, joint effusion, synovitis and raised inflammatory markers are common features in both diseases, although the inflammation in rheumatoid disease is more severe.

As degenerative diseases, both RA and OA weaken the joint capsule and Baker's cyst formation may occur in either condition, although rupture is classically associated with active RA. Muscle wasting occurs as a consequence of local inflammation and reduced use of the joint secondary to pain. The vastus medialis muscle is the first to atrophy with disuse and its bulk is best assessed by measuring the thigh circumference 15–20 cm proximal to the tibial tuberosity. The key difference between RA and OA is that the former is a systemic connective tissue disorder, therefore the presence of extra-articular manifestations are only associated with RA. The nodules in OA are bony and periarticular, not subcutaneous.

Rheumatoid arthritis

6 E   Emphysema

The extra-articular manifestations of RA are truly numerous and are beyond the scope of this text. As well as patterns of joint involvement candidates should familiarize themselves with the cutaneous, ocular, pulmonary, cardiovascular and haematological complications complicit with this complex and common disease.

Rheumatoid lung is a term used to describe a restrictive deficit secondary to fibrosis and accounts for 20% of pulmonary complications associated with RA. Pleuritis is also common (5%) presenting with chest pain and (exudative) pulmonary effusions. Pulmonary nodules are histologically similar to cutaneous nodules; they are typically peripherally placed and asymptomatic, but may cavitate. In the presence of pneumoconiosis, pulmonary nodules may cause large cavitating lesions (Caplin's syndrome) with associated respiratory compromise, but this is becoming increasingly rare in the UK following the collapse of the mining industry and improved health and safety on industrial sites.

However, the most common pulmonary manifestation in RA is an obstructive lung disease, which accounts for 35%–50% of all RA pulmonary disease. Patients present with wheeze and exertional dyspnoea similar to COPD, however the underlying pathology is bronchiolitis, and not emphysema.

Systemic manifestations of rheumatoid arthritis

7 B   Erythema nodosum

Dermatological manifestations of systemic diseases are beloved of examiners almost as much as they are hated by those sitting the exam. The question lists some of the most commonly asked about cutaneous

signs associated with systemic conditions, and candidates should know
the appearance and be able to list a differential diagnosis for each.
Erythema nodosum is the only one which is not seen in association
with RA.

Dupuytren's contracture

8   E   Syphilis

Dupuytren's contracture is a deformity caused by thickening of the
palmer fascia, which results in finger flexion. The differential diagnosis
includes skin fibrosis (look for previous scarring), tendon fibrosis and
ulna nerve palsy. Tendon contracture and Dupuytren's may be differentiated clinically by passively flexing the fingers; in tendon contracture
the thickened area will move with flexion, in Dupuytren's it will not.
Also look for Garrod's pads, thickened subcutaneous tissue over the
dorsal aspect of the PIPJs. The exact cause is unknown, but it is 10
times more prevalent in men, most commonly occurring in middle age.
It is associated with repetitive trauma in manual workers. Dupuytren's
is also associated with various systemic conditions which makes it a
common exam subject, although it is important to remember idiopathic
Dupuytren's is more common. The following mnemonic (ABCDEF) may
be of use:

- AIDS
- Bent penis – Peyronie's disease disease is fibrosis of the corpus
  cavernosum, seen in 3% of Dupuytren's
- Cirrhosis – Particularly alcoholic liver disease
- Diabetes mellitus
- Epilepsy and anti-epileptic medication (particularly phenytoin)
- Familial (autosomal dominant)
- Fibromatoses – A group of disorders characterized by dif-
  fuse fibrosis. A patient may develop each in isolation, or may
  develop several over the course of their life. Such conditions
  include Reidel's thyroiditis, retroperitoneal fibrosis, Ledderhose
  disease and desmoid tumours.

Fracture patterns

9   A   The fifth metacarpal

A boxer's fracture is a fracture of the fifth metacarpal bone, so called
because it typically occurs when a closed fist strikes a solid surface.
Although required knowledge of fracture patterns is limited in most
medical schools, the commonest should be familiar to finals candidates.
The most commonly asked about fractures at the author's own school
are Colles', Smith's, Barton's, Monteggia's and Galeazzi's fractures, as
well as boxer's fracture.

The carpal tunnel

10 D Adductor pollicis

The anatomy of the nervous supply to the hand is an extremely common examination topic throughout medical school, and especially in finals examinations. Put simply, the ulnar nerve supplies all intrinsic muscles of the hand, except the 'LOAF' muscles:

- First and second lumbricals
- Opponens pollicis
- Abductor pollicis brevis
- Flexor pollicis brevis

These LOAF muscles are supplied by the median nerve. In reality it can be difficult to isolate between median and ulnar function, as the lumbricals are difficult to test, the action of opponens pollicis is supplemented by other muscles such as adductor pollicis, and is therefore impossible to isolate, and flexor pollicis has a variable innervation. Therefore, in an exam, the only way of truly isolating median nerve function is to test abductor pollicis brevis (raise thumb to the ceiling while the palm is facing up); this muscle is therefore said to have an autonomous motor supply.

Similarly, to truly isolate ulnar motor function, test the palmar interossei (finger adduction) and the radial nerve by assessing finger extension at the MCPJ.

Carpal tunnel syndrome (1)

11 C Alcoholism

Carpal tunnel syndrome is a palsy secondary to nerve compression within the narrow confines of the carpal tunnel. Chronic compression impairs the blood supply to the nerve fibres, which results in fibrosis and impaired conduction. The clinical syndrome is one of altered sensation, aching pain (especially at night) and muscle weakness and wasting affecting the thenar eminence. It occurs more commonly in women than men and the cause is most commonly idiopathic. Secondary causes are all conditions where the space within the carpal tunnel becomes compromised. These include:

- Anatomical abnormalities – Deformity following previous fracture
- Soft tissue proliferation – Obesity, lipoma, ganglion, acromegaly, amyloidosis
- Inflammation – RA, gout
- Diabetes – Due to abnormal collagen proliferation within the endoneurium.
- Fluid balance aberration – Pregnancy, menopause, hypothyroidism, renal failure

Peripheral neuropathies due to alcoholism, vitamin B_{12} deficiency, etc. may mimic carpal tunnel syndrome but since their mechanism is not compressive, they cannot be considered as causes of carpal tunnel syndrome.

Arthritis and the hand

12 C Squaring of the thumb

This easy question is assessing basic knowledge of a common condition in clinical practice and examinations. Squaring of the thumb is a feature of OA of the hands along with Bouchard's nodes (PIPJ) and Heberden's nodes (DIPJ).

Signs of rheumatoid disease of the hand are more numerous:

- Z thumb – Flexion of the interphalangeal joint with hyperextension of MCPJ
- Fixed ulnar deviation of fingers – As opposed to Jaccoud's deformity in SLE, where fingers appear normal in extension but ulnar deviation occurs on flexion
- Swan-neck deformity – Due to fibrosis of the interosseous and lumbrical muscles, forcing a hyperextension of PIPJ and flexion of DIPJ
- Boutonnià re deformity – Due to trapping of a flexed PIPJ through a rupture in the central portion of the extensor tendon expansion, resulting in fixed flexion of the PIPJ and hyperextension of DIPJ.
- Radial deviation of the wrist
- Volar subluxation of the wrist
- Volar subluxation of the MCPJs

Soft tissue pathology

13 C Ganglion

The lump in question is not fixed to the skin, therefore sebaceous cyst can effectively be excluded as a possible diagnosis. Similarly, fixation to the tendon excludes lipoma as a possible diagnosis, as there is no fatty tissue in tendons. The three remaining entities may be difficult to differentiate clinically, but fibroma and giant cell tumours are extremely rare and therefore ganglion is the best answer in this case.

A ganglion is a cystic degeneration of fibrous tissue. They therefore occur most commonly around joints and tendon sheaths. Candidates should be clear that they are not degenerations or projections of synovial membranes. Ninety per cent of ganglia occur in association with the wrist joint and tendons of the hand.

Carpal tunnel syndrome (2)

14 D   Reduced two-point discrimination

As alluded to in Question 11, carpal tunnel syndrome is caused by compression of the median nerve within the carpal tunnel. This compression damages the nerve by inducing a state of chronic ischaemia, the consequences of which include fibroblast proliferation and impairment of nerve function.

Night pain and pins and needles are two common early symptoms which occur due to ischaemia of the nerve axon. They are, however, reversible and patients learn various tricks to alleviate their discomfort, such as hanging the affected hand out of the bed or shaking it, which re-establishes perfusion through the vasa nervorum. A positive Phalen's test demonstrates the medial nerve is susceptible to pressure, but does not indicate the presence of lasting damage. Reduced two-point discrimination, however, indicates a loss of nerve fibres which is rarely entirely reversible. Muscle wasting is a late sign of irreversible nerve damage and permanent loss of function.

Anatomy of the shoulder

15 A   Pectoralis minor

The shoulder joint actually comprises four joints: the sternoclavicular joint, the acromioclavicular joint, the glenohumeral joint and the scapulothoracic joint. The joint is highly reliant on supporting ligaments and muscles for stability, which is compromised for the sake of greater mobility. The rotator cuff is the assembly of muscles largely responsible for retaining the head of the humerus within the glenoid fossa, whilst also allowing free rotational movement in all planes. Of the muscles listed above, the pectoralis minor is the only one that does not contribute to the rotator cuff.

Common shoulder pathology (1)

16 E   Diabetes

Adhesive capsulitis is an uncommon condition where fibrotic contracture around the glenohumeral joint restricts movement. The diagnosis is clinical, and the disease is classically described as occurring in three stages: an initial painful phase, a painless 'locked' phase and a resolution phase, typically occurring sequentially over a period of several months. The fibrotic proliferation is similar in histology to that seen in Dupuytren's contracture, and there is a strong correlation between the two conditions. The classic association with adhesive capsulitis is diabetes mellitus although the underlying reasons are not known.

Common shoulder pathology (2)

17 B Supraspinatus

The coracoacromial arch is formed by the coracoid process, the anterior third of the acromion and the coracoacromial ligament which bridges between the two. Through this space run the ligaments of the four muscles of the rotator cuff, with the subacromial bursa providing some protection from friction. However, degenerative joint diseases commonly narrow this space, causing rubbing of tendons against bony structures and resultant inflammatory pain.

The most commonly affected tendon is that of supraspinatus; this classically results in pain on resisted shoulder abduction. The other muscles can be similarly isolated. Infraspinatus tendon impingement causes pain on resisted lateral rotation, subscapularis causes pain on resisted medial rotation. Teres minor is only rarely involved. Pain on all ranges of movement is suggestive of a subacromial bursitis.

Muscle lumps

18 C Muscle hernia

An intramuscular haematoma is a collection of blood around an injured muscle, which is typically painful and restricts movement. On examination, tensing the muscle will cause pain and the haematoma will become less prominent due to overlying muscle tissue. Intermuscular lipomata are lipomas occurring within the bulk of the muscle; they may be painful or painless, and may become more or less prominent on contraction depending on their position within the muscle, but they rarely occur in the limbs and most commonly are found on the back or trunk. Muscle rupture occurs in two main groups: athletes following injury when it is typically painful, and the elderly, in whom it occurs due to innate weakening of the tissue (the original incident may or may not be noticed). Typically, the muscle tear will not be palpable with the muscle relaxed, but a lump will become prominent on contraction. A muscle hernia is an extrusion of muscle fibres through a defect in its fibrous sheath. The most common site is the thigh. The hernia becomes more prominent on muscle contraction and less so on relaxation. The fascia defect may occasionally be palpable with the lump reduced. Primary muscle tumours (rhabdomyosarcoma = striated, leiomyosarcoma = smooth) are rare and are predominantly diseases of old age. Most soft tissue sarcomas are fibrosarcomas derived from fibrous tissue such as fascia, tendons and aponeuroses.

Bone pathology

19 E Osteomyelitis – mid-shaft long bone

Enchondromas and ecchondromas are benign cartilage growths occurring in the centre or the surface of a bone, respectively. They most commonly occur in the hands and feet, and rarely affect long bones. Osteomas are benign bone tumours of the cranial vault. Malignant bone tumours grow in characteristic sites which helps to define the likely diagnosis; osteosarcomas are the most common primary bone tumours and their most common sites (in order of prevalence) are distal femur, proximal tibia and proximal humerus. Giant cell tumours (also known as osteoclastoma) have a similar distribution. Ewing's sarcoma occurs in the centre of long bones, which aids its clinical distinction from other primary bone tumours. Osteomyelitis is a disease predominantly of childhood. This is because of the rich blood supply to the growth plate which allows bacterial seeding of the metaphysis and subsequent infection affecting the ends of long bones. The mid-shaft is rarely affected.

Disorders of bone

20 B   Exostosis

The key features of this history are that the lump is slow growing and asymptomatic; this effectively rules out a sarcoma. Osteosarcomas typically occur in the long bones, the most common site being the femur, just above the knee. Presentation is with bone pain and rapid growth, neither of which feature in the history. Examination reveals a firm mass which is often warm to palpation due to vastly increased vasculature; a bruit may also be heard. Enchondroma is a benign cartilage growth within a bone, which most commonly affects the hands and feet; the position of the lesion and radiographic features therefore preclude this diagnosis. Osteomas are benign, slow-growing bone tumours which most commonly occur on the forehead and the vault of the skull. The quadriceps tendon inserts into the patella, and therefore calcification of this structure cannot be considered a sensible diagnosis.

The radiographic findings, the positioning and the history are all consistent with the diagnosis of the exostosis. An exostosis is a developmental aberration caused when a small piece of metaphyseal cartilage becomes separated from the main growth plate. It continues to grow in its aberrant position on the side of the bone, and forms a bony knob, which typically points away from the adjacent joint. They are usually asymptomatic, but may interfere with muscle or tendon function.

Paget's disease of the bone

21 B   It most commonly affects a single bone

Paget's disease of the bone is a common (3%) condition which is largely underdiagnosed as the majority of those affected are asymptomatic. Features in those who are symptomatic include bony pain, fracture and deformity. Deformity occurs due to bone overgrowth, and may manifest as head enlargement (osteoporosis circumscripta) and long bone bowing and enlargement (sabre tibia). Complications include nerve compression within bony channels (particularly cranial nerves, spinal cord), fracture, high-output cardiac failure (due to increased bone vasculature necessitating increased cardiac output) and sarcomatous change, which will affect 1% of cases.

[handwritten margin note: affects multiple bones.]

Only 15% of cases are restricted to a single bone (mono-ostotic); the vast majority of cases are polyostotic, affecting (in order of sites most commonly involved) pelvis, lumbar spine, femur, thoracic spine, sacrum, skull and tibia. Diagnosis is based on characteristic biochemical and radiological findings.

Bone disease

22 A Osteomalacia *[handwritten: →pseudofractures]*

The majority of medical schools will expect their graduates to be able to differentiate metabolic bone pathology on plain radiographs and also in a viva scenario. Most candidates should at least be able to name the characteristic abnormalities of each of the conditions listed in the question.

[handwritten margin note: T < −25]

Osteoporosis is an age-related loss of bone mass with cortical thinning and loss of trabeculae. It is difficult to identify from plain films alone, but certain fracture patterns typify the weakness inherent in the abnormal bone, including vertebral crush fractures. Confirmation of the diagnosis requires DEXA scanning. Gout is typified by soft tissue gouty tophi, with plain films showing punched-out lesions away from the joint line. Paget's disease is a disorder of bone turnover; the radiographic features are variable, but include sclerotic and lytic lesions, with coarse irregular trabeculae. Osteomyelitis may show no abnormalities on radiographs; 50% will show periosteum lifting, which represents a subperiosteal abscess formed by pus tracking from the medullary canal. Later a sclerotic reaction may be seen on plain films. Osteomalacia is a disease of reduced bone quality, the mass is normal. It occurs secondary to the ineffective mineralization of the bone matrix, which may be due to dietary deficiency, abnormal uptake (gastrointestinal disease), abnormal metabolism (secondary to renal or liver failure) or the actions of certain drugs. The loss of cortical bone and failure of mineralization results in the radiographic appearance of Looser's zones: these are radiolucent lines through the cortex, which have the appearance of non-displaced partial fractures (pseudofractures).

Management of osteoporosis

23 A Any patient with a fracture over the age of 65

Osteoporosis is an extremely common condition; 1 in 3 women and 1 in 12 men will sustain a fracture secondary to osteoporosis by the age of 90. Investigation of bone density is by DEXA scanning, the result of which is expressed as a T score. A T score of −1 represents a BMD of 1 standard deviation below the mean of a normal population. The WHO definition of osteoporosis is a BMD less than 2.5 standard deviations below the mean (T score less than –2.5). Individuals with a T score between –1 and –2.5 meet the WHO criteria for osteopenia, but are not classed as having osteoporosis.

Current best practice regarding the use of bisphosphonates to treat osteoporosis is covered by NICE guidelines published in 2011. All of the above options are correct except for option A; the guidance states any individual over 75 who sustains a fracture should be offered bisphosphonates irrespective of their T score. Treatment of those under the age of 75 should be guided by DEXA scans. Bisphosphonates are also indicated in the prophylactic treatment of patients receiving steroid therapy of >7.5 mg daily for longer than 3 months.

In those under 65, bisphosphonates are only indicated if T score is less than –3.0 *or* less than –2.5 *with* an identified risk factor for osteoporosis. Risk factors include smoking, steroids, sedentary lifestyle, poor diet, alcohol, liver cirrhosis, hyperthyroidism/hyperparathyroidism, early menopause, amenorrhoea >6 months in women and hypogonadism in men. Anorexia nervosa is another common risk factor, with risk increasing once BMI <19 kg/m^2.

Acute limb pain

24 C Bony infarct

The clue is in the question; note that the question specifies the ethnic origin of the child and the full blood count shows he is anaemic. All candidates should identify that this boy may have sickle cell disease and that this may be a bony crisis. The question is made easier by the given scenario in which the infection markers are broadly normal making septic arthritis and osteomyelitis extremely unlikely; often diagnosis is clouded since infection is the most common trigger for a sickle crisis, and inflammatory markers will be raised. This makes the clinical distinction between bone or joint infection and bone infarction more difficult, and aspirates and MRI may be required. Gout in a child of this age is extremely rare, and would indicate an enzyme deficiency and hereditary disease. Juvenile arthritis is, again, rare and presents most commonly with polyarthropathy, systemic upset and raised inflammatory markers.

Septic arthritis

25 E *Staphylococcus aureus*

Septic arthritis is an infection of a synovial joint. Diagnosis is by clinical suspicion. In cases where uncertainty exists joint aspiration may be useful, but if history and examination are suggestive nothing should delay immediate arthroscopic washout in an effort to save the joint. Intravenous antibiotics should be started immediately once cultures of blood and synovial fluid are acquired and the joint should be splinted for 48 hours and analgesia given. Always look for a focus of infection; joint sepsis occurs secondary to bacteraemia from another source. Common culprits are UTI, LRTI, cellulitis/abscess or intravenous drug use.

The most commonly implicated organism is *Staphylococcus aureus*, which accounts for 60% of septic arthritis. β-haemolytic streptococci account for an additional 15%. Gram-negative organisms collectively account for 17% and are usually secondary to gastrointestinal infection, biliary sepsis or urinary tract infection. *Streptococcus pneumoniae* is relatively uncommon (3%), but when it does occur, 50% of patients also have a streptococcal pneumonia. *Haemophilus influenzae* is more common in children less than 3 years, but it is uncommon in adults.

Crystalline arthropathy

26 D **Xanthine oxidase deficiency**

Uric acid is the breakdown product of purine metabolism. At physiological pH, uric acid is 98% ionized, however raised levels of uric acid predispose to formation of monosodium urate, which has a low solubility and deposits in joints, soft tissues and the renal tubules. There are several genetic disorders which affect purine metabolism with various clinical manifestations; Lesch–Nyhan syndrome is due to complete deficiency in hypoxanthine-guanine phosphoribosyl transferase which normally reduces urate production through recycling of metabolic intermediates. Deficiency causes hyperuricaemia and severe physical and mental disorders.

[margin note:] purine salvage pathway

Conditions which increase cell turnover will also predispose to hyperuricaemia. Such conditions include psoriasis, haemolytic anaemias, malignancy and cytotoxic drugs. Certain drugs influence uric acid handling; thiazide diuretics and aspirin both inhibit secretion into the renal tubules and therefore impair excretion. Alcohol interferes with ADP/ATP metabolism and predisposes to hyperuricaemia.

Xanthine oxidase is an enzyme which converts xanthine to urate. It is the target for allopurinol, which inhibits the enzyme's function in order to lower urate levels. Therefore, its deficiency would not predispose to gout.

Acutely hot joint

27 B **Septic arthritis**

The scenario describes an excruciating painful limb associated with severely limited movement. This is consistent with all the listed diagnoses, as is erythema and effusion. Answering this question correctly requires correct interpretation of the aspirate results.

Osteomyelitis is rare outside childhood, particularly in the long bones. When it does occur in adults, it is usually in association with other co-morbidities such as diabetes or systemic sepsis, intravenous drug use or endocarditis. Osteomyelitis may also be seen in severely debilitated patients, and may complicate severe pressure ulceration in paralysed, elderly, or ITU patients. The high white cell count with predominant neutrophils is highly suggestive of an infective process. White cell counts in joint aspirates in crystalline or inflammatory arthropathy may also be high, approaching 50,000 cells/mm³, but white cell counts over this should definitely raise the suspicion that the cause is septic arthritis. A neutrophil count >90% of the total is also not typical of non-infective causes.

Candidates should not be lured into the trap of assuming a high urate level implies gout; asymptomatic hyperuricaemia is 10 times more common than gout. In addition, urate levels are often normal in an acute gout attack and therefore serum urate levels should not be used to confirm or exclude gout as a diagnosis.

Spinal cord injury

28 B   Radiculopathy

This patient presents with lower motor neurone signs localized to the C5 level. There are no deficits below the level of C5 and therefore spinal cord compression and Brown–Séquard syndrome can be safely excluded as possible diagnoses. Deltoid weakness and loss of sensation over the badge area is classically associated with axillary nerve injury, which may occur following a shoulder dislocation or fractures of the proximal humerus. However, the loss of biceps strength and absence of biceps reflex implicates a lesion of the musculocutaneous nerve. The unifying diagnosis is therefore a lesion of the C5 nerve root, i.e. an isolated C5 radiculopathy.

Compression of nerve roots is common and results in lower motor neurone signs and dermatomal loss of sensation at the levels affected. It is most common in the lumbar spine, but also complicates cervical spine disease. Causes of root compression are varied, but the two most common mechanisms are disc prolapse and narrowing of the intervertebral foramina, which may be due to osteoarthritis, Paget's or another degenerative disease.

Spinal cord compression

29 A   Cauda equina syndrome

Suspected cord compression is a common clinical scenario which is encountered repeatedly in practice. Distinguishing the level of the lesion is an important skill. The spinal cord in an adult terminates at

No & cord Compression

level L1–2, therefore there is no such thing as S1 cord compression. The signs described are pure LMN with no UMN component, therefore anterior cord syndrome can be discounted.

A conus syndrome occurs when the tail end of the cord and the nerve roots surrounding it become compressed by a lesion, typically at the L1–2 level. Compression of nerve roots causes LMN signs, compression of the end of the spinal cord causes localized UMN signs at the level of compression. The syndrome is one of mixed modality patchy sensory loss, with patchy LMN signs combined with spasticity of the anal and urinary sphincters, causing urinary retention and constipation, plus or minus additional UMN signs depending on the level of the lesion. The lack of UMN signs in the scenario makes this diagnosis unlikely.

Cauda equina syndrome occurs when compression occurs within the spinal canal, below the level of the cord. It is a syndrome of pure LMN signs as no spinal cord is involved. Compression of the nerve roots causes patchy sensory and motor losses with considerable case-to-case variability. Loss of urinary continence and anal tone are, however, relatively consistent. Typically, urinary incontinence occurs over a background of bladder atony, therefore patients will have grossly distended bladders and incontinence is an overflow phenomenon. The distinguishing feature from nerve root compression is that the sensorimotor deficit involves multiple levels and is bilateral, whereas root compression will be unilateral and confined to a single dermatome and myotome, unless root compression is occurring at multiple levels.

Lumbar disc herniation

30 C L4/5

The sensory loss elicited implicates an L5 nerve root compression. This is backed by weakness in dorsiflexion of the foot (tibialis anterior and peroneus tertius) with sparing of the ankle (S1, S2) and knee (L3, L4) reflexes.

Candidates often struggle with the derivation of the level of prolapse from the nerve root signs as it appears counter-intuitive. It is important to remember that lumbar disc protrusion does not usually affect the nerve exiting above the disc. Therefore, lateral protrusion of the L4/5 disc spares the L4 spinal nerve, but compresses the L5 spinal nerve which exits the spinal canal one vertebral level below the level of disc herniation. Similarly, herniation of the L3/4 disc compresses the L4 spinal nerve, and the L5/S1 disc compresses the S1 spinal nerve. Another important point to remember is that straight leg raising causes pain in L4/5 and L5/S1 disc herniation, whereas a positive femoral stretch test indicates L3/4 disc herniation.

SECTION 13:
NEUROSURGERY

Questions

1. Cranial anatomy (1)   282
2. Cranial anatomy (2)   282
3. Foramina of the skull base   282
4. Cerebral blood supply   282
5. Cerebrospinal fluid   283
6. Lumbar puncture   283
7. Anatomy of the spine   283
8. Trauma (1)   283
9. Trauma (2)   284
10. Disc prolapse   284
11. Head injury (1)   284
12. Head injury (2)   285
13. Basal skull fracture   285
14. Epilepsy   285
15. Meningitis   286
16. Pituitary disease (1)   286
17. Pituitary disease (2)   286
18. Vasculitis   287
19. Intracranial tumour (1)   287
20. Intracranial tumour (2)   287

Answers   289

QUESTIONS

1. Cranial anatomy (1)

Which one of the following forms the innermost layer of the scalp?

A. Loose connective tissue
B. Aponeurotic layer (galea)
C. Skin
D. Pericranium
E. Dense connective tissue

(handwritten annotations, right side)
S Skin
C Connective tissue (dense)
A Aponeurosis (galea)
L Loose connective tissue
P Pericranium

(handwritten annotations, left side)
contains
blood supply to scalp. → br of int and ext. carotid . a.

2. Cranial anatomy (2)

All of the following bones contribute to the formation of the pterion, except

A. Frontal bone
B. Parietal bone
C. Temporal bone
D. Greater wing of sphenoid bone
E. Lesser wing of sphenoid bone

(handwritten) ↓ weakest point of skull.

3. Foramina of the skull base

A 61-year-old teacher presents with a 3-month history of intermittent, right-sided facial pain affecting the area between his chin and lower eyelid. He reports that it occurs at any time of the day and has frequently disrupted his teaching sessions and daily activities such as brushing his teeth or having a meal. On examination, there is no obvious abnormality demonstrated. The admitting physician suspects trigeminal neuralgia in the distribution of the maxillary and mandibular branches. A specialist review is requested and appropriate treatment started. Through which of the following basal skull foramina does the mandibular branch of the trigeminal nerve (cranial nerve V$_3$) pass?

A. Superior orbital fissure *CN III, IV, VI and V$_1$*
B. Foramen rotundum *V$_2$*
C. Foramen ovale *V$_3$*
D. Foramen lacerum *ICA*
E. Foramen spinosum *Middle meningeal artery.*

4. Cerebral blood supply

Which of the following vessels supplying the brain is derived from the vertebral artery?

A. Posterior cerebral artery
B. Posterior communicating artery
C. Middle cerebral artery

D. Ophthalmic artery
E. Anterior cerebral artery

5. Cerebrospinal fluid

In which layer does cerebrospinal fluid circulate?

A. Subdural space
B. Subarachnoid space
C. Extradural space
D. Between pia mater and spinal cord
E. Spinal canal

6. Lumbar puncture

As the emergency department doctor on call, you are asked to perform a lumbar puncture. The mid-point at the level of the iliac crests is identified as your point of insertion of the puncture needle. Which intervertebral space does this represent?   * Spinal cord ends at L2

A. L1/L2
B. L2/L3
C. L3/L4
D. L4/L5
E. L5/S1

7. Anatomy of the spine

While explaining the procedure of a lumbar puncture to a junior colleague, you are asked about the layers through which the lumbar puncture needle must pass before reaching the area containing cerebrospinal fluid. After piercing the skin and subcutaneous tissues, which anatomical structure would be traversed next during a tap?

A. Interspinous ligament
B. Supraspinous ligament
C. Dura mater
D. Ligamentum flavum
E. Epidural space

Handwritten annotation:
Skin
subcutaneous tissue
supraspinous ligament
Interspinous ligament
Ligamentum flavum
Epidural space
Dura mater
Arachnoid mater
Subarachnoid space (CSF)

8. Trauma (1)

A 28-year-old male motorcyclist is brought into the emergency department where you, as the doctor on call, are asked to assess his consciousness as part of the primary survey. He is unresponsive when you speak to him, but, on rubbing his sternum, opens his eyes and tries to push your hand away. During your assessment he also mutters something that you are unable to understand. His Glasgow Coma Scale score is

A. 7
B. 8
C. 9
D. 10
E. 11

9. Trauma (2)

A 21-year-old female student presents to the emergency department following a fall from a ledge approximately 1.5 m high while walking home. She has been drinking heavily and her friends report that she is now drowsier following her fall. She opens her eyes when her name is mentioned and is talking about her studies tomorrow. She also winces when you press her nail bed. Her score according to the Glasgow Coma Scale will be

A. 3
B. 5
C. 7
D. 9
E. 11

10. Disc prolapse

A healthy 34-year-old builder presents to his general practitioner having fallen 4.5 m from a ladder 4 days previously, while working at a construction site. Although no major injuries were sustained, since his accident, he has been having near constant lower backache, which radiates down his right leg and is worse on coughing. On examination, the pain is noted to be particularly worse on the outer aspect of the right leg. In addition, there is reduced sensation over this area and the dorsum of the foot. Ankle and big toe dorsiflexion also appear to be weak in comparison to the left side. The patient is referred to the local hospital for an MRI scan, which shows a lateral disc protrusion in the lumbar spine. Which nerve root is likely to be affected in this individual?

A. L2
B. L3
C. L4
D. L5
E. S1

11. Head injury (1)

A 20-year-old university cricketer is hit in the side of his head by a cricket ball while fielding close to the bat during a varsity match. He is reported to have briefly lost consciousness, but at the time of examination in the emergency department his Glasgow Coma Scale score is 15/15. In addition, he complains of severe headache and blurred vision since regaining consciousness. A neurological examination reveals that his right pupil is dilated, but no other focal neurology is elicited. A CT scan is performed on the basis of these findings, which shows a lenticular-shaped collection suggestive of an extradural haematoma. Damage to which one of the following vessels would classically be associated with this pathology?

[handwritten: Lenticular shaped - epidural]

[handwritten: Crescent shaped - subdural]
[handwritten: ↳ due to venous hemorrhage]

A. Maxillary artery
B. Middle meningeal artery
C. Cerebral veins
D. Middle cerebral artery
E. Anterior communicating artery

[handwritten left margin: pterion]

12. Head injury (2)

An 85-year-old pensioner is brought to the emergency department by her family who are concerned that she has become increasingly confused and drowsy in the past 3 weeks. She is pleasantly confused and unable to recall events clearly but oriented to time and person and complains only of occasional frontal headache. Her family informs you that she may have fallen while climbing from the bathtub some weeks previously. She has also started sleeping for long periods of time, which is not her normal habit. A head CT scan is performed, which shows mild generalized atrophy and a crescent-shaped collection. This presentation is consistent with

*[handwritten: * Subdural → gradual presentation.]*

A. Intracerebral haemorrhage
B. Subarachnoid haemorrhage
C. Extradural haemorrhage
D. Subdural haemorrhage
E. None of the above

13. Basal skull fracture

Which of the following sets of clinical signs are usually associated with a basal skull fracture?

A. Periorbital ecchymoses, otorrhoea, retroauricular ecchymoses, cranial nerve III palsy *[handwritten: → raccoon eyes.]* *[handwritten: CN VII not VI ✓]*
B. Periorbital ecchymoses, rhinorrhoea, anosmia, cranial nerve VI palsy
C. Rib fracture, otorrhoea, rhinorrhoea, anosmia
D. Rib fracture, otorrhoea, rhinorrhoea, retroauricular ecchymoses
E. Periorbital ecchymoses, otorrhoea, rhinorrhoea, retroauricular ecchymoses

[handwritten: Bottle sign → ecchymoses of mastoid process also hemotympanum, CN VII palsy, anosmia]

14. Epilepsy

A 29-year-old nurse is referred to the neurology outpatient clinic with a 6-month history of intermittent upper limb jerking, in which a digit on the left hand jerks initially, extending to the hand, arm and eventually the face. She reports being aware of these movements and feeling weak in the same arm for several hours after. This type of seizure could be described as being

A. Jacksonian
B. Temporal lobe
C. Grand mal (tonic–clonic)
D. Absence (petit mal)
E. Status epilepticus

15. Meningitis

A 21-year-old male medical student presents with a 14-day history of intermittent fever, rigours, headache, neck stiffness and a single episode of vomiting just prior to attending his appointment. On questioning, he admits to a visit to rural east Africa 2 months ago as part of a university outreach group and is up to date on all vaccinations. Furthermore, he had not had unprotected sexual intercourse over the past several months. On examination, he is noted to be tachycardic with a pulse rate of 100 beats/min and appears slightly dehydrated. Routine blood tests show moderately raised inflammatory markers. The admitting team suspects meningitis and conducts a lumbar puncture. The tap reveals a white cell count of $995/mm^3$ with a neutrophilia and lymphocytosis, 2.5 g/L of protein and 3.0 mmol/L of glucose. Samples are additionally sent for Gram staining and virological examination and appropriate therapy started pending final confirmation. Which one of the following micro-organisms is most likely causing meningitis in this patient?

A. *Treponema pallidum*
B. Epstein–Barr virus → usually self limiting
C. *Mycobacterium tuberculosis*
D. *Neisseria meningitides* → acute rapid onset
E. Human immunodeficiency virus (HIV)
 → did not have unprotected sex.

blotchy rash
run

16. Pituitary disease (1)

All of the following are secreted by the adenohypophysis, except

A. Follicle-stimulating hormone (FSH)
B. Oxytocin
C. Adrenocorticotropic hormone (ACTH)
D. Growth hormone (GH)
E. Prolactin

17. Pituitary disease (2)

A 28-year-old solicitor presents to the neurosurgery clinic with a 1-year history of increasing tiredness, sweatiness, difficulty concentrating and pain and numbness in his hands at night. Further questioning reveals that his shoes have become tight in the past year, while examination reveals moderate hypertension, a protruding jaw and slightly coarse features. The admitting clinician suspects a growth-hormone-secreting pituitary tumour and requests several tests to confirm this diagnosis. Which one of the following tests is most appropriate to investigate this condition?

A. Dexamethasone suppression test
B. Short Synacthen test
C. Fasting blood glucose
D. Glucose tolerance test
E. Fasting lipids

18. Vasculitis

A 72-year-old woman presents with a throbbing headache of 1 week's duration. Further questioning reveals the increasing difficulty in combing her hair, which causes pain over the scalp and jaw pain while eating. She is known to suffer from muscle aches and was diagnosed with polymyalgia rheumatica approximately 1 year ago. Physical examination reveals little else of note. The admitting physician suspects giant cell (temporal) arteritis and requests a full blood screen and temporal artery biopsy. An increase in which one of the following blood markers would be diagnostic of this condition?

A. Neutrophil count
B. Erythrocyte sedimentation rate → diagnostic of polymyalgia and TA if
C. C-reactive protein   >100 mm/h.
D. D-dimer → venous thromboembolism
E. Bradykinin

19. Intracranial tumour (1)

Cancers arising in the following organs commonly metastasize to the brain, except

A. Lung
B. Bowel
C. Kidney
D. Endometrium
E. Skin

20. Intracranial tumour (2)

A 62-year-old cleaner presents with multiple episodes of uncontrolled right arm jerking, unsteadiness while walking, difficulty seeing objects to one side and occasional headaches over the past several weeks. She is otherwise fit and well without any significant past medical history. Examination reveals increased lower limb tone, reduced power in the legs and papilloedema on fundoscopy. In addition, there appears to be a bony protuberance overlying the right parietal bone. A head CT scan with contrast is performed which shows a dense, homogeneous lesion in the right parasagittal area. This lesion is likely to represent what type of cranial tumour?

A. Astrocytoma
B. Oligodendroglioma
C. Meningioma
D. Craniopharyngioma
E. Medulloblastoma

ANSWERS

Cranial anatomy (1)

1 D Pericranium

The scalp is formed by five layers denoted by the acronym SCALP from the outermost to innermost layer these are:

- Skin
- Connective tissue (dense)
- Aponeurotic layer (galea)
- Loose connective tissue
- Pericranium

The outer surface (periosteum) of the skull bones provides nutrition and the ability to repair the bones. It can be lifted surgically during craniotomy.

Blood supply to the scalp is provided by branches of the external and internal carotid arteries, which run in the dense connective tissue layer of the scalp and anastomose freely with each other. The nerve supply to the scalp varies according to region. The anterior scalp is supplied by the supratrochlear and supraorbital branches of cranial nerve V_1 (ophthalmic division of the trigeminal nerve). The posterior scalp is supplied by the posterior rami of the C2/C3 nerve roots and the lateral scalp is supplied by the auriculotemporal branch of cranial nerve V_3 (mandibular division of the trigeminal nerve).

Cranial anatomy (2)

2 E Lesser wing of sphenoid bone

The pterion is a point at the posterior end of the sapheno-parietal junction, 3 cm superoposterior to the mid-point of the zygomatic process of the frontal bone. It marks the convergence of the frontal, parietal, temporal and sphenoid (greater wing) bones in an 'H'-shaped suture. It is the thinnest part of the skull and overlies the anterior division of the middle meningeal artery, which runs on the inner aspect of the skull.

The middle meningeal artery is a branch of the maxillary artery, which itself is a branch of the external carotid artery. It is the largest of three branches supplying the meninges (the others being the anterior and posterior meningeal arteries). This artery can potentially be damaged if there is injury, such as a blow to the side of the head, and result in the collection of blood between the dura mater and the skull (an epi/extradural haematoma). The lesser wing of the sphenoid contains the optic canal, anterior clinoid process and superior orbital fissure, which transmit a number of cranial nerves. It forms the posterior aspect of the anterior fossa at the base of the skull and does not contribute to the formation of the pterion.

Foramina of the skull base

3   C   Foramen ovale

All of the options in this question are found in the middle cranial fossa and transmit the following structures:

- Superior orbital fissure – Oculomotor, trochlear and abducens nerves (cranial nerves III, IV and VI), ophthalmic division of trigeminal nerve (cranial nerve V_1 as the lacrimal, frontal and nasociliary nerves) and ophthalmic veins.
- Foramen rotundum – Maxillary division of trigeminal nerve (cranial nerve V_2) supplies sensation to the cheek and nose. It passes through the foramen rotundum into the pterygopalatine fossa and enters the orbit via the inferior orbital fissure.
- Foramen ovale – Mandibular division of trigeminal nerve (cranial nerve V_3), accessory meningeal artery and lesser petrosal nerve.
- Foramen lacerum – Internal carotid artery.
- Foramen spinosum – Middle meningeal artery, which can be damaged as a result of pterion fractures, causing an extradural haematoma.

The trigeminal nerve (cranial nerve V) is a mixed sensory and motor nerve with three branches: ophthalmic (V_1), maxillary (V_2) and mandibular (V_3).

Trigeminal neuralgia is a condition defined by brief episodes of intense, stabbing facial pain usually affecting one side of the face in a maxillary and mandibular distribution (the area supplied by the ophthalmic branch, i.e. skin of upper nose, eyelid, forehead and scalp are only occasionally affected). The attacks can be frequent and precipitated by a touch to the skin, washing, shaving, eating and talking. The cause is usually unknown, but can occasionally be the result of a vascular abnormality or cerebello-pontine angle tumour. Medical treatment is with carbamazepine, phenytoin and alcohol injection of the nerve, while surgical intervention to explore the nerve root can reveal tortuous blood vessels compressing it on entering the brainstem.

Cerebral blood supply

4   A   Posterior cerebral artery

Blood supply to the brain is derived from two main supplies: the internal carotid and vertebral arteries. The two vessels anastomose at the base of the brain to form the circle of Willis, branches of which supply different areas of the cerebrum.

The internal carotid artery is a branch of the common carotid artery. On the right, the latter begins as a bifurcation of the brachiocephalic trunk, whereas the left common carotid is a direct branch of the aortic arch. The vessel has no branches in the neck, which it traverses within the carotid sheath, together with the vagus nerve and internal jugular vein. The skull base is entered via the carotid canal, in the petrous part of the temporal bone, and intracranial branches are given off. Intracranial branches of the internal carotid are the ophthalmic artery, branches to the hypophysis and meninges, anterior cerebral artery and middle cerebral artery.

The vertebral artery meanwhile forms as a branch of the first part of the subclavian artery, ascending though the transverse foramina of the first six cervical vertebrae (C1–C6). After leaving the C1 foramen, the artery winds around the superior articular process of the atlas and passes through the foramen magnum into the cranium. Here it gives off intradural branches (the anterior and posterior spinal arteries and the posterior inferior cerebellar arteries), and joins its opposing vessel to form the basilar artery. Several vessels are also derived from the basilar artery. These are the anterior inferior cerebellar artery, pontine and labyrinthine branches and the superior cerebellar artery. The last two branches of the vertebral artery are formed by its division into two posterior cerebral arteries (which contribute to the formation of the circle of Willis). The posterior communicating artery joins the posterior cerebral artery to the internal carotid artery in the circle of Willis.

Cerebrospinal fluid

5 B   Subarachnoid space

The meninges are three membranous layers surrounding the spinal cord. From inner to outermost they are the pia mater, arachnoid mater and dura mater. The subdural space is on the inner side of the dura, separating it from the arachnoid. The epidural/extradural space lies above the dura mater, containing the internal vertebral venous plexus and epidural fat.

The CSF is a clear, watery fluid that surrounds the spinal cord and brain, cushioning the latter from contact with the skull and reducing its weight. It is produced by the choroids plexus in the lateral, third and fourth ventricles and circulates there, in the central canal and in the subarachnoid space (the space between the arachnoid and pia mater layers). It is absorbed by the arachnoid villi that project into the superior sagittal sinus. The CSF will normally have a clear appearance, a white cell count of <5 cells/mm^3 (predominantly mononuclear cells), glucose level of 2.8–4.2 mmol/L (approximately half to two-thirds of the blood glucose level) and a protein content of 0.15–0.45 g/L.

Lumbar puncture

6 C L3/L4

The spinal cord is part of the central nervous system and involved with transmission of neural impulses from the brain to the body peripheries. It is found in the upper two-thirds of the vertebral canal, terminating in a conical end (the conus medullaris) at the level of the second vertebral level (L2) in adults.

A lumbar puncture (or spinal tap) is a diagnostic technique used to enter the subarachnoid space in order to measure the pressure of the CSF that flows within (8–14 mmHg in an adult) and to withdraw a sample for chemical analysis. The most common site of lumbar puncture is the L3/L4 vertebral space, found at the level of the iliac crests. Spinal tap above the conus medullaris can cause spinal cord injury and subsequent paralysis. Below this level is the filum terminale and cauda equina, which floats freely in cerebrospinal fluid and is not damaged by lumbar puncture. As a result, any space from L2/L3 to L5/S1 provides a safe entry point for puncture, but it is vitally important to identify the surface landmarks prior to a tap being performed.

Lumbar puncture is contraindicated in the presence of a bleeding diathesis, cardiorespiratory compromise, infection at the site of needle insertion and in cases of suspected raised ICP as indicated by very severe headache, reduced consciousness, rising blood pressure, vomiting, focal neurology and papilloedema. Withdrawal of CSF in the presence of raised ICP creates a pressure gradient, which can cause tentorial herniation and death.

Anatomy of the spine

7 B Supraspinous ligament

As discussed previously, lumbar puncture is an important diagnostic technique used to enter into the subarachnoid space to measure CSF pressure and obtain a sample for analysis. Understanding the anatomy of the lumbar region (where the tap is commonly performed) is essential to avoid (potentially dangerous) complications such as post-puncture headache, nerve root trauma, bleeding, infection and coning, i.e. herniation of cerebellar tonsils with compression of the medulla.

The layers encountered from superficial to deep while performing a lumbar puncture are skin; subcutaneous tissue; supraspinous ligament and interspinous ligament (both ligaments form a connection between adjacent spinous processes); ligamentum flavum (a strong, yellow coloured ligament that extends between adjacent vertebrae in the interlaminar space which can be up to 1 cm thick); epidural/extradural space (containing internal vertebral venous plexus); dura mater; arachnoid mater; and the subarachnoid space (contains CSF).

Trauma (1)

8 C 9

The GCS is a tool used to rapidly assess the consciousness and neurological function of a patient, particularly (but not exclusively) in the trauma setting. See Section 3, answer to Question 19 for the GCS. The patient in this scenario will score 9/15 (E2, V2, M5).

Trauma (2)

9 E 11

The patient in this scenario will score 11/15 (E3, V4, M4). (See Section 3, answer to Question 19 for the GCS.)

Disc prolapse

10 D L5

The intervertebral disc is a structure found between spinal vertebrae where it forms a cartilaginous joint to stabilize and allow slight movement of the vertebrae. The disc is composed in its inner aspect of the nucleus pulposus, a jelly-like substance, which is surrounded by the annulus fibrosus on the outer aspect.

With age, the nucleus can dehydrate and the annulus becomes weaker at the same time. This process, together with trauma, can result in tearing of the annulus fibrosus, through which the nucleus pulposus can extrude or herniate and impinge on spinal roots, as they exit the intervertebral foramen of their corresponding vertebrae. It is the tearing process which causes the acute backache that patients may present with an impingement that produces mostly unilateral symptoms of leg pain, numbness, reduced function and areflexia in the region of distribution of a particular nerve root.

Posterolateral herniation will compress the root exiting the foramen below the affected level, i.e. L5/S1 will compress the S1 root. Ninety-five per cent of lumbar disc prolapses are at the level of L4/L5 and L5/S1. L4 compression can cause quadriceps wasting/weakness, reduced sensation over the medial calf and impaired knee jerk. L5 compression produces signs and symptoms as described in the scenario above, and S1 compression leads to wasting/weakness of plantar flexors, sensory impairment over the lateral aspect of the foot and sole and an impaired ankle jerk.

Treatment of lateral disc protrusion is usually conservative with bed rest, avoiding heavy lifting, analgesia and muscle relaxants. The development of severe and recurrent leg pain and neurological signs, particularly foot drop, is worrying and may need further imaging, e.g. MRI, with a view to surgical treatment. Operative intervention involves removal of the prolapsed disc.

Whereas lateral disc prolapse is a relatively benign condition, central disc prolapse can result in compression of the cauda equina (cauda equina syndrome), causing backache, bilateral sciatica, urinary retention and saddle anaesthesia. It is a neurosurgical emergency that requires urgent decompression to prevent paralysis and permanent sphincter damage.

Head injury (1)

11 B   Middle meningeal artery

The middle meningeal artery is a branch of the maxillary artery, itself a branch of the external carotid artery, and the largest of three branches supplying the meninges. This artery runs beneath the pterion, the thinnest part of the skull, and can be damaged if there is injury, such as a blow to the side of the head, and result in the collection of blood between the dura mater and skull (an epi/extradural haematoma).

Clinically, extradural haematomas present with a history of trauma followed by a brief loss of consciousness from which the patient recovers, seemingly without any lasting effect (the lucid interval). This is followed by steady and often dramatic neurological deterioration and ultimately death. More than 50% of cases of extradural haematoma are associated with an ipsilateral dilated pupil. A CT scan of the head is the imaging technique of choice and demonstrates a lenticular (lens) shaped collection within the extradural space. Treatment aims to prevent secondary brain damage and if affecting the patient's consciousness the haematoma can need urgent evacuation in a neurosurgical unit.

The anterior communicating and middle cerebral arteries form part of the circle of Willis. The middle cerebral and anterior cerebral arteries are derived from the internal carotid artery as its two terminal intracerebral branches. The anterior communicating artery acts as a bridge connecting the two anterior cerebral arteries, which are the two circulatory branches derived from the pair of internal carotid arteries.

Extradural haematomas can occasionally be caused by damage to the sagittal or transverse sinuses. Along with the cavernous sinus, these structures form the dural venous sinuses into which the venous blood drains after running in the subarachnoid space. In addition, subdural haematomas form when a cerebral vein ruptures as it passes through the arachnoid into the subdural space.

Head injury (2)

12 D   Subdural haemorrhage

Subdural haematoma is a collection of blood between the dura and arachnoid mater, caused by tearing of bridging veins, which leak into the subdural space. It is most commonly associated with increasing age, alcohol misuse, dementia and brain atrophy. Subdural haematoma can be an acute, subacute or chronic process. However, as the leak of blood is at a low pressure, signs and symptoms commonly take many days to weeks to develop.

Presentation can be non-specific and confused by the age of the patient. Clinical features include dementia, deteriorating and/or fluctuating consciousness with increasing drowsiness, as well as symptoms and signs of raised intracranial pressure, i.e. headache, seizures, irritability and papilloedema. The investigation of choice is a head CT scan, the findings of which will vary according to the stage of the disease process. A CT taken early in the pathological process will show a hyperdense crescentic fluid collection while in the later stages a hypodense collection with a thick membrane is seen.

Treatment of chronic subdural haematoma is by surgical drainage, which involves burr holes in the posterior frontal and posterior parietal positions. The dura is then incised and the haematoma irrigated, after which the brain should re-expand. The burr holes are plugged with haemostatic foam and different layers sutured over. Prophylactic antibiotics are also given.

Extradural and subarachnoid haemorrhage are discussed elsewhere in this chapter.

Basal skull fracture

13 E **Periorbital ecchymoses, otorrhoea, rhinorrhoea, retroauricular ecchymoses**
Basal (or basilar) skull fractures are linear fractures that can be caused by head injury due to a blow at the back of the head or sudden deceleration, as occurs in traffic accidents. Classically, clinical features of this injury are:

- Periorbital ecchymoses (raccoon or panda eyes)
- Retroauricular ecchymoses (Battle's sign is ecchymosis of the mastoid process)
- Otorrhoea and rhinorrhoea (the leak of cerebrospinal fluid into the ears and nose respectively)
- Haemotympanum
- Anosmia
- Cranial nerve VII (facial nerve) palsy
- Depressed skull fracture ('step off') – this is associated with an increased incidence of intracranial injury, early seizures and a risk of intracranial injury

Hospital guidelines for investigation and treatment vary, but in general treatment is mainly supportive as for any head injury, i.e. maintain

ABC, treat raised intracranial pressure, treat seizures and give anti-biotic prophylaxis in cases of penetrating head injury. Most patients with basilar skull fractures are admitted for observation and supportive management only.

Epilepsy

14 A **Jacksonian**

Epilepsy is a neurological condition occurring as a result of sudden, uncontrolled neuronal discharge in the CNS that is usually self-terminating. It has a wide range of presentations from mild 'absences', in which there is no awareness of a preceding period of time, to convulsions or seizures lasting many minutes.

The condition is classified as partial/focal (i.e. originating in one part of the brain) or generalized (i.e. multiple foci of uncontrolled activity in the brain). Partial seizures are subdivided as simple, complex (i.e. associated impaired consciousness) and those that lead to tonic–clonic convulsions. Generalized seizure types include periods of absence and generalized tonic–clonic seizures.

Simple partial seizures are the most common seizure type of which Jacksonian motor seizure or 'march' is a variety. It is characterized by involuntary movements beginning in the hand or face and progressively involving larger muscle groups, i.e. a march. Patients are usually aware of these movements and have no loss of consciousness. They may experience weakness in the limb once the seizure subsides – Todd's paralysis.

Temporal lobe epilepsy is a complex partial seizure characterized by an initial aura (e.g. visual, auditory or gustatory hallucination) followed by change in consciousness, such as a feeling of depersonalization, flashbacks and mood changes. Attacks usually last several seconds and can be followed by headache and confusion. In cases refractory to medical intervention, surgical lobectomy is an infrequently used treatment option. Most commonly, this will involve removal of the hippocampus and amygdala, which can act as foci of epileptic activity.

Absence seizures are usually confined to childhood and consist of multiple seizures a day lasting several seconds, manifesting as blank stares, with or without eye blinking and occasional muscle jerks. Patients are commonly not aware of their seizures and usually suffer no residual effects.

Grand mal seizures occur as episodes of sudden loss of consciousness, followed by jerking of all limbs for up to several minutes. This may be associated with urinary and/or faecal incontinence and injuries associated with falling at the time when consciousness is lost. Patients will usually be confused and drowsy in the post ictal phase. There may be an inducing stimulus and classically EEG recordings will demonstrate generalized spike and wave activity in the 3–5 Hz range.

Status epilepticus is a medical emergency in which seizures are either prolonged (lasting for more than 30 minutes) or an individual suffers repeated seizures without regaining full consciousness in between. It most commonly presents as a tonic–clonic event in known epileptics. Treatment is medical, but patients may need anaesthetic intervention in order to paralyse and artificially ventilate, with the hope of gaining control over seizure activity and thereby preventing cerebral damage.

Meningitis

15 C *Mycobacterium tuberculosis*

Meningitis is inflammation of the meninges, usually due to microorganisms that reach the meninges as a result of extension from the ears and nasopharynx, cranial/spinal injury and haematogenous spread. Non-infectious causes include disseminated carcinoma and drugs that cause inflammation of the meninges.

The typical triad of presentation is headache, neck stiffness and fever. Photophobia, vomiting, drowsiness and the presence of cranial nerve lesions are suggestive of the development of complications such as hydrocephalus and cerebral abscess. Examination may reveal the following:

- Petechial or blotchy rash suggestive of meningococcal meningitis (due to *Neisseria meningitides*)
- Evidence of septic shock
- Kernig's sign – Inability to straighten the leg at the knee when the thighs are held at a right angle to the body (due to reflex spasm of spinal muscles)
- Brudzinski's sign – Hip flexion on tilting the head forward

Additionally, duration of the symptoms, travel history, sexual history, occupational history and co-morbidities contribute to determining the causative agent. Viral meningitis is usually a benign and self-limiting illness. Acute bacterial meningitis can present suddenly and progress rapidly, while chronic illness (as caused by tuberculosis and syphilis) can have a more insidious onset. Immunocompromised individuals are most at risk from fungal infection.

Although blood tests and cultures are a useful adjunct, the investigation of choice is a lumbar puncture. The description of findings in this question combined with the history of travel is typical of tubercular meningitis. Viral meningitis will result in little change of CSF except for the presence of an increased number of cells, while acute bacterial meningitis will produce a turbid appearance of CSF, together with an increased presence of polymorphs and growth of micro-organisms on a smear.

Treatment is dependent on the cause, but will include appropriate resuscitation and commencement of intravenous antibiotics, if the clinical suspicion of bacterial meningitis in particular is high. Tubercular meningitis is treated with standard anti-tuberculosis medication and the patient is monitored for signs of relapse and complications, given the high mortality rate.

Pituitary disease (1)

16 B   Oxytocin

The following table lists hormones released by the adenohypophysis and the neurohypophysis.

Site of hormone	Hormone	Target	Action release
Adenohypophysis (anterior pituitary)	FSH	Ovaries/testes	Follicle development and spermatogenesis
	LH	Ovaries/testes	Oestradiol, testosterone and progesterone production (women only)
	ACTH	Adrenal cortex	Activates release of corticosteroids
	TSH	Thyroid gland	T3/T4 (thyroxine) release
	Growth hormone	Liver, muscle, bone, fat cells	Anabolic action and growth
	Prolactin	Breast	Breast hyperplasia and post-partum milk production
Neurohypophysis (posterior pituitary)	ADH	Distal tubule, collecting ducts, arteriolar muscle	Water reabsorption, smooth muscle vasoconstriction
	Oxytocin	Uterus, breast	Uterine contraction, milk expression

Pituitary disease (2)

17 D   Glucose tolerance test

Growth hormone is an anterior pituitary hormone involved in anabolism and growth. It can occasionally be produced in excess, most commonly as a result of a pituitary adenoma (benign growth-hormone-secreting tumour). Excess growth hormone in infancy results in gigantism, while in adults it causes acromegaly. The symptoms are the result of (i) a mass effect of tumour expansion such as headache and visual disturbance due to compression of the optic chiasm (resulting in bitemporal hemianopia) and (ii) physical effects of excess growth hormone. The effects of excess hormone can be insidious, and as a result, it can take many months and years for classical signs and symptoms to occur. The physical effects of excess growth hormone secretion include:

- Soft tissue swelling with enlarged hands, feet, lips, ears and nose (ask for changes in glove/hat size if worn)
- Protruding lower jaw from mandibular growth (prognathism)
- General coarseness of the features
- Barrel chest due to increased curvature of the spine and hunching of the back (kyphosis)
- Cardiomegaly and heart failure
- Hypertension
- Thick, deep voice due to vocal cord swelling
- Carpal tunnel syndrome due to thickening of the flexor retinaculum
- Diabetes mellitus
- Kidney failure

Classically, the condition is diagnosed by conducting a glucose tolerance test. A baseline measurement is made of the growth hormone level followed by oral administration of 75 g glucose orally. The growth hormone level is then recorded at 30-minute intervals. If, by 2 hours, the level is not less than 1 µg/L, as would be expected in normal individuals (due to the suppression effect of glucose on growth hormone), acromegaly is virtually diagnostic. More recently, IGF-1 levels have also been used to gauge GH secretion, but assays must be refined enough to account for conditions which may naturally increase or decrease IGF-1 levels. Imaging modalities such as MRI and CT (particularly for imaging of the chest, abdomen and pelvis for evidence of tumours which might produce ectopic growth hormone e.g. pancreatic, ovarian and adrenal tumours) can also be used.

Treatment of the condition is either medical or surgical. Medical therapy involves using radiotherapy, lareotide/octreotide (somatostatin analogues), pegvisomant (a growth hormone receptor antagonist) and bromocriptine (a dopamine agonist), which reduce the level of growth hormone. Surgical treatment is via the trans-sphenoidal (most common), transcranial or transethmoidal approaches to the sella turcica (in which the pituitary gland is found). Surgical removal results in rapid regression of soft tissue changes, but can be associated with a hormonal imbalance, which may need to be addressed in the long term.

The dexamethasone suppression test is used for diagnosis of Cushing's disease. The short Synacthen test is used to diagnose adrenal insufficiency (Addison's disease). Fasting blood glucose is used to diagnose suspected cases of type 2 diabetes mellitus. Fasting lipids are used to check serum levels of various fats, but are not diagnostic of any specific condition.

Vasculitis

18 B   Erythrocyte sedimentation rate

Giant cell or temporal arteritis is a vasculitic condition of the temporal artery associated with polymyalgia rheumatica in a large proportion of patients. It usually occurs in more elderly individuals and presents with headache, scalp and temporal artery tenderness, jaw claudication (as jaw pain while eating) and occasional visual disturbance such as amaurosis fugax. Although several inflammatory markers can be raised, an ESR >100 mm/h is virtually diagnostic. The gold standard test is a temporal artery biopsy, which will show a granulomatous inflammatory infiltrate of the media and adventitia. However, it is only positive in 60% of individuals. Treatment is immediate with high-dose steroids, as there is a risk of permanent visual loss, and should not be delayed if the diagnosis is clinically suspected.

Erythrocyte sedimentation rate (ESR) is a test that measures the rate at which blood cells fall in an upright tube. It has a limited value as a marker of inflammation, but is particularly useful for diagnosis of temporal arteritis and polymyalgia rheumatica (which may co-exist), particularly at values >100 mm/h.

Neutrophil count is a frequently used marker of infection, especially if bacterial in origin. C-reactive protein is an acute-phase protein produced by the liver and is a marker of general inflammation. The D-dimer is a product of fibrinolysis. It is used mainly in cases of suspected venous thromboembolism, e.g. DVT and pulmonary embolus. A negative value is highly predictive of the absence of a clot whereas a high value suggests either the presence of a clot or some other inflammatory process. Bradykinin is a vasoactive protein, which induces vasodilation, increases vascular permeability and causes smooth muscle contraction. It is not a marker of inflammation.

Intracranial tumour (1)

19 D   Endometrium

Almost half of all brain tumours are the result of metastases. Cerebral metastases account for almost 20% of presentations in individuals with carcinoma. The most common sites of origin for cerebral metastases are the lungs, breast, bowel, skin (malignant melanoma) and kidney (especially renal cell carcinoma). Endometrial carcinoma is not frequently associated with metastases to the brain.

Intracranial tumour (2)

20 C Meningioma

Astrocytoma is the commonest primary cerebral tumour, affecting mainly middle-aged individuals, and occurring in the frontal, temporal, parietal and thalamic areas. Tumours may be 'low grade' or 'malignant', with symptoms developing slowly. Patients may present with epilepsy, signs of focal brain damage (i.e. personality change, hemiparesis) and signs of raised intracranial pressure (i.e. headache, projectile vomiting, depression and reduced consciousness). Presentation on CT and MRI depends on the tumour grade, while treatment depends on many factors, including lesion site, degree of malignancy, patient's age and wishes and absence/presence of raised ICP. Treatment modalities include steroids for relief of raised ICP, surgical resection and chemoradiotherapy.

Oligodendrogliomas are rare tumours of oligodendrocytes (glial cells that innervate axons of CNS neurones), affecting mainly the frontal lobe of patients aged 30–50 years. They are usually well-demarcated, calcified cystic tumours of gelatinous consistency and may involve the ventricular wall, resulting in metastatic spread via the CSF. Treatment is dependent on tumour stage, but as with astrocytomas, surgical resection and chemoradiotherapy are the main modalities.

Meningioma is an intracranial tumour arising from the arachnoid granulations, characterized by slow and expansile growth. They are more prevalent in middle-aged women and are most commonly found around the venous sinuses, but can involve any meningeal site, including the cerebral convexity, parasagittal area, sphenoid wing, olfactory groove, cerebellopontine angle, foramen magnum and spinal cord. Many patients present with focal epilepsy while the remainder develop slow pressure effects, i.e. evidence of raised ICP followed by focal neurological signs (depending on the site involved). For example, parasagittal tumours near the vertex of the skull can affect foot and leg motor and sensory function, while posteriorly located tumours can cause a homonymous hemianopia. Imaging may reveal hyperostosis (bone thickening) of the parietal bone and sagittal suture, while CT and MRI will reveal the lesion directly. Treatment involves removing the tumour completely where possible or irradiating it in non-resectable cases.

Craniopharyngioma is a cystic, suprasellar cranial tumour with surrounding ring calcification, occurring most commonly in children and middle-aged adults. It can result in growth retardation in children, diabetes insipidus due to pituitary gland compression, bitemporal hemianopia from optic chiasm compression, and signs of raised intracranial pressure (projectile vomiting, headache, papilloedema) due to obstructive hydrocephalus. Treatment is with surgical resection and radiotherapy.

Medulloblastoma is an extracranial tumour of primitive neuroecto-dermal origin, occurring most commonly in childhood. It is a malig-nant tumour originating in the cerebellar vermis, from where it spreads into the fourth ventricle and throughout the CSF. Patients can present with truncal and gait ataxia as a result of cerebellar involve-ment, which develops over several weeks, or symptoms of raised ICP secondary to blockage of CSF flow. Treatment is once again dependent on tumour stage, but involves the modalities previously described. Prognosis is variable, with a 5-year survival of 50%–85%.

SECTION 14:
ENT SURGERY

Questions

1. Ear pain (1)   304
2. Management of ear pain   304
3. Pathogens involved in ear disease   304
4. Management of ear disease   305
5. Ear pain (2)   305
6. Complications of otitis media   305
7. Ear disease   305
8. Causative pathogens in ear infections   306
9. Decline in hearing   306
10. Diagnosis of ear disease (1)   306
11. Difficulty hearing   307
12. Diagnosis of ear disease (2)   307
13. Dizziness   307
14. Sore throat (1)   307
15. Facial trauma   308
16. Nasal obstruction   308
17. Epistaxis (1)   308
18. Epistaxis (2)   309
19. Sore throat (2)   309
20. Parotid swelling   310

Answers   311

QUESTIONS

1. Ear pain (1)

A 19-year-old Caucasian woman attends the outpatient clinic with a 2-day history of left-sided earache. The pain has worsened in the past 24 hours and she describes some seepage from the affected ear. Over the past few weeks her left ear has felt 'blocked' and she has been using cotton wool buds to clean them. Her hearing is not impaired. She is afebrile (36.7°C). On examination, the pain is worsened on superior movement of the auricle. There is a scanty discharge emerging from the left ear. Which of the following is the most likely diagnosis?

  A. Acute otitis externa
  B. Chronic otitis externa
  C. Acute otitis media
  D. Mastoiditis
  E. Chronic otitis media

2. Management of ear pain

The patient in Question 1 is due to undergo treatment for her 2-day history of ear pain. Which of the following is most appropriate therapy?

  A. Discharge with advice to stop using cotton wool buds
  B. Discharge with combination of acidifying and antibiotic ear drops
  C. Discharge with oral analgesics
  D. Referral to ENT specialist for myringotomy
  E. None of the above as the ear canal is 'self-cleaning'

3. Pathogens involved in ear disease

A 6-year-old Asian boy is brought to the paediatric emergency department by his mother. She is worried because the boy is lethargic and has been complaining of right-sided earache all day. There have been no similar attacks in the past. On examination, he looks unwell, and his temperature is 39.0°C, pulse rate is 110 beats/min and blood pressure is 90/40 mmHg. There is no cervical lymphadenopathy. Otoscopic examination reveals a bright red right tympanic membrane. You decide to take a microbiology swab. Which one of the following is the most likely pathogen?

  A. Group B streptococcus
  B. *Haemophilus influenzae*
  C. *Mycobacterium tuberculosis*
  D. *Moraxella catarrhalis*
  E. None of the above

4. Management of ear disease

The patient is Question 3 is to undergo treatment for his ear infection. Which one of the following options is most appropriate therapy?

    A. Immediate myringotomy
    B. Advice on hygiene and antipyretics
    C. Refer to ENT for tympanostomy tube
    D. Oral antibiotics (amoxicillin) for 5 days
    E. Antibiotic (amoxicillin) ear drops

5. Ear pain (2)

You are asked to review a 34-year-old Caucasian male patient in the clinic. He describes a long history of problems in his right ear as a child. He also describes a 10-day history of pain in and behind the same ear. There has been a continuous discharge from the ear and he has been feeling 'under the weather'. He has a low-grade fever (37.5°C). Clinical examination reveals tenderness behind the right ear. Otoscopic examination reveals a bulging, red tympanic membrane. Select the most appropriate statement regarding the management of this patient from the list below.

    A. The patient should be discharged on high-dose oral antibiotics for 7 days
    B. Admit the patient for intravenous antibiotics and investigation
    C. The condition cannot be treated by myringotomy and a tympanostomy tube
    D. Mastoidectomy should be performed as soon as practically possible
    E. None of the above

6. Complications of otitis media

The following may all complicate acute otitis media, except

    A. Facial paralysis
    B. Extradural abscess
    C. Mastoiditis
    D. Cavernous sinus thrombosis
    E. Labrynthitis

7. Ear disease

You are asked to review a 75-year-old female patient in the emergency department. She describes a 1-week history of severe left-sided earache, which is especially profound at night. She has taken to carrying tissues with her to clean up copious exudate discharging from the ear. Of note her past medical history includes controlled diabetes mellitus. Physical examination reveals granulation tissue in the external auditory canal. The erythrocyte sedimentation rate is elevated. Which one of the following is the most likely diagnosis?

A. Chronic secretory otitis media
B. Acute mastoiditis
C. Malignant otitis externa
D. Bullous myringitis
E. None of the above

8. Causative pathogens in ear infections

Regarding the same patient in Question 7, which one of the following pathogens is most likely to be responsible?

A. *Pseudomonas aeruginosa*
B. *Streptococcus viridans*
C. *Staphylococcus aureus*
D. *Escherichia coli*
E. *Moraxella catarrhalis*

9. Decline in hearing

A 22-year-old Caucasian man presents to the ENT clinic complaining that he is unable to hear properly in the right ear. A week earlier, he received a blow to the right ear while playing rugby. Rinne's test is negative on the right (bone conduction greater than air conduction). On Weber's test, sound is heard best on the right side. Which one of the following is the most appropriate, regarding the likely cause?

A. Left-sided sensorineural deafness
B. Right-sided conductive deafness
C. Right-sided sensorineural deafness
D. Left-sided conductive deafness
E. None of the above

10. Diagnosis of ear disease (1)

Regarding the same patient in Question 9, otoscopic examination reveals a limited amount of cerumen and a defect in the tympanic membrane. Which one of the following is the most likely diagnosis?

A. Otosclerosis
B. Excess wax
C. Eustachian tube obstruction
D. Perforated tympanic membrane
E. None of the above

11. Difficulty hearing

A 65-year-old Caucasian woman attends the clinic complaining of gradual progressive difficulty hearing in her left ear. She has noticed that she is having to ask her friends and relatives to speak up in public places. This is causing her some social embarrassment. Weber's test localizes to the right ear. Rinne's test is positive bilaterally. Which one of the following is the most appropriate statement regarding the likely cause?

A. Left-sided sensorineural deafness
B. Right-sided conductive deafness
C. Right-sided sensorineural deafness
D. Left-sided conductive deafness
E. None of the above

12. Diagnosis of ear disease (2)

Regarding the patient in Question 11, which one of the following is the most likely diagnosis?

A. Otosclerosis
B. Sudden idiopathic hearing loss
C. Ossicular discontinuity
D. Presbycusis
E. None of the above

13. Dizziness

A 60-year-old Caucasian woman presents to the emergency department complaining of new-onset 'dizziness'. She noticed it in the morning when she turned her head around to talk to her children. She felt the room was spinning around her for a few minutes and she had to go and rest in bed. She denies any deafness, tinnitus, otalgia or otorrhoea. She describes a less severe attack happening two months earlier. On examination she appears comfortable at rest, her pulse is 90 beats/min, blood pressure is 133/68 mmHg and respiratory rate is 12 beats/min. Otoscopic assessment is within normal limits. What will you do next?

A. Request a head computed tomography scan
B. Request magnetic resonance imaging of the brain
C. Perform positional testing
D. Prescribe betahistine
E. Prescribe cyclizine

14. Sore throat (1)

A 4-year-old girl is brought to the paediatric emergency department by her father. He is concerned that she is finding it painful to swallow her saliva. She describes a 1-week history of sore throat and feeling unwell. On examination she is febrile (39.0°C) and dribbling her saliva. A faint high-pitched sound is heard on inspiration from the end of the bed. What will you do next?

  A. Call for senior help and an ENT specialist
  B. Immediately set up an adrenaline nebulizer
  C. Start oral third-generation cephalosporins
  D. Request a neck radiograph
  E. Site a surgical airway

15. Facial trauma

A 17-year-old boy is transferred to the emergency resuscitation bay following a serious road traffic accident. He was not wearing a seat belt and 'bulls-eyed' the windscreen on impact with another car. No life-threatening injuries were detected on primary survey. On secondary survey you notice major bruising to the front and right side of his forehead and face. His right eye is also badly bruised. He has multiple superficial cuts and some blood is trickling from the right nostril. Which one of the following statements is the most appropriate regarding facial trauma?

  A. An orbital fracture may be responsible for the epistaxis
  B. Cerebrospinal fluid rhinorrhoea does not complicate facial injury
  C. Zygomatic fracture may narrow the oropharyngeal isthmus
  D. Inhalation injury should not be suspected
  E. Sensory loss involving the infraorbital nerve is unlikely

16. Nasal obstruction

A 40-year-old Caucasian man presents to the outpatient clinic complaining of progressively severe nasal obstruction. His wife has noticed that he has started to snore at night. He also describes a recent history of clear discharge from his nose. He suffers from recurrent attacks of sinusitis. Physical examination does not reveal any tenderness across the paranasal sinuses. What will you do next?

  A. Request magnetic resonance imaging
  B. Request allergy testing
  C. Request plain radiographs of the sinuses
  D. Examine the nose with a light and mirror
  E. Refer for rhinomanometry

17. Epistaxis (1)

A 50-year-old Asian woman attends the emergency department complaining of a nose bleed that has persisted for more than 10 minutes at home. She is pinching her nose tightly and placed a towel under her mouth to catch any blood. A friend is holding an ice pack on her forehead. She describes several previous attacks which have resolved spontaneously. She is not in any respiratory distress. Her pulse rate is 100 beats/min, blood pressure is 130/70 mmHg and respiratory rate is 12 breaths/min. Physical assessment reveals an anterior bleeding point. What is the next procedure to control the bleeding?

A. Anterior nasal packing
B. Anterior and postnasal packing
C. Silver nitrate cautery
D. Arterial ligation of the sphenopalatine artery
E. None of the above

18. Epistaxis (2)

A 10-year-old boy presents with a history of multiple episodes of moderately severe epistaxis that resolve with conservative management. The most recent attack required hospital admission. He also describes multiple episodes of having a 'stuffy noise' associated with mild headaches. During these episodes his mother thinks he looks 'puffy'. There is no history of foreign body inhalation or nasal trauma. He does not suffer from easy bruising. Which one of the following is the most likely diagnosis?

A. Leukaemia
B. Juvenile nasal angiofibroma
C. Trauma to Little's area
D. Allergic rhinitis
E. Nasal polyps

19. Sore throat (2)

You review a 33-year-old Afro-Caribbean woman in the minors bay of the emergency department. She describes a 4-day history of a sore throat (being worse on the right side) and pain on swallowing. Today, she is unable to even swallow her own saliva. She feels unwell and describes 'ache' in all her muscles and joints. On examination she is febrile (37.9°C), pulse rate is 100 beats/min, blood pressure is 144/90 mmHg and respiratory rate is 12 breaths/min. She is reluctant to open her mouth due to pain. Examination of the oropharynx reveals asymmetric tonsillar enlargement (right more than left) with marked tonsillar exudate. The uvula is deviated to the left. She has bilateral cervical lymphadenopathy. Which one of the following is the most appropriate management?

A. Oral amoxicillin 500 mg four times daily
B. Aspiration of abscess in the emergency department
C. Chlorhexidine mouthwash four times daily
D. Regular oral analgesia and discharge to general practitioner
E. None of the above

20. Parotid swelling

A 68-year-old Caucasian man presents with a 3-week history of a swelling at the angle of the right jaw. He denies pain or any other symptoms of note. On further enquiry, he has felt lethargic for the past few months but denies weight loss. On physical examination, he has a 4 cm × 3 cm firm irregular swelling arising from the right parotid gland. He has an asymmetrical smile and is unable to purse his lips to whistle. The most likely diagnosis is

- A. Benign pleomorphic adenoma
- B. Warthin's tumour (adenolymphoma)
- C. Parotid carcinoma
- D. Salivary gland calculus
- E. None of the above

ANSWERS

Ear pain (1)

1 A Acute otitis externa

Acute otitis externa is a condition caused by inflammation of the outer ear canal. It is particularly common in people who regularly clean their ears with cotton wool buds and in swimmers. The overriding feature is pain, which is worsened by superior elevation of the pinna. The signs may be minimal and therefore the diagnosis is easily missed.

Chronic otitis externa is a low-grade condition commonly associated with dermatitis, which may or may not be associated with pain. Acute otitis media causes deep seated pain, deafness and fever coupled with copious mucoid discharge. Classical mastoiditis should be suspected if there are signs of acute otitis media with mastoid tenderness.

Management of ear pain

2 B Discharge with combination of acidifying and antibiotic ear drops

Topical therapy is the mainstay of treatment in this case. Acidifying drops may prevent the build-up of cerumen (ear wax) and create a more hostile environment for pathogens. Antibiotic drops will usually treat infection in the ear canal. Advice on prevention is important, which includes refraining from swimming, and refraining from using cotton wool buds, headphones or ear plugs. Removal of ear debris and cerumen will aid contact with therapeutic medications and impregnated wicks/gauzes are available for this purpose. Myringotomy is not required. The 'self-cleaning' mechanism (migration of skin toward the external meatus) may not be functioning effectively in patients with otitis externa.

Pathogens involved in ear disease

3 B *Haemophilus influenzae*

Acute otitis media is commonly caused by *Haemophilus influenzae* or *Streptococcus pneumonia* (beta-haemolytic streptococcus). Less commonly, infection may be due to *Moraxella catarrhalis* and *Mycobacterium tuberculosis*. Group B streptococcus species are more commonly found in pregnant women (who are usually asymptomatic) and can infect neonates, causing conditions such as pneumonia and meningitis.

Management of ear disease

4 D Oral antibiotics (amoxicillin) for 5 days

Acute otitis media should be treated with systemic antibiotics, particularly if systemic features are present or there is no improvement in the condition of otherwise asymptomatic children after 72 hours of conservative management. A 5-day course of oral amoxicillin is effective against most of the common pathogenic organisms, but can be replaced with co-amoxiclav if there is no improvement after the first 48 hours of treatment. Analgesics and warm olive oil drops may also be soothing. Myringotomy (fashioning a hole in the tympanic membrane) is reserved for treatment of recurrent otitis media or for otitis media with effusion (glue ear). If a child has multiple infections which are not controlled with medical therapy or there is a significant build-up of fluid, then it may be necessary to insert a grommet (tympanostomy) to enable adequate drainage.

Ear pain (2)

5 B   Admit the patient for intravenous antibiotics and investigation
This patient needs hospital admission as there should be a high index of suspicion of classic mastoiditis. This results from the breakdown of the bony partition between the mastoid air cells. A CT scan will usually confirm fluid-filled middle ear and mastoid and demineralisation of the mastoid trabeculae. A CT scan will exclude any intracranial involvement. The patient should be given high-dose IV antibiotics. Initial procedures may include myringotomy and a tympanostomy tube. If these procedures fail only then is simple or radical mastoidectomy indicated.

Complications of otitis media

6 D   Cavernous sinus thrombosis
All of the options are rare but recognized complications of acute suppurative otitis media with the exception of cavernous sinus thrombosis, which may complicate dental infection or abscess.

Ear disease

7 C   Malignant otitis externa
Malignant otitis externa should be suspected in any patient presenting with severe otalgia which is worse at night, otorrhoea and granulation tissue at the bone–cartilaginous junction. The latter feature is the hallmark of the condition. It is more common in elderly patients and those who are immunocompromised (diabetes mellitus, steroid use, HIV-positive, etc.). Osteitis of the base of the skull may ensue. Cranial nerve involvement indicates a poor prognosis, whilst death may occur as a result of intracranial complications.

Causative pathogens in ear infections

8 A   *Pseudomonas aeruginosa*
The most common pathogen responsible for malignant otitis externa is *Pseudomonas aeruginosa*, followed by *Staphylococcus epidermidis*,

Gram-negative bacteria and fungi. Anti-pseudomonal antibiotics such as piperacillin and tazobactam should be used to treat the condition.

Decline in hearing

9 B Right-sided conductive deafness

These findings suggest a right-sided conductive deafness. Sound is normally heard better by air than bone conduction (Rinne-positive). Conductive deafness reverses Rinne's test (Rinne-negative). In the normal setting, in Weber's test, sound should be heard equally in both ears. A conductive deficit causes the sound to be heard best on the same side as the hearing loss.

Diagnosis of ear disease (1)

10 D Perforated tympanic membrane

Perforation of the ear drum impairs the transmission of sound waves. Traumatic perforations are more common following a blow to the ear with the flat of the hand. These heal spontaneously provided the ear is kept clean and dry. Excess wax can cause conductive deafness, but is less likely given the history and signs. Otosclerosis is a disease involving new bone growth in the inner ear, which may fix the footplate of the stapes, impeding its motion. Eustachian tube obstruction is more common in children.

Difficulty hearing

11 A Left-sided sensorineural deafness

This patient has the clinical features of a left-sided sensorineural deafness. Examination using Weber's test (tuning fork held on the forehead) localizes to the opposite side.

Diagnosis of ear disease (2)

12 D Presbycusis

This patient has a sensorineural hearing loss in the left ear. The most likely cause is presbycusis (age-related hearing loss), a common condition affecting people from the age of 60–65 years onwards. It is caused by progressive loss of the hair cells in the cochlea with age. It affects amplification and discrimination of words. The social implications can lead to embarrassment and isolation if not properly detected. It is treated with an amplification hearing aid device. Sudden hearing loss is rare and unlikely from the history. The latter is thought to be caused by viral infection or vascular ischaemia. Otosclerosis and ossicular discontinuity result in conductive hearing loss.

Dizziness

13 C   Perform positional testing
This patient has benign paroxysmal positional vertigo (BPPV), one of the commonest causes of vertigo. It is typically provoked by certain head movements. The vertigo lasts for a few seconds, but this can seem longer to the patient. The condition is thought to be due to detachment of calcium carbonate crystals from the otolith organ of the affected utricle. The diagnosis may be confirmed by positional testing. It usually resolves spontaneously. A CT scan and MRI would not help in diagnosing this condition but may help differentiate it from other disorders of balance (e.g. transient ischaemic attack, CVA, mass lesions, Ménière's disease). Betahistine (a vasodilator) may help to reduce the endolymphatic fluid imbalance in the inner ear in patients suffering from Ménière's disease. Cyclizine may help to control associated nausea, but will not help to establish a cause.

Sore throat (1)

14 A   Call for senior help and an ENT specialist
This patient has stridor secondary to epiglottitis (also known as acute supraglottitis). This is an emergency not to be missed. You should call immediately for senior help and ENT opinion. The time from stridor to complete respiratory compromise may be very short. In most cases a paediatric anaesthetist will be successful in intubating the child, but the ENT surgeon will be on standby in case a surgical airway is required. Adrenaline nebulizers may buy time, but should not delay expert opinion and treatment. Intravenous cephalosporins should be started and later changed depending on the results of cultures.

Facial trauma

15 A   An orbital fracture may be responsible for the epistaxis
Facial trauma may be complicated by an orbital fracture which may tear the anterior ethmoidal artery resulting in epistaxis. Facial injury may be complicated by CSF rhinorrhoea, especially if it involves the frontal sinus and/or the cribriform plate. Maxillary and mandibular injuries may narrow the oropharyngeal isthmus leading to airway compromise. Inhalation of foreign bodies (teeth and blood) should always be suspected. Sensory loss resulting from damage to the infraorbital nerve may complicate facial injuries.

Nasal obstruction

16 D   Examine the nose with a light and mirror
This patient requires complete ENT assessment to determine the cause for his symptoms. Examination with a head light and mirror may help to exclude any masses or polyps which can commonly occur following

recurrent sinusitis. Plain radiographs of the sinuses are of limited value. Computed tomography and MRI scans may be required to differentiate secretions from soft tissue masses in patients with sinus disease, but should not be requested until a proper physical assessment has been conducted. Rhinomanometry measures nasal airflow, and is an objective method for quantifying the degree of nasal obstruction.

Epistaxis (1)

17 C   **Silver nitrate cautery**

Ninety per cent of epistaxis occurs in Kiesselbach's plexus, which is localized to the anterio-inferior portion of the nasal septum (Kiesselbach's triangle/Little's area). If an obvious bleeding point is seen, attempts to control it with silver nitrate cautery is first-line management. Nasal packs are used only if bleeding continues and no clear bleeding source is identifiable. If anterior packing fails, it may be necessary to pack the postnasal space, but specialist ENT opinion should be sought. If these measures fail to control the bleeding, assessment under a general anaesthetic is required, at which time it may become necessary to ligate the sphenopalatine or maxillary arteries to control ongoing haemorrhage.

Epistaxis (2)

18 B   **Juvenile nasal angiofibroma**

Juvenile nasal angiofibroma is the most likely diagnosis in this patient. This condition presents with episodes of nasal obstruction and epistaxis. However, otological (hearing loss), ocular (diplopia) and facial symptoms (swelling) can also occur. The mass may be seen on indirect mirror, rigid endoscope or rhinoscopy. A biopsy may cause severe haemorrhage and is therefore deferred. The extent of the lesion can be delineated by MRI, CT and angiographic assessment. Surgical excision is the mainstay of treatment. Minor trauma and allergic rhinitis should not lead to facial symptoms. Nasal polyps are rare in children under 10 years. This patient should have a full work-up to exclude haematological causes for repeated epistaxis.

Sore throat (2)

19 E   **None of the above**

This patient has a peritonsillar abscess (quinsy). The appropriate management is referral to an ENT specialist for formal incision and drainage in the operating theatre. Intravenous antibiotics and chlorhexidine mouthwash will not treat a peritonsillar abscess. Regular analgesia may soothe pain following the procedure, but will not treat the quinsy abscess or be suitable as a standalone treatment.

Parotid swelling

20 C   Parotid carcinoma

Parotid carcinoma should be suspected in any patient presenting with a parotid tumour and facial nerve involvement. The parotid gland accounts for approximately 80% of salivary gland tumours, and 80% of them are benign. Common examples of benign salivary gland tumours are pleomorphic adenoma and adenolymphoma (Warthin's tumour). Salivary gland calculi tend to present with intermittent episodes of pain and swelling and do not involve the facial nerve.

SECTION 15:
OPHTHALMIC SURGERY

Questions

1. Diagnosis of eye pain   318
2. Red eye (1)   318
3. Red eye (2)   318
4. Ophthalmic emergencies   319
5. Paediatric ophthalmology   319
6. Nerve palsy and the eye   319
7. Foreign bodies (1)   320
8. Foreign bodies (2)   320
9. Foreign bodies (3)   320
10. Ocular trauma (1)   320
11. Ocular trauma (2)   321
12. Ocular trauma (3)   321
13. Acute visual disturbance (1)   321
14. Acute visual disturbance (2)   322
15. Acute visual disturbance (3)   322
16. Neurovascular visual disturbance   322
17. Investigation of visual field deficit   323
18. Headache   323
19. Eye infection   323
20. Glaucoma   324

Answers   325

QUESTIONS

1. Diagnosis of eye pain

A 40-year-old woman presents complaining that her right eye hurts and that she cannot tolerate the bright light in the room. She is protecting her right eye with her hand. There is no history of trauma or foreign body. Visual acuity is reduced in the right eye. Examination reveals redness at the junction between the cornea and sclera of the right eye. The right pupil appears small. Slit lamp examination reveals a collection of cells in the anterior chamber of the eye. What is the most likely cause of this woman's symptoms?

    A.   Conjunctivitis
    B.   Acute closed angle glaucoma
    C.   Corneal ulceration
    D.   Iritis
    E.   Trauma

2. Red eye (1)

A 22-year-old Caucasian man presents with a 1-day history of discomfort and a 'weepy' left eye. His brother recently had similar symptoms. He denies any previous trauma. His vision is entirely unaltered and has normal acuity on formal testing. Physical examination reveals a red eye with uniform engorgement of all the conjunctival blood vessels. What is the most likely diagnosis?

    A.   Conjunctivitis
    B.   Trauma
    C.   Iritis
    D.   Glaucoma → ↑ IOP
    E.   Keratitis

3. Red eye (2)

A 64-year-old Caucasian man presents with a 1-week history of an erythematous vesicular rash on the right side of his face and forehead. He also complains of a painful red right eye. His visual acuity is reduced on the right. Slit lamp assessment with fluorescein stain reveals a discrete green patch under blue light. What is the most likely cause for the acute red eye in this patient?

    A.   Acute closed angle glaucoma
    B.   Herpes simplex corneal ulcer
    C.   Varicella zoster corneal ulcer
    D.   Iridiocyclitis
    E.   Conjunctivitis

4. Ophthalmic emergencies

A 72-year-old Asian man presents complaining of sudden severe pain in his right eye. The pain is associated with nausea and vomiting. His vision is mildly impaired on the right side. On examination, the eye is inflamed and acutely tender. The pupil is semi-dilated and fixed. The intraocular pressure is raised. What is the most likely diagnosis?

- Ⓐ Acute closed angle glaucoma
- B. Viral conjunctivitis
- C. Iritis — pupil constricted
- D. Episcleritis ? IOP not raised
- E. Keratitis

[handwritten margin note:] Unwell
Sinus tender rest
restricted painful
eye movements

5. Paediatric ophthalmology

A 9-year-old boy is brought to the hospital by his father because he noticed that his right eye was 'red, bulging and not moving very well'. The boy describes a headache and pain on moving his right eye. He has had multiple previous attacks of sinusitis. On examination, his temperature is 39.0°C, blood pressure 100/60 mmHg, pulse 94 beats/min, and respiratory rate 20 breaths/min. Physical assessment reveals proptosis and ophthalmoplegia of the right eye with pain to gentle palpation. The sinuses are tender, his eyelids are erythematous and the conjunctiva is markedly injected, but visual acuity is intact bilaterally. A purulent nasal discharge is additionally noted by the examining clinician. What is the most appropriate next step?

- A. Needle aspiration of the orbit
- B. Oral amoxicillin 500 mg four times daily for 10 days
- C. Topical steroid eye drops
- Ⓓ Admit for high-dose intravenous antibiotics
- E. None of the above

6. Nerve palsy and the eye

A 64-year-old Caucasian woman presents to the emergency department complaining of a 'droopy left eyelid'. She has been a smoker since her twenties (with a 40 pack year history) and drinks between 20 and 25 units of alcohol each week. There is no prior history of neuromuscular disorder. Physical examination reveals clubbing, and a small reactive left pupil. Visual acuity is unaltered and eye movements are normal. An absence of sweating is noticed across the left side of the forehead. Which of the following diagnoses is most likely?

- Ⓐ Horner's syndrome secondary to an apical lung tumour
- B. Horner's syndrome secondary to syringomyelia
- C. Myasthenia gravis
- D. Third nerve palsy
- E. Pseudoptosis

7. Foreign bodies (1)

A 40-year-old Caucasian man presents complaining of pain in his left eye. Earlier that day he was working in his house, attempting to put up a shelf with nails. He felt a sensation of 'some material entering his eye'. He does not wear contact lenses. His eye has been extremely watery and he has been unable to open it properly. All of the following statements regarding assessment are correct, except

- A. It is vital to assess visual acuity
- B. Local anaesthesia may be required to formally assess the eye
- C. The use of fluorescein is required to exclude an abrasion
- D. Laceration to the margin of the eyelid can be sutured in the emergency room
- E. It is important to identify and remove any foreign bodies

8. Foreign bodies (2)

Regarding the same patient as in Question 7, fluorescein assessment under the blue light slit lamp reveals a discrete green region at the lateral corneal margin. Which one of the following statements best describes the management for corneal abrasion following foreign body injury?

- A. An eye pad should not be prescribed
- B. Topical steroids should be prescribed
- C. Chloramphenicol may help prevent infection
- D. Cycloplegic drops may speed healing
- E. Surgery has no role in the management

9. Foreign bodies (3)

Regarding the same patient as in Questions 7 and 8, following clinical assessment and thorough irrigation, the assessing clinician removes all the foreign bodies, which are sent for culture. Which one of the following pathogens is most likely to be responsible for infection?

- A. *Streptococcus* →
- B. *Pseudomonas* Contact lens wearer
- C. *Candida* → Immuno Compromised
- D. *Chlamydia* → conjuctivitis or trachoma
- E. *Staphylococcus*

10. Ocular trauma (1)

A 12-year-old Caucasian boy is brought to the emergency department by his mother on a Sunday afternoon. He was playing squash and the ball 'flew and hit his left eye'. The boy complains of double vision and his visual acuity is reduced on the left side. Physical examination reveals an irregular left pupil that reacts poorly to light. Eye movements are restricted. There is reduced sensation below the left eye and blood is spotted from the ipsilateral nose. Slit lamp assessment reveals a subconjunctival haemorrhage. What is the most likely diagnosis?

A. Extradural haemorrhage
B. Orbital 'blow out' fracture
C. Third nerve palsy — opthalmoplegia , dilation , ptosis
D. Retinal detachment
E. Lacerated levator muscle

11. Ocular trauma (2)

Which one of the following is the most accurate statement regarding chemical ocular injury?

A. Alkali are especially damaging
B. The severity of injury is unrelated to the substance
C. Specialist referral can be delayed
D. Irrigation is unnecessary
E. None of the above

12. Ocular trauma (3)

A 20-year-old man is brought into the resuscitation bay of the emergency department having been involved in a road traffic accident. He is immediately intubated and ventilated as he has a Glasgow Coma Scale score of 4/15 on arrival. You are asked to review his ocular injuries as part of the secondary survey just prior to the computed tomography scan. On inspection, you see a deep horizontal laceration at the inferior aspect of the lower eyelid. Which structure is most likely to be damaged given the pattern of injury?

A. Nasolacrimal duct
B. Levator palpebrae superioris
C. Inferior oblique muscle
D. Lacrimal canaliculi
E. Lateral rectus muscle

13. Acute visual disturbance (1)

A 54-year-old Caucasian man presents to the eye clinic complaining of experiencing 'flashes of light', heaviness around his right eye and the sensation of 'floaters' in the right visual field. He is concerned as the symptoms have not resolved spontaneously. Examination reveals loss of peripheral vision over the right visual fields. What is the most likely diagnosis?

A. Arterial occlusion
B. Macular degeneration
C. Posterior vitreous detachment
D. Migraine
E. Retinal detachment

14. Acute visual disturbance (2)

An 80-year-old African American man presents to the emergency department as he has noticed a sudden loss of central aspects of his visual fields. On
examination, visual acuity is mildly reduced bilaterally. The central lines on an
Amsler chart (grid line chart) appear distorted. The peripheral fields are normal.
Fundoscopy reveals multiple retinal infiltrates, but the macula appears normal
in size and shape. What is the most likely diagnosis?

  A. Retinal detachment
  B. Migraine
  C. Age-related macular degeneration
  D. Arterial occlusion
  E. None of the above

15. Acute visual disturbance (3)

A 48-year-old Caucasian man presents to the emergency department complaining of sudden-onset loss of vision in his left eye which has now resolved. A few
hours ago, he experienced the sensation of a 'curtain falling down over his left
eye'. He is a smoker with a 40 pack year history and also has a past history
of transient ischaemic attacks and angina. Fundoscopy reveals retinal infarcts
and a cherry-red spot at the macula. The most appropriate management for this
patient is

  A. Treatment with steroids
  B. Laser treatment to the ischaemic retina
  C. Oral sumatriptan
  D. Carotid duplex and oral aspirin
  E. None of the above

16. Neurovascular visual disturbance

An 80-year-old Caucasian man comes to the emergency department because
of sudden-onset, transient visual loss in his right eye. He is currently
asymptomatic, and denies any other new symptoms. His past medical history includes hypertension and peripheral vascular disease. His medications
include aspirin and ramipril. On examination, his temperature is 36.7°C,
blood pressure 170/80 mmHg, pulse rate 70 beats/min and respiratory rate 12
breaths/min. Which one of the following is most likely to be found on clinical examination?

  A. Carotid bruit
  B. Pansystolic heart murmur
  C. Irregularly irregular heart beat
  D. Papilloedema
  E. Haemorrhagic exudates in the retina

17. Investigation of visual field deficit

A 40-year-old Caucasian man presents with visual disturbance in both temporal visual fields. He works as a taxi driver and is finding he cannot notice customers on the street as well as he used to. His appetite is reduced. He has a 2-week history of morning headache. Clinical examination reveals bitemporal hemianopia. Which of the following is the best diagnostic investigation?

- A. Fundoscopy
- B. Serum thyroid-stimulating hormone
- C. Angiogram
- D. Skull radiograph
- E. None of the above

18. Headache

You are asked to see a 77-year-old Caucasian woman on the ward by the admitting medical team. She describes a 1-week history of a constant ache on the right side of her head. This area is especially tender when she touches it or combs her hair. She describes suffering a similar series of symptoms approximately a year before the present admission on the left side, which resulted in complete blindness in her left eye. She has no visual disturbance in the right eye and acuity is normal. What would you recommend the team to do next?

- A. Refer immediately to an ophthalmologist
- B. Start high-dose steroids immediately
- C. Perform a temporal artery biopsy
- D. Perform erythrocyte sedimentation rate
- E. None of the above

19. Eye infection

An 18-year-old Caucasian man presents with a 2-day history of a unilateral sore, red, right eye. He describes 'gum sticking the eyelids together'. He also describes dysuria and a painful right knee. His visual acuity is normal and examination reveals a diffusely injected conjunctiva. What is the pathogen most likely to be causing this man's symptoms?

- A. *Staphylococcus*
- B. *Chlamydia*
- C. *Streptococcus*
- D. *Escherichia coli*
- E. *Proteus*

20. Glaucoma

Regarding the management of chronic/primary open angle glaucoma, all the following statements are true, except

- A. Older patients are at increased risk
- B. People with diabetes and those of African Caribbean origin are at higher risk
- C. Symptoms may not be present despite significant pathology
- D. Can be treated by carbonic anhydrase inhibitors
- E. Laser trabeculoplasty is rarely indicated

ANSWERS

[handwritten: Topical corticosteroids]

Diagnosis of eye pain

[handwritten: hypopyon — anterior chamber (pus)]

1 D   Iritis

This patient has anterior uveitis or iritis. This condition leads to eye pain, redness, excessive tearing, photophobia, visual loss in late stages and a constricted pupil due to spasm of the papillary sphincter. The presence of a hypopyon (pus deposition from leucocytes) in the anterior chamber on slit lamp assessment helps differentiate iritis from other causes of acute red eye. Approximately 50% of cases are primary and of unknown origin whilst the remainder may be associated with certain sexually transmitted infections, tuberculosis and autoimmune disorders such as systemic lupus erythematosus (SLE) and sarcoidosis. If an underlying cause is found, it must be treated but due to the frequent inability to identify a precipitating factor, management consists largely of symptomatic control. Treatment with topical corticosteroids may reduce inflammation and prevent adhesion formation and visual loss.

Red eye (1)

[handwritten: viral self limiting; Bacterial → Chloramphenicol]

2 A   Conjunctivitis

Conjunctivitis is an inflammation of the conjunctiva, the connective tissue layer that covers the eyeball and inner layer of the eyelid. It is one of the most common causes of an uncomfortable red eye in clinical practice. Conjunctivitis is primarily a diagnosis of exclusion, made in instances of red eye and discharge where there is neither visual loss nor evidence of glaucoma, iritis or keratitis. It is typically bilateral, but the recent family history with discharge from the eye suggests an infective cause in the patient described by the scenario. It is also worth remembering that conjunctivitis may be viral (which is generally self-limiting) or bacterial in nature. Bacterial conjunctivitis is treated according to clinical severity. Classical therapy consists of instilling chloramphenicol eye drops to the affected eye; initially hourly for the first 24 hours, gradually decreasing the frequency to four times per day. General advice on hygienic measures may also be appropriate.

Red eye (2)

3 C   Varicella zoster corneal ulcer

When reactivation of dormant varicella zoster virus (herpes zoster/shingles) affects the nasociliary division of the trigeminal nerve, herpetic eruptions can occur on the nose tip. The presence of these lesions is highly suggestive of present or imminent corneal involvement by the viral process (also known as Hutchinson's sign/rule). Ophthalmic zoster (herpes zoster ophthalmicus) can cause multiple ophthalmic conditions, including scleritis, iritis, corneal ulceration (which can be detected by fluorescein staining) and, in severe cases, blindness. Patients with corneal ulceration should be referred on to specialist care as there is a high risk of visual loss. Treatment is with acyclovir eye ointment and oral aciclovir (800 mg, five times daily) for 7–10 days. In cases of corneal ulceration, intensive treatment is started in the form of antibiotic eye drops whilst cycloplegic drops may additionally be used to relieve pain resulting from ciliary muscle spasm.

Ophthalmic emergencies

4 A Acute closed angle glaucoma

Acute closed angle glaucoma (or primary angle closure glaucoma) is an ophthalmic emergency that occurs when the iris is pressed against the trabecular meshwork at the angle of the anterior chamber of the eye, thereby blocking the outflow of aqueous humour. This blockage, and subsequent aqueous accumulation, precipitates a dangerous elevation of the intra-ocular pressure (IOP) which must be reduced to prevent optic nerve damage and preserve sight. In cases where it is not possible to immediately transfer the patient to a specialist unit for definitive surgical treatment, pilocarpine 4% (to constrict the pupil) and acetazolamide, as a stat dose of 500 mg IV followed by 500 mg orally, should be given. Mannitol 20% (500 mL) given by slow IV infusion is also proven to effectively reduce IOP. The pupil is usually constricted in iritis and an examination will confirm hypopyon. Intraocular pressure is not elevated in cases of conjunctivitis, episcleritis and keratitis.

[handwritten margin note: Closed angle glaucoma → refer to specialist to decompress]

Paediatric ophthalmology

5 D Admit for high-dose intravenous antibiotics

The scenario suggests a diagnosis of orbital cellulitis, a potentially blinding and life-threatening condition that must not be missed. It most commonly results from the spread of infection from the adjacent paranasal sinuses and is especially important to diagnose promptly in children, in whom it occurs more frequently than adults and can lead to rapid loss of sight. The typical triad suggestive of infection is that

- The patient is unwell
- There is tenderness over the sinuses
- There is painful restriction of eye movements

Owing to the seriousness of the condition, affected individuals should be admitted to hospital and given intravenous broad-spectrum antibiotics (e.g. amoxicillin or cephalosporin) unless cultures identify a causative agent for which specific treatment can be administered. The duration of intravenous therapy is dependent on the clinical course but typically lasts 1–2 weeks. Once the condition settles, intravenous antibiotics are replaced with oral antibiotics for a further 2 weeks at which point the patient is usually reviewed in the outpatient clinic. Topical steroid application and needle aspiration is not indicated in this scenario, although formal surgical drainage may be necessary in the presence of an orbital abscess refractory to intravenous therapy.

Nerve palsy and the eye

[handwritten margin note: ptosis, miosis, anhydrosis]

6 A   **Horner's syndrome secondary to an apical lung tumour**
The features indicative of Horner's syndrome include ptosis or drooping of the eyelid, a small reactive pupil and the absence of sweating on the same side of the face. Horner's syndrome is caused by damage to the sympathetic nerve supply to the eye, in this case most likely due to a Pancoast/apical lung tumour. Ptosis can also be caused by general muscular disorders such as dystrophia myotonica and myasthenia gravis, but these are less likely in the absence of typical facies and without wider abnormalities of muscular tone. Third nerve palsy may present with ptosis, but the pupil is usually dilated and the affected eye may assume the classic 'down and out' position.

Foreign bodies (1)

7 D   **Laceration to the margin of the eyelid can be sutured in the emergency room**
Lacerations to the eyelids generally need specialist attention, especially if

- The lid margins are torn – as accurate approximation is important
- Lacrimal ducts have been damaged
- There is suspicion of a foreign body or penetrating eyelid injury

It may be necessary to use local anaesthesia to assess the eye and fluorescein is required to exclude an abrasion. Foreign bodies should be removed and visual acuity should always be tested to establish a baseline of function. However, normal visual acuity does not rule out the possibility of serious ophthalmic injury.

[handwritten margin note: cycloplegic —relieve muscle spasm.]

Foreign bodies (2)

8 C   **Chloramphenicol may help prevent infection**
In the management of corneal abrasion, an eye patch may help to speed healing. Chloramphenicol drops are commonly prescribed as a prophylactic agent against infection. Cycloplegic drugs may help relieve pain, but there is no evidence that they aid healing. Topical steroids

are contraindicated since they increase the risk of infection. Surgery is undertaken in cases of recurrent abrasion to enhance adhesion between the epithelium and underlying basement membrane.

Foreign bodies (3)

9 E   *Staphylococcus*
Studies have revealed that coagulase-negative *Staphylococcus* is the most common pathogen isolated from ocular foreign bodies. *Pseudomonas* is more common in contact lens wearers. *Chlamydia* can cause conjunctivitis or trachoma, but can be more difficult to culture. *Candida* may be cultured from the ocular surface of the eye in immunocompromised patients.

Ocular trauma (1)

10 B   Orbital 'blow out' fracture
Orbital 'blow out' fracture should be suspected following blunt ocular injury when the patient has diplopia, a recessed eye, defective eye movements, ipsilateral epistaxis and diminished sensation over the distribution of the infra-orbital nerve. Any disturbance in visual acuity following blunt ocular trauma should prompt early specialist referral. Pupillary abnormalities are common and can mask a dilated pupil caused by acute extradural haemorrhage; a high index of suspicion is therefore required. Third nerve palsy presents with ophthalmoplegia, ptosis and pupillary dilatation, however the history in this scenario is more consistent with a bony orbital injury.

Ocular trauma (2)

11 A   Alkali are especially damaging
Alkaline chemicals that have a high pH can penetrate the surface of the eye and cause severe injury to both external structures such as the cornea and internal structures such as the lens. In general, more damage occurs with higher pH chemicals than with acids. The severity of the injury is dependent on the nature of the substance and degree of contamination. Thorough irrigation is essential and may be all that is required in cases of minimal contamination. Specialist advice should always be sought in cases of chemical ocular injury.

Ocular trauma (3)

12 C   Inferior oblique muscle
Horizontal injuries of the lower eyelid may involve the inferior tarsal plate, inferior oblique muscle and infra-orbital nerve. Horizontal lacerations of the upper lid may penetrate the septum and injure the

levator palpebrae superioris. Lateral ocular injuries may damage the lateral rectus. The lacrimal duct, canal and gland are more susceptible to medial ocular injury.

Acute visual disturbance (1)

13 E   Retinal detachment

Retinal detachment should be suspected from the clinical history. Advanced detachment affects the visual fields. Sudden onset of floaters indicates pigment or blood in the vitreous, whilst flashing lights (photopsia) are caused by retinal traction. The condition is a medical emergency and requires immediate specialist referral. There is characteristically no field loss in posterior vitreous detachment. Migrainerelated field defects usually resolve within a few hours. Peripheral fields are often normal in cases of macular degeneration.

Acute visual disturbance (2)

14 C   Age-related macular degeneration

Macular degeneration of old age is one of the leading causes of blindness. The macula is the central region of the retina, which can atrophy over time leading to the loss of central vision. Yellow retinal deposits or drusen are commonly observed. The macula may look entirely normal. Central visual field loss is not a typical ophthalmic feature of migraine or arterial occlusion. Retinal detachment may result in peripheral visual field loss.

Acute visual disturbance (3)

15 D   Carotid duplex and oral aspirin

The scenario describes a case of amaurosis fugax, a transient monocular visual loss. The extent of visual field loss depends on the size of the affected retina. The retinal artery may become blocked due to atherosclerosis, thrombosis or emboli. Episodes may occur in conjunction with transient ischaemic attacks. Carotid arterial duplex will identify flow abnormalities and/or the source of an embolus. Risk factors for arterial disease should be treated and the patient prescribed aspirin or clopidogrel. Steroid treatment is reserved for acute visual disturbance associated with optic neuritis. Laser treatment to ablate the retina may be indicated in venous occlusion to prevent secondary glaucoma, whilst oral sumatriptan is used to treat ocular manifestations of migraine.

Neurovascular visual disturbance

16 A   Carotid bruit

The patient has amaurosis fugax, a common cause for transient visual loss in patients with previous arterial disease. A carotid bruit is the most likely examination finding, TIAs and amaurosis fugax are caused by platelet microthrombi from the surface of atherosclerotic disease. Atrial thrombi are too large to present in this manner and therefore atrial fibrillation is a less common cause. A pansystolic murmur is more likely to be due to mitral or tricuspid regurgitation, but may also be caused by an atrial or ventricular septal defect which may allow emboli to cross from the right heart to the left. So-called paradoxical emboli are, however, a rare cause of TIA.

Papilloedema is seen in cases of raised intracranial pressure. Occlusion of the posterior ciliary arteries may lead to ischaemia of the optic nerve head (ischaemic optic neuropathy) but this should not be mistaken for papilloedema. Retinal 'flame haemorrhages' are seen in cases of venous occlusion.

Investigation of visual field deficit

17 E   None of the above
The scenario suggests the presence of a pituitary tumour impinging on the optic chiasm. Other causes for bitemporal hemianopia include nasopharyngeal carcinoma and sphenoid sinus mucocele. If a pituitary tumour is suspected, further assessment with an MRI and occasionally a CT scan (to detect calcification secondary to tumour growth) is indicated. Fundoscopy cannot be considered a valid answer here. Although fundoscopy may help identify disc atrophy, it does not constitute a diagnostic investigation in this case.

Headache

18 B   Start high-dose steroids immediately
This patient has giant cell (temporal) arteritis. Giant cell arteritis has several serious complications, most notably blindness, which may occur in 10%–15% of untreated or inadequately treated patients. Blindness may not be preceded by visual symptoms. High dosages of steroids (40–60 mg per day of prednisone) are used for giant cell arteritis. Clinical suspicion should guide commencing steroid treatment, which should not be delayed whilst awaiting a formal tissue diagnosis. The ESR is almost always elevated, but should not delay treatment. Where the history is uncertain, temporal artery biopsy should be undertaken. Referral to an ophthalmologist can often be avoided.

Eye infection

19 B   *Chlamydia*
Reiter's syndrome is characterized by the triad of urethritis, arthritis of large joints and conjunctivitis. The most likely pathogen involved

in the process is *Chlamydia*. It is important to include a detailed sexual history during initial assessment and urethral swabs should be taken during clinical work-up so as to culture the causative organism and treat the patient with appropriate pharmacological agents. Eye involvement occurs in about 50% of men with urogenital reactive arthritis. Conjunctivitis and uveitis can present as redness of the eyes, eye pain and irritation, or blurred vision. Eye involvement typically occurs early in the course of reactive arthritis, and symptoms may come and go. *Staphylococcus* is more commonly cultured from ocular foreign bodies. *E. coli* and *Proteus* may be cultured from urinary specimens in patients with urinary tract infections.

Glaucoma

20 E **Laser trabeculoplasty is rarely indicated**
Primary (chronic) open angle glaucoma is the commonest form of glaucoma and the third leading cause of blindness in the UK. It is caused by a gradual resistance to the outflow of aqueous humour through the trabecular network. There is an increased risk as a result of advancing age, diabetes, being a first-degree relative of sufferers, African Caribbean ethnicity and myopia. Symptoms may be absent despite ongoing gradual increases in intraocular pressure. Central visual fields are spared until quite late on in the disease process. The condition is treated with β-blockers such as timolol to reduce secretion of aqueous, carbonic anhydrase inhibitors (acetazolamide) which also reduce aqueous secretion and pilocarpine (para-sympathomimetic agent) to constrict the pupil and increase the outflow of aqueous. If these measures fail patients often require laser trabeculoplasty – a procedure that applies laser energy to regions around the trabecular network to improve drainage.

SECTION 16:
LUMPS, BUMPS, SKIN AND HERNIAS

Questions

1. Neck lumps (1) — 334
2. Neck lumps (2) — 334
3. Neck lumps (3) — 334
4. Complications of thyroid surgery — 334
5. Neck lumps (4) — 335
6. Thyroid carcinoma — 335
7. Thyroid disease — 335
8. Neck swellings — 336
9. Neck anatomy — 336
10. Salivary gland swellings (1) — 336
11. Salivary gland swellings (2) — 336
12. Facial swelling — 337
13. Parotid gland pathology — 337
14. Lumps around the body (1) — 337
15. Lumps around the body (2) — 338
16. Anatomy of the abdominal wall and hernia — 338
17. Gynaecomastia — 338
18. Hernias (1) — 339
19. Hernias (2) — 339
20. Groin swelling — 339

Answers — 340

QUESTIONS

1. Neck lumps (1)

An 18-year-old school student of East African origin presents with a 2-week history of lethargy, myalgia, rigours with hot flushes and intermittent pyrexia. Neither she nor any close contacts have been travelling recently. Examination reveals enlarged anterior and posterior chain lymph nodes in the neck. A blood film reveals the presence of Downey bodies, thrombocytosis and an increase in the lymphocyte count to 50% of total leucocytes. This girl is likely to have

[handwritten: Pfeiffer's disease]
[handwritten: EBV infection]

A. Tuberculosis
B. Toxoplasmosis
C. Human immunodeficiency virus (HIV) infection
D. Lymphoma
E. Infectious mononucleosis   *[handwritten: Monospot / Paul-Bunnell test.]*

2. Neck lumps (2)

A 16-year-old girl presents with a smooth, round and painless lump in the midline of the neck, of which she feels very self-conscious. On examination, it is firm, transilluminates and is painless to touch. In addition, it moves up when the patient is asked to take a sip of water. This is likely to be a

A. Papillary carcinoma of the thyroid
B. Goitre
C. Thyroglossal cyst
D. Lingual thyroid
E. Sebaceous cyst

3. Neck lumps (3)

A 45-year-old female business executive presents with a swelling in the midline of the neck and features of hyperthyroidism secondary to Graves' disease. Following a course of antithyroid medication, a subtotal thyroidectomy is performed. Raised titres of which immunoglobulin would be expected in this individual?

A. Anti-thyroglobulin antibody
B. Rheumatoid factor
C. Antinuclear antibody
D. Antineutrophil cytoplasmic antibody
E. Anti-thyroid-stimulating hormone receptor antibody

4. Complications of thyroid surgery

You are asked to assess a 25-year-old patient who returned from theatre 2 hours ago following a thyroidectomy for a large, hyperplastic goitre and is now complaining of difficulty swallowing sips of water. On examination you note that she

is very short of breath with a respiratory rate of 30 breaths/min, using her accessory muscles of respiration and only able to answer your questions in two or three
words. In addition, there appears to be a fluctuant mass in the midline of the neck
underlying the surgical clips. Immediate management of this patient would be

A. High-flow oxygen via Hudson mask
B. Removal of surgical clips at the bedside
C. Intravenous access with two large-bore cannulae and fluid
   resuscitation
D. Removal of surgical clips in theatre under general anaesthesia
E. Call your senior and wait for him/her to remove the clips

5. Neck lumps (4)

A 28-year-old secretary presents with a lump in the midline of the neck that has
grown progressively larger over the past several months. On examination, there is a
palpable lymph node in the left submandibular region. An aspirate is taken, confirming a malignant cancer of the thyroid gland. The origin of this is most likely to be

Papillary → Lymphatic Spread

A. Follicular
B. Anaplastic
C. Medullary
D. Lymphoma
E. Papillary

6. Thyroid carcinoma

→ offects parofollicularcells

A 37-year-old patient is diagnosed with medullary carcinoma of the thyroid
gland. The concentration of which electrolyte could be reduced in this patient?

↓ secretes Calcitonin.

A. Sodium
B. Potassium
C. Chloride
D. Calcium
E. Magnesium

7. Thyroid disease

A 68-year-old man presents with a 10-week history of a rapidly growing swelling in the midline of the neck. Prior to this problem developing he has been in
excellent health. Over the past 10 weeks, he has begun to feel more worn out
and is unable to complete his daily 3-mile walk without getting short of breath,
which he was previously able to manage comfortably. His wife also reports that
his voice has become increasingly hoarse in the last 2 weeks. The presentation is
likely to be consistent with

A. Recurrent laryngeal nerve damage
B. Tracheal trauma

C. Medullary carcinoma of the thyroid
D. Anaplastic carcinoma of the thyroid — *rapidly growing with compression symptoms.*
E. Papillary carcinoma of the thyroid

8. Neck swellings

A 59-year-old fisherman presents with longstanding weight loss, anorexia and lethargy. Physical examination reveals a palpable swelling in the left supra-clavicular fossa. A disseminated adenocarcinoma of the stomach is diagnosed following a gastroscopy and computed tomography scan of the thorax and abdomen. This patient has presented with

A. Virchow's node
B. Battle's sign
C. Cloquet's node
D. Troisier's sign
E. Trousseau's sign

9. Neck anatomy

Which of the following structures does not form a border of the anterior triangle of the neck?

A. Midline of the neck
B. Anterior border of sternocleidomastoid muscle
C. Lower border of the mandible
D. Investing fascia
E. Middle third of the clavicle

10. Salivary gland swellings (1)

A 45-year-old woman is diagnosed with a submandibular calculus, having presented with a tender lump below the jaw on eating. Which structure is likely to be obstructed?

A. Warthin's duct
B. Stensen's duct → *duct of parotid gland*
C. Biliary duct
D. Lingual nerve → *passes through submandibular gland*
E. Facial nerve → *passes through parotid gland*

11. Salivary gland swellings (2)

A 40-year-old man presents with a month-long history of intermittent, left-sided pain and swelling in the anterior neck under the left jaw. His symptoms are associated with meal times and regress shortly after completing each meal. In recent days however, the pain appears to have become more intense and the swelling more firm. On examination a firm lump is palpable in the left submandibular region, bimanual palpation of which causes the patient to complain of a foul taste in his mouth. The most appropriate diagnostic investigation will be

A. Plain radiographs of the mouth
B. Blood calcium level
C. Biopsy of submandibular tissue
D. Sialogram
E. None of the above

12. Facial swelling

A 54-year-old builder attends your outpatient clinic with his wife, reporting an 8-month history of a lump on the left side of his face, in front of his ear. It is painless and does not trouble him. He has attended on the insistence of his wife, who is worried that it may be growing larger. On examination, the swelling appears to lie anterior to the angle of the jaw on the left side. It is non-tender and approximately 5 cm in diameter with a clear edge. The skin is easily moved on top of it and the lump itself feels rubbery to touch. There is no cervical lymph-adenopathy or facial droop evident on examination. An aspirate is taken which shows cells of many different types. A decision is made at a follow-up appointment to excise the lump under anaesthesia. This is likely to be

A. Pleomorphic adenoma
B. Adenolymphoma (Warthin's tumour) → soft, usually bilateral
C. Mikulicz's syndrome
D. Sjörgen's syndrome
E. Carcinoma of the parotid gland

13. Parotid gland pathology

A 6-year-old boy presents with his mother to the general practice at which you are based, with a 3-week history of bilateral cheek swelling. The family is newly registered and medical records have not yet been transferred to the practice. His mother informs you that the young boy has not received any of his childhood vaccinations, as she has been worried about their possible detrimental effects. The clinical suspicion is of mumps parotitis. Which class of infectious agent is responsible for mumps?

A. RNA viruses
B. DNA viruses
C. Gram-negative bacteria
D. Gram-positive bacteria
E. Fungi

14. Lumps around the body (1)

A 39-year-old man of Italian origin presents complaining of an exquisitely tender area over his right buttock, which has been present for several weeks. Within the past few days, the area has begun to weep profusely and his temperature at home prior to admission was 38°C. He reports having had this problem previously and was operated on during a previous admission. On examination you note that the man is extremely hairy and that there is an irregular, erythematous, warm and exquisitely tender shallow lump overlying the top of the right buttock. A small scar is seen over the lump and, on palpation, it is fluctuant and discharges purulent fluid. A pilonidal abscess is suspected. Definitive management would consist of

A. Advising to shave the affected area
B. Intravenous antibiotics
C. Drainage of the abscess under local anaesthesia
D. Drainage of the abscess under general anaesthesia
E. Oral antibiotics

definitive treatment ← D

15. Lumps around the body (2)

A 56-year-old priest presents with a lump at the back of his hand that has been getting larger over the past year. Although it does not trouble him, his parishioners are increasingly commenting on it after his Sunday service. On examination, there is a soft, non-tender, irregular lump on the dorsum of the hand 3 cm × 5 cm in size. It is fluctuant on movement and transilluminates, but does not reduce when pressed down. The skin moves freely over it and no other such lumps are to be found on either arm. An aspirate produces a dark gelatinous material. This is most likely a

A. Sebaceous cyst
B. Ganglion
C. Bursa
D. Rheumatoid nodule → *Rheumatoid arthritis*
E. Cystic hygroma

16. Anatomy of the abdominal wall and hernia

Which one of the following muscles lies closest to the peritoneal cavity?

A. Rectus abdominis
B. External oblique
C. Internal oblique
D. Transversus abdominis
E. Cremaster → *from internal oblique.*

17. Gynaecomastia

A 55-year-old man with known atrial fibrillation presents to his general practitioner with a 3-month history of gynaecomastia. Which of his following medications is not associated with gynaecomastia?

A. Digoxin
B. Cimetidine *H₂-blocker*

C. Spironolactone Ald. antagonist
D. Furosemide
E. Metronidazole

18. Hernias (1)

Regarding hernias in females, the most common is
↳ Inguinal for both males and females

A. Epigastric
B. Umbilical
C. Femoral
D. Inguinal
E. Incisional

19. Hernias (2)

Which of the following structures form a part of both the inguinal and femoral canals?

A. Transversalis fascia
B. Internal oblique muscle
C. Transversus abdominis muscle
D. Inguinal ligament
E. Pectineal ligament

20. Groin swelling

A 35-year-old professional weightlifter presents with a red and swollen lump in the left groin. An inguinal hernia is suspected and, at the time of operation, the lump is found to contain a small loop of necrotic bowel. This type of hernia is best described as

A. Irreducible
B. Strangulated
C. Obstructed
D. Sliding
E. Richter's

ANSWERS

Neck lumps (1)

1 E   Infectious mononucleosis

Lymph nodes are the most common neck swellings in clinical practice, accounting for some 85% of all such presentations. Cervical lymphadenopathy itself can be local or occur as part of a generalized, systemic lymphadenopathy.

Infectious mononucleosis (Pfeiffer's disease/glandular fever) is a viral illness resulting from EBV infection. It commonly occurs in young adults and teenagers, presenting with fever, sore throat, lethargy and myalgia. A blood film typically shows a reactive lymphocytosis of between 35% and 70% of the total leucocyte count and atypical T cells known as Downey bodies. Infectious mononucleosis is usually definitively diagnosed by a positive Monospot/Paul Bunnell test. Treatment involves simple analgesics and bed rest.

Neck lumps (2)

2 C   Thyroglossal cyst

The description is that of a thyroglossal cyst. These are persistent remnants of the thyroglossal duct, which guides the passage of the thyroid gland during development. Typically, these cysts are smooth, round and 2–3 cm in diameter. They occur more commonly in females, especially teenagers and young adults. On examination the lump tends to move up with swallowing and tongue protrusion. Definitive management is by excision of the lump. Lingual thyroid occurs when residual tissue is left on the base of the tongue as the thyroid migrates along its tract during development.

Neck lumps (3)

3 E   Anti-thyroid-stimulating hormone receptor antibody

Graves' disease is an autoimmune disorder that occurs most commonly in women (10:1) between the ages of 20 and 50 years. It is associated with signs of hyperthyroidism including the following:

- Weight loss
- Heat intolerance
- Sweating
- Diarrhoea
- Tremor
- Irritability
- Increased activity
- Emotional lability

- Psychosis
- Exophthalmos
- Tremor
- Ophthalmoplegia
- Diffuse thyroid enlargement

↑ T₃/T₄
TSH suppression

Most commonly there is an increase in antibodies against TSH receptors, resulting in a reduced level of TSH and increased free T4 and T3. It is also associated with other autoimmune disorders such as pernicious anaemia, type 1 diabetes mellitus and Addison's disease. Treatment is medical with carbimazole, propylthiouracil, propranolol and radioiodine therapy, or surgical with a partial/total thyroidectomy.

Anti-thyroglobulin antibody, although raised in some patients with Graves' disease, is most commonly associated with Hashimoto's thyroiditis, an autoimmune inflammatory disease of the thyroid gland resulting in thyrotoxicosis. Rheumatoid factor is commonly raised in patients with rheumatoid arthritis, Sjögren's syndrome and Felty's syndrome. Raised antinuclear antibody titres occur in SLE, RA, chronic active hepatitis and systemic sclerosis. Antineutrophil cytoplasmic antibody (ANCA) is a marker of vasculitis and occurs in two forms: cANCA directed against serine protease 3 is usually elevated in patients with Wegener's disease, whereas pANCA is directed against myeloperoxidase and elevated in systemic vasculitides such as microscopic polyangiitis.

TPO
+G

Complications of thyroid surgery

4 B Removal of surgical clips at the bedside

The scenario is one of haemorrhage following a thyroidectomy and formation of a tension haematoma, resulting in a compromised airway. This is a surgical emergency and requires immediate removal of the surgical clips at the bedside, followed by returning the patient to theatre to explore the area and control the haemorrhage. Although all of the other management routes are possible, it is reasonable to proceed with clip removal at the bedside as waiting for senior colleagues could result in this patient's death. Other complications of thyroidectomy are as follows:

- Immediate – Haemorrhage, laryngeal oedema, recurrent/superior laryngeal nerve damage, tracheal damage and thyroid storm
- Early – Reactionary haemorrhage, hypocalcaemia (secondary to parathyroid insufficiency) and infection
- Late – Hypothyroidism, keloid scar, disease recurrence → *Leftover tissue ?*

Neck lumps (4)

5 E Papillary

[handwritten: papillary]
[handwritten: most common]
[handwritten: lymphatic spread]
[handwritten: → majority]
[handwritten: young people]

Thyroid cancers can be either primary or secondary in origin. Papillary carcinoma of the thyroid accounts for approximately 70% of primary thyroid cancers. They occur commonly in women aged 20–40 years and are usually multifocal. They are locally invasive, spreading via the lymphatic system and causing enlarged cervical lymph nodes. Prognosis is usually good with 10-year survival in patients with extra-thyroid disease at 55%.

[handwritten left margin: follicular 30%]
[handwritten left margin: less common and haematogenous spread]
[handwritten left margin: older age group]

Follicular carcinoma makes up 15% of thyroid malignancy, occurring again more commonly in women in the 45- to 70-year age group. It is more common in areas of endemic goitre, with tumours usually being solitary and encapsulated. They metastasize by haematogenous spread to lungs and bones. Medullary carcinoma makes up less than 10% of thyroid cancers and occurs equally in men and women. These cancers arise from the parafollicular C cells, which secrete calcitonin and can occur as part of the MEN 2 syndrome. Metastasis is via the lymph nodes. Anaplastic thyroid carcinoma occurs in the elderly and is typified by a rapidly growing aggressive tumour which infiltrates locally and spreads via both lymphatic and haematogenous systems. It can present with symptoms of tracheal compression and laryngeal nerve involvement. Lymphoma is rare and usually associated with Hashimoto's thyroiditis.

Thyroid carcinoma

6 D Calcium

Medullary carcinoma of the thyroid gland makes up less than 10% of all thyroid cancers and occurs equally in men and women. These cancers arise from the parafollicular C cells, which secrete calcitonin. Calcitonin acts to reduce the serum calcium and phosphate level. As a result, the calcium level could be low in this patient. Medullary carcinoma also occurs as part of the MEN 2 syndrome. Metastasis is via the lymphatic system.

Thyroid disease

7 D Anaplastic carcinoma of the thyroid

Anaplastic thyroid carcinoma occurs in the elderly (50–70 years) and is typified by a rapidly growing, aggressive tumour, which infiltrates locally early on and spreads via both lymphatic and haematogenous systems. It can present with symptoms of tracheal compression and laryngeal nerve involvement, resulting in a hoarse voice and shortness of breath.

Treatment is with radiotherapy and chemotherapy, but rarely curative given the rapid progression of the disease process. A tracheostomy may be needed, as a palliative procedure, should the patient's airway become compromised. Five-year survival is extremely poor at 14%.

Neck swellings

8 D Troisier's sign

Eponymous conditions are an exam favourite and knowledge of some of the more common eponyms is useful in both written and clinical examinations. Virchow's node (signal node) is an enlarged, hard, left supraclavicular lymph node which can contain metastasis of an intra-abdominal mass, e.g. gastric malignancy. Battle's sign is bruising over the mastoid process following a base of skull fracture involving the petrous temporal bone. Cloquet's node refers to the most superior of the deep inguinal lymph nodes, which passes through the femoral canal. There are approximately three to five deep inguinal nodes in the body. Enlarged inguinal lymph nodes can be a sign of localized lower limb infection, systemic infection or metastases from distal carcinomas, e.g. carcinoma of the anus and vulva. Troisier's sign is the term given to enlargement of the left supraclavicular lymph node (Virchow's node), usually secondary to advanced metastatic gastric carcinoma. Trousseau's sign of malignancy is phlebothrombosis of the superficial veins due to cancer induced blood hypercoagulability. Trousseau also gives his name to Trousseau's sign of latent tetany which may be elicited in individuals with a low serum calcium level.

Neck anatomy

9 E Middle third of the clavicle

Borders of the anterior triangle of the neck are as follows:

- Medial: midline of the neck
- Lateral: anterior border of SCM
- Superior: lower border of mandible
- Roof: investing fascia
- Floor: prevertebral fascia

Borders of the posterior triangle of the neck are as follows:

- Anterior: posterior border of the SCM
- Posterior: anterior border of trapezius muscle
- Base: middle third of the clavicle
- Floor: prevertebral fascia overlying the prevertebral muscles: (splenius capitis, levator scapulae, scalenus anterior/middle/posterior)

Neck anatomy, particularly that of the anterior and posterior triangles, is frequently tested in both written and practical examinations. A good working knowledge of their borders is therefore useful.

Salivary gland swellings (1)

10 A Warthin's duct

80%. Eighty per cent of salivary gland calculi occur within the submandibular glands. Calculi usually occur in young to middle-aged adults and present with pain and swelling under the jaw, following obstruction of Warthin's duct, which runs through the submandibular gland and opens on the floor of the mouth. Symptoms tend to occur before, during and after eating. Pressing on the gland can produce a foul tasting fluid in the mouth, but can occasionally relieve symptoms.

The calculi are often composed of calcium pyrophosphate or calcium carbonate, which is thought to be secondary to fragments of toothpaste acting as a focus for stone formation. Partial obstruction of the duct will result in swelling and pain lasting from several minutes to hours, whereas complete obstruction will cause persistent swelling and infection. Treatment for stones within the intraoral part of the duct involves removal under general anaesthesia, whereas stones within the substance of the gland can require removal of the entire gland.

Stensen's duct passes through the parotid gland. The lingual nerve also passes through the submandibular gland. The trunk of the facial nerve lies between the deep and superficial parts of the parotid glands.

Salivary gland swellings (2)

11 D Sialogram

Sialogram consists of taking a baseline radiograph of the affected salivary gland followed by injection of a radio-opaque contrast into Warthin's duct. Multiple radiographs are then taken to show any underlying obstructions within the duct. The flushing effect of the contrast is also considered to be therapeutic and may help to remove stones from within the duct. Plain radiographs of the mouth include the following:

- Tangential view of the cheek (to visualize the parotid gland)
- Mandibular occlusal radiograph (to visualize the submandibular gland)
- Lateral oblique radiograph of the mandible (to visualize the submandibular gland)

See also the explanation in the answer to Question 13.

Facial swelling

12 A Pleomorphic adenoma

Pleomorphic adenoma is the most common salivary neoplasm and consists of several different types of tissue. Ninety per cent of these tumours occur in the parotid gland and grow slowly over many years. They can invade locally and can recur. Treatment is by superficial parotidectomy.

Adenolymphoma (Warthin's tumour) is a benign cystic tumour that contains epithelial lymphoid elements. It occurs in middle to old age, causing a soft cystic lump in the parotid gland, in a similar location to a pleomorphic adenoma. The epithelial element is thought to arise from embryonic parotid ducts that have become separated from the main duct system of the gland, whereas the lymphoid element arises from normal lymph tissue close to the developing gland.

Mikulicz's and Sjögren's syndrome are autoimmune diseases that result in slow, progressive and usually painless enlargement of the salivary glands as a result of lymphoid tissue replacing the glandular tissue. The syndromes consist of enlargement of parotid/submandibular glands, enlargement of lacrimal glands causing a bulge at the outer end of the upper eyelids and narrowing of the palpebral fissures, dry mouth, dry eyes and generalized arthritis (the last two symptoms are more common in Sjögren's syndrome).

Carcinoma of the parotid gland can arise anew or in a longstanding pleomorphic adenoma. Men and women are equally affected and there is a rapid enlargement of the swelling, which is painful with pain radiating to the side of the face and ear. There may be mouth asymmetry and difficulty closing the mouth, as well as involvement of the facial nerve (which passes through the parotid gland), suggesting cancer invasion into the gland.

Parotid gland pathology

13 A RNA viruses

The mumps virus is an RNA paramyxovirus spread by droplet infection. It has an incubation period of 2–3 weeks. Affected individuals are infective for 7 days before and after onset of parotid swelling. Parotid swelling is bilateral in 70% of cases. In addition to a viral prodrome, complications of mumps can include orchitis (enquiry about testicular pain is necessary), arthritis, meningitis, pancreatitis and myocarditis. Treatment is symptomatic.

An immunization programme exists in the United Kingdom, in which the MMR vaccine (combining measles, mumps and rubella – all RNA viruses) is given as a single injection at 13 months and a booster at 3–5 years of age. The use of the MMR vaccine became controversial in the late 1990s due to a speculative link with autism (although this was later discredited in the medical press). This resulted in a reduced uptake of the MMR vaccine and a subsequent increase in the number of cases of mumps and associated complications.

Lumps around the body (1)

14 D **Drainage of the abscess under general anaesthesia**
Pilonidal abscesses occur as a result of infection of one or more pilonidal sinuses. These are short tracts leading from an opening in the skin near the top of the buttocks or natal cleft into the body. The tract is lined with granulation tissue and can get filled with hair debris and bacteria to act as a site of infection and result in abscess formation and/or recurrent sepsis. Pilonidal sinuses are more common in males (4:1), particularly among those who are more hairy and of Middle Eastern/Mediterranean origin (although the condition is not exclusive to these populations). Pilonidal sinuses present with persistent discharge of purulent or clear fluid, and recurrent infection. They can be exquisitely tender.

A number of surgical techniques exist, but definitive treatment generally involves drainage of the abscess cavity and wide excision of the natal cleft. The recurrence rate after surgery can be as high as 15%. Encouraging good hygiene and advising individuals at risk to shave the affected area and back in particular reduces this risk. Antibiotics may stop an early infection but, in this scenario, drainage under general anaesthesia would be the most appropriate treatment.

Lumps around the body (2)

15 B **Ganglion**
A ganglion is a cystic, myxomatous degeneration of fibrous tissue that most commonly occurs around joints, where there is a large amount of fibrous tissue. They present mostly between the ages of 20 and 60 years, growing slowly over many months. They are non-tender, spherical and smooth on the surface. They may slip between deeper structures when pressed, suggesting that the contents have reduced into a joint. The overlying skin is also freely mobile, while aspiration reveals a thick, gel-like material.

Traditional therapy consists of striking the swelling with a heavy book such as a bible. However, this tends to be only a temporary measure (and also painful!), resulting in recurrence in many cases. It can also be aspirated and injected with hydrocortisone (again resulting in recurrence), but surgical excision is the definitive management. A bursa is a fluid-filled cavity occurring between tendons, bones and skin to allow easier movement between them. Rheumatoid nodules commonly occur in relation to rheumatoid arthritis, a symmetrical inflammatory disease of the joints. The presenting history is not suggestive of this condition.

Anatomy of the abdominal wall and hernia

16 D **Transversus abdominis**
The abdomen is demarcated on the surface of the body by the xiphoid process, lower six costal cartilages and anterior ends of the lower six

ribs. Inferior markings are the pubic symphysis, pubic crest, tubercle, ASIS and the iliac crest. Muscles of the anterior abdominal wall from most superficial to deep are:

- External oblique
- Internal oblique
- Rectus abdominis – A straight muscle lying between the linea alba and linea semilunaris, coated in its own protective sheath, formed at various levels by the external/internal oblique aponeuroses, transversus abdominis aponeurosis and transversalis fascia
- Ttransversus abdominis

Cremaster muscle arises in the middle of the inguinal ligament from the internal oblique muscle and inserts into the pubic crest and pubic tubercle. It is involved in testicular retraction.

Gynaecomastia

17 D Furosemide

Gynaecomastia is the development of breast tissue in men. Oestradiol is the growth hormone of the breast, and an increase in serum concentration results in increased breast tissue. In men, oestradiol is a derivative of the peripheral conversion of testosterone and adrenal oestrone. Gynaecomastia can be regarded as the result of reduced androgen and increased oestrogen production. There are many causes, which are classified as follows:

- Physiological:
    - Neonatal – Secondary to ingestion of maternal oestrogens.
    - Pubertal – Up to 50% of pubertal boys may develop asymmetrical gynaecomastia, secondary to a relative oestrogen excess during this period, which resolves spontaneously in the majority of individuals. Some patients may need surgical removal of the tissue.
    - Old age.
    - Hyperthyroidism can cause an increase in oestrogen levels.
    - Liver disease results in a reduced breakdown of oestrogen-derived compounds and as a result can cause gynaecomastia in patients with advanced disease.
    - Oestrogen-producing tumours, e.g. testicular and adrenal carcinomas (these can cause increased levels of androstenedione, which is converted by aromatase into oestrone, a type of oestrogen).
    - hCG-producing tumours, e.g. testicular (Leydig cell tumour) and bronchial carcinoma.
    - Starvation/refeeding.
    - Carcinoma of the male breast.

- Drugs account for 10%–20% of clinically significant gynaeco-mastia in men and include:
  - Oestrogenic drugs which increase the level of serum oestrogen, e.g. oestrogens, digoxin (digitalis), cannabis, diamorphine, omeprazole, androstenedione and imatinib mesylate.
  - Anti-androgens which reduce serum testosterone, e.g. spironolactone, cimetidine, cyproterone, ketoconazole, metronidazole and finasteride.
- Others: Gonadotrophins (GnRH analogues used for treating prostate cancer), cytotoxic agents, methyldopa, isoniazid.

Furosemide is a loop diuretic used for the treatment the following:

- Oedema associated with heart failure
- Nephrotic syndrome
- Liver cirrhosis
- Hypertension

Hernias (1)

18 D Inguinal

A hernia is a protrusion of a viscus through a defect in the wall of the cavity containing it into an abnormal position. Hernias occur more commonly in men than in women (9:1). Overall, abdominal wall hernias account for 80%–90% of hernias. Inguinal hernias remain the commonest type of hernia in both men and women, although femoral hernias occur 4 times more commonly in women than in men. The approximate incidence of various hernias is as follows:

- Inguinal: 78% – of which direct inguinal hernias account for approximately 25% and indirect inguinal hernias 75%
- Incisional: 10%
- Femoral: 7%
- Umbilical: 3%
- Eepigastric: 1%

Hernias (2)

19 D Inguinal ligament

Boundaries of the femoral canal:

- Anterior: Inguinal ligament
- Medial: Lacunar part of inguinal ligament (lacunar/Gimbernat's ligament)
- Lateral: Femoral vein
- Inferior: Pectineal ligament (of Astley Cooper) – this is involved in hip flexion and thigh adduction

Boundaries of the inguinal canal:

- Anterior: External oblique aponeurosis, reinforced by the internal oblique aponeurosis in the lateral third of its structure
- Posterior: The transversalis fascia forms the lateral portion and the medial portion is formed by the merging of the pubic attachments of the internal oblique and transversus abdominis aponeurosis (the conjoint tendon)
- Roof: Arching fibres of the internal oblique and transversus abdominis muscles
- Floor: Inguinal ligament and lacunar ligament (deep reflection of inguinal ligament) on its medial aspect

Groin swelling

20 B Strangulated

Although this lump can be described as irreducible, i.e. the hernia sac cannot be returned to its containing cavity, the description is really one of a strangulated hernia. This is when the blood supply to the bowel is permanently compromised and the affected segment becomes necrotic. Obstructed hernia means that the sac contains bowel through which faeces cannot pass. However, the blood supply is usually intact and the bowel is therefore salvageable at the time of repair. Sliding hernia occurs when part of the hernia sac is formed by an intra-abdominal structure, e.g. sigmoid/descending colon on the left side or caecum/ascending colon on the right side. In a Richter's hernia, only a part of the bowel herniates, of which the blood supply can also become compromised causing necrosis.

SECTION 17:
PRACTICE EXAM

Questions

1. Anticoagulation in surgical patients   354
2. Postoperative care in upper gastrointestinal surgery   354
3. Systemic inflammatory response syndrome   354
4. Consent   355
5. Management of general surgical patients   355
6. Electrolyte replacement strategies (1)   355
7. Electrolyte replacement strategies (2)   356
8. Electrolyte imbalance in special circumstances   356
9. Fluid replacement   356
10. Urine output monitoring   357
11. Paediatric trauma   357
12. Paediatric resuscitation   357
13. Trauma in the elderly patient   358
14. Trauma in pregnancy (1)   358
15. Trauma in pregnancy (2)   358
16. Chronic pancreatitis   358
17. Pancreatic malignancy   358
18. Tumour markers   359
19. Peptic ulcer disease   359
20. Management of peptic ulcer disease   359
21. Hepatomegaly   359
22. Surgery for ulcerative colitis   360
23. Perianal disease   360
24. Fistula *in ano*   360
25. Pilonidal sinus   360
26. Right iliac fossa mass (2)   361

27. Management of diarrhoea   361
28. Surgical anatomy of appendicectomy   361
29. Mechanical bowel obstruction   362
30. Vascular anatomy of the gallbladder   362
31. Colorectal surgical resections   362
32. Abdominal distension   362
33. Metastatic breast carcinoma   363
34. Hormone therapy for breast carcinoma   363
35. Endocrine disorders   363
36. Investigation of endocrine disease   363
37. Hunter's canal   364
38. Lipodermatosclerosis   364
39. Fontaine's classification   364
40. Subclavian steal syndrome   365
41. Upper limb pain   365
42. Scrotal swellings (1)   365
43. Urological emergencies   365
44. Complications of urological procedures (1)   366
45. Complications of urological procedures (2)   366
46. Nephrotic syndrome   366
47. Median nerve neuropathy   367
48. Upper limb nerve palsy   367
49. Supracondylar fractures   367
50. Colles' fracture   368
51. Neck of femur fracture   368
52. Fractures of the proximal femur   368
53. Operative complications   368
54. Fractures   369
55. Fracture complications   369
56. Autoimmune neurological disease   369
57. Inherited neurological disease   370
58. Lumbar puncture   370
59. Neurological infection   370
60. Spinal cord injury   371
61. Neck lumps (1)   371
62. Neck lumps (2)   371
63. Thyroid disease   371
64. Hoarse voice   372
65. Tongue pathology   372
66. Systemic disease and the eye   373
67. The diabetic eye (1)   373
68. The diabetic eye (2)   373
69. Thyroid eye disease   374
70. Dry eye   374

71. Neck lumps (3)   374
72. Neck lumps (4)   374
73. Neck lumps (5)   375
74. Groin swelling   375
75. Complications of inguinal hernia repair   375
76. Inguinal hernia surgical anatomy   376
77. Anatomy of the spermatic cord   376
78. Umbilical swelling   376
79. Skin lumps (1)   376
80. Skin lumps (2)   377
81. Malignant melanoma   377
82. Skin lesions   377
83. Scrotal swellings (2)   378
84. Scrotal swellings (3)   378
85. Testicular pain (1)   378
86. Scrotal swellings (4)   379
87. Testicular pain (2)   379
88. Breast lumps   379
89. Treatment of breast lumps   380
90. Investigation of breast lumps   380
91. Ureteric constrictions   380
92. Complications of mechanical ventilation   381
93. Subclavian vein cannulation   381
94. Central venous pressure monitoring   381
95. Posterior approach to the hip joint   381
96. Systemic effects of epidural analgesia   382
97. Complications of axillary lymph node surgery   382
98. Acid–base disorders   382
99. Branches of the external carotid artery   382
100. Cardiogenic shock   383

Answers   384

QUESTIONS

This practice exam consists of 100 single best answer questions, and, under standard examination conditions, candidates are expected to complete this paper in 95 minutes.

1. Anticoagulation in surgical patients

A 73-year-old woman is seen in the outpatients department. She complains of altered bowel habit and weight loss. A colonoscopy is performed which identifies a large polyp. Polypectomy was not possible due to the patient being on warfarin for a metal heart valve. You are asked to re-book the patient for definitive management. Which one of the following statements pertaining to this scenario is correct?

A. Admission is required to monitor the patient while warfarin is stopped   *if indication is atrial fibrillation*

B. Warfarin should be replaced with therapeutic doses of low-molecular-weight heparin for 5 days prior to the procedure   *no, cannot run LMWH during operation*

C. An echocardiogram is required prior to the procedure to exclude valve thrombus

D. Conversion to unfractionated heparin infusion is required   *IV*

E. A computed tomography pneumocolon should be performed to identify/exclude further disease before a management decision is made   *↳ need an intervention not further confirmation*

2. Postoperative care in upper gastrointestinal surgery

NGT→ to protect anastomosis and prevent dilation of esophagus

A patient who underwent an oesophagectomy in an attempt to cure stage 1 cancer becomes confused 4 days postoperatively and pulls out his nasogastric tube. What is the best course of action?

A. Attempt reinsertion   *→ Contraindicated once tube is removed*

B. Endoscopic insertion of nasojejunal tube   *→ will damage anastomosis*

C. Restrict oral intake

D. Computed tomography to identify complications of removal

E. Sedation

3. Systemic inflammatory response syndrome

Systemic inflammatory response syndrome is a term used to describe the disseminated response to an inflammatory insult such as sepsis, pancreatitis or severe trauma. Which one of the following is not a manifestation of systemic inflammatory response syndrome?

A. Temperature <36°C

B. Heart rate >90 beats/min

C. Respiratory rate >20 breaths/min

D. Blood pressure <90 mmHg
E. White cell count >12 × 10⁹/L

4. Consent

Your registrar asks you to consent a patient for insertion of a central line. You counsel the patient through the reasons for the procedure as well as intended benefits and complications. What is the most common immediate complication of central line insertion?

A. Infection
B. Thrombus
C. Haemorrhage
D. Pneumothorax
E. Air embolism

5. Management of general surgical patients

A 69-year-old man is admitted, complaining of right upper quadrant pain and fever. A correct diagnosis of acute cholecystitis is made and antibiotics prescribed. The option of immediate surgery is discussed, but the patient opts to wait for 6 weeks. Ten days later the patient phones to ask advice; his pain has not improved and his fevers have returned following completion of the antibiotics, with rigors and night sweats now a problem. In addition, he is concerned regarding itching the previous day, which he ascribed to his antibiotics. The most appropriate advice for this patient is

rigors → indicate abscess formation

A. This is normal, paracetamol should relieve the fevers
B. Surgery is now not possible for 6 weeks, attend general practitioner for further course of antibiotics and analgesics
C. Book an outpatients appointment for review
D. Attend the emergency department
E. Patient requires urgent cholecystectomy

6. Electrolyte replacement strategies (1)

A 43-year-old patient is being managed following presentation with perfuse diarrhoea and profound dehydration secondary to an exacerbation of Crohn's colitis. Your initial bloods come back showing sodium 137 mmol/L, potassium ↓2.9 mmol/L, urea 9.2 mmol/L, creatinine 134 μmol/L. He has a peripheral cannula in situ only. Which one of the following statements regarding potassium replacement in this patient is the most correct? *

A. 40 mmol potassium chloride can safely be given over 1 hour → *in certain cases only.*
B. Central line insertion is advisable
C. Bolus potassium is safe, provided a central line is used

↳ never → k⁺ is cardioplegic ↳ leads to cardiac arrest.

D. Maximum concentration of potassium to be given peripherally is 20 mmol/500 mL

E. Maximum rate of potassium infusion peripherally is 20 mmol every 4 hours

7. Electrolyte replacement strategies (2)

A postoperative patient is being managed on a high-dependency unit following a subtotal colectomy. Blood results show the phosphate level is 0.25 mmol/L. Which one of the following statements regarding intravenous phosphate is incorrect?

→ no hypocalc. → binds to s. Calcium
→ deposits in tissues

A May cause hypercalcaemia
B. Should never be given at a rate greater than 30 mmol over 6 hours
C. Should preferentially be given via a central line
D. May cause metastatic calcification
E. Should be used even if the patient is asymptomatic

8. Electrolyte imbalance in special circumstances

A 34-year-old patient is admitted intoxicated. He appears neglected and smells strongly of alcohol. The third day following his admission, he develops alcohol withdrawal and is managed with chlordiazepoxide. On day 5 of his admission, he has the following blood results: haemoglobin 11.2 g/dL, white cell count 7.9×10^9/L, mean corpuscular volume 103 fL, sodium 137 mmol/L, potassium 2.3 mmol/L, urea 3.4 mmol/L, creatinine 69 mmol/L, amylase 930 IU/L, phosphate 0.17 mmol/L, calcium 2.25 mmol/L, C-reactive protein 8 mg/L. Which test should be done urgently?

A. Group and save
B. Septic screen
C Serum magnesium Mg
D. B_{12} and folate levels
E. Urinary electrolytes

9. Fluid replacement

A patient is admitted complaining of central abdominal pain. On assessment the patient is thought to have subacute small bowel obstruction secondary to adhesions. He is managed with a nasogastric tube and 6 hourly bags of Hartmann's solution. His arterial blood gases the following day show the following:

- pO_2 = 10.5 (on 28% oxygen)   Metabolic   alkalosis
- pCO_2 = 5.2
- pH = 7.46 ↑
- Base excess = 7.5 ↑

Which one of the following statements is the most correct?

A. This patient has a respiratory acidosis
B. This patient has chronic obstructive pulmonary disease
C. This patient should have their fluid rate reduced
D. This patient requires ventilation
Ⓔ This patient has a metabolic alkalosis

10. Urine output monitoring

You are asked to see a patient by the ward staff after a postoperative patient's urine output becomes low. On review, the patient appears comfortable with a urinary catheter *in situ*. Observations are stable at blood pressure 118/67 mmHg, pulse rate 98 beats/min and respiratory rate 18 breaths/min. Over the previous 3 hours the urinary output has been 55 mL, 43 mL and 35 mL. Currently, in the last hour no urine has been passed. Which one of the following statements is the most correct?

A. The first course of action should be a colloid fluid challenge
B. This patient requires central venous pressure monitoring
C. The first course of action should be a crystalloid fluid challenge
D. This patient is in acute renal failure
Ⓔ The most likely cause is catheter occlusion

11. Paediatric trauma → Physiological reserve more. S/s of shock appear late.

Which one of the following is the first appreciable sign of shock in the paediatric patient?

A. Narrowed pulse pressure
B. Hypotension → >45% volume loss → impending cardiac arrest
Ⓒ Tachycardia
D. Reduced urinary output
E. Reduced pain response

12. Paediatric resuscitation

A 4-year-old child is admitted following a road traffic accident. She is tachycardic and you wish to administer fluid and blood. The child is peripherally shut down and it has not been possible to gain access after two attempts at peripheral cannulation. Your next option is

Ⓐ Intraosseous infusion
B. Femoral line insertion ←
C. External jugular cannulation ← alternatives to interosseous
D. Saphenous vein cut-down ←
E. Internal jugular central line insertion ← avoided in children
        + subclavian vein

13. Trauma in the elderly patient

Which one of the following mechanisms is the most common traumatic cause of death in the elderly (over 65)?

- (A) Falls
- B. Motor vehicle accidents
- C. Burns
- D. Assault
- E. Non-accidental injury

14. Trauma in pregnancy (1)

Of the following, which parameter is typically unchanged from its adult normal range during the third trimester of pregnancy?

- (A) Blood pressure
- B. Heart rate ↑ due to ↑ plasma volume
- C. pCO$_2$ ↓ due to ↑ tidal volume.
- D. Haematocrit ↓ dilutional anemia
- E. White cell count ↑

15. Trauma in pregnancy (2)

Blunt abd trauma → Commonest cause of uterine rupture.

3rd trim
wall is thin
stretched to maximum point

A patient is admitted following a car accident where she was a restrained passenger. The patient is 32 weeks pregnant. She is shocked with a rigid and tender abdomen. An abdominal radiograph is performed which shows air under the diaphragm and the fetus's left leg appears extended. The most appropriate next course of action is

minimize

- A. Ultrasound examination
- B. Diagnostic peritoneal lavage
- C. Computed tomography scan of the abdomen → Should not be done in any
- D. Caesarean section → not enough exposure   pregnant women.
- (E) Explorative laparotomy

16. Chronic pancreatitis

The most common cause of chronic pancreatitis is

- A. Gallstone disease
- B. Hyperlipidaemia
- (C) Alcohol
- D. Hypercalcaemia
- E. Cystic fibrosis

17. Pancreatic malignancy

Which one of the following statements regarding pancreatic cancer is correct?

- A. Predominantly a disease of the developing world
- (B) Incidence is increasing

C. male
D. head
E. CA 19.9
a. developed

C. Female predominance
D. Majority occur in the neck and tail of the pancreas
E. Associated with raised serum CA125

18. Tumour markers

Which of the following tumour markers are most commonly associated with pancreatic cancer?

A. Carcinoembryonic antigen
B. Cancer antigen (CA)125
C. CA19–9
D. α-fetoprotein (AFP)
E. β-human chorionic gonadotrophin

19. Peptic ulcer disease

The most common cause of a peptic ulcer is

A. Non-steroidal anti-inflammatory drugs
B. Cigarette smoking
C. Frequent intake of caffeinated drinks
D. *Helicobacter pylori*
E. High levels of emotional stress

20. Management of peptic ulcer disease

A 29-year-old city worker is diagnosed with a duodenal ulcer which was visualized with upper gastrointestinal endoscopy. A tissue biopsy of the ulcer was taken and a Campylobacter-like organisms (CLO) test revealed the presence of *Helicobacter pylori*. Which one of the following treatment regimens will offer the highest chance of cure?

A. Omeprazole, amoxicillin, clarithromycin
B. Ranitidine, amoxicillin, metronidazole
C. Omeprazole, clarithromycin
D. Ranitidine, amoxicillin
E. Amoxicillin, clarithromycin

21. Hepatomegaly

A 50-year-old man, who has come on holiday from India, presents with a 10-day history of aching abdominal pain and recent weight loss. On examination, his abdomen is tender in the right hypochondrium and distended with a positive shifting dullness. The liver is enlarged with a hard nodular consistency. The most likely diagnosis is

A. Haemochromatosis
B. Hepatocellular carcinoma

C. Pyogenic liver abscess

D. Alcoholic cirrhosis

E. None of the above

22. Surgery for ulcerative colitis

Which of the following is an absolute contraindication for pan-proctocolectomy?

A. Dysplastic change in the rectal mucosa

B. Toxic megacolon

C. Intractable anaemia

D. Previous pelvic surgery *— complicates surgery but if surgery is life saving → carried on.*

E. Young woman with concerns regarding fertility

Indication for surgery

23. Perianal disease

A 45-year-old patient presents to the outpatient department following referral by his general practitioner for rectal bleeding. The patient reports that as well as the bleeding in the past few days he has experienced increased pain in the perianal area. On examination you identify thrombosed haemorrhoids. The appropriate management is

A. Admit, analgesia, haemorrhoidectomy

B. Oral ánd local analgesia and discharge with follow-up

C. Outpatient department banding

D. 5% phenol in arachis oil injection above the dentate line

E. Discharge to general practitioner for management

24. Fistula *in ano*

Goodsall's Rule

A patient is being prepared for treatment of a fistula in the operating theatre. The consultant asks you to examine the patient and from your findings predict the course the tract is likely to have taken. You note a sinus in the 8 o'clock position with the patient in the lithotomy position. Where is the most likely point at which you may find the corresponding internal opening within the anal canal?

A. 12 o'clock

B. 8 o'clock

C. Along the transverse line bisecting the anal canal

D. 6 o'clock

E. It is not possible to predict

ant

anal canal.

post

lithotomy position

25. Pilonidal sinus

Which one of the following is *not* an independent risk factor for development of pilonidal sinus?

A. Family history

B. Poor personal hygiene

C. Obesity
D. Male sex
E. Professional driver

26. Right iliac fossa mass (2)

A 40-year-old patient presents with abdominal pain. He appears unkempt and gives only a vague history. On examination, he is tender over his right iliac fossa where a mass can be felt. The mass is soft and boggy. Compression is possible, which accentuates a similar swelling found below the level of the inguinal ligament. The swelling is not hot or erythematous. On mobilization, the patient complains of severe back pain. The diagnosis is

A. Ureteric abscess
B. Appendix mass
C. Femoral hernia
D. Psoas abscess
E. Spigelian hernia

27. Management of diarrhoea

A 46-year-old patient is seen in the outpatient department for follow-up of Crohn's disease. He reports intractable diarrhoea, but does not report any systemic symptoms or abdominal pain. Contrast follow-through fails to show any evidence of active disease or fistulation. He is otherwise well. His maintenance medications include mesalazine and 6-mercaptopurine. The most appropriate choice of drug is

A. Loperamide hydrochloride
B. Ispaghula husk
C. Methotrexate
D. Cholestyramine ? diarrh due to malabsorption
E. Codeine phosphate

28. Surgical anatomy of appendicectomy

You are asked to assist in theatre during an emergency appendicectomy. The consultant asks you to locate McBurney's point. From the list below, which answer best describes the location of McBurney's point?

A. Two-thirds of the distance from the umbilicus to the right anterior superior iliac spine
B. The midpoint between the anterior superior iliac spine and the pubic symphysis
C. The midpoint between the anterior superior iliac spine and the pubic tubercle
D. Two-thirds the distance from the right anterior superior iliac spine to the umbilicus
E. One-third the distance from the umbilicus to the right anterior superior iliac spine

29. Mechanical bowel obstruction

The most common cause of mechanic intestinal obstruction is

    A. Inflammatory bowel disease
    B. Volvulus
    C. Neoplasia
    D. Adhesions
    E. Hernias

30. Vascular anatomy of the gallbladder

A patient is sent for emergency laparoscopic cholecystectomy after being diagnosed with acute cholecystitis, which failed to resolve after 48 hours. One step of this procedure entails clamping and dividing the arterial blood supply to the gallbladder to facilitate its resection. From the list of answers below, select the artery that supplies the gallbladder.

    A. Cystic artery
    B. Right hepatic artery
    C. Common hepatic artery
    D. Left hepatic artery
    E. Gastroduodenal artery

31. Colorectal surgical resections

A patient with a perforation of the sigmoid colon, secondary to diverticulitis, is sent for an emergency colonic resection. From the list below, select the most appropriate colonic resection that should be performed in this patient.

    A. Right hemicolectomy
    B. Left hemicolectomy
    C. Anterior resection
    D. Abdominoperineal resection
    E. Hartmann's procedure

32. Abdominal distension

A 55-year-old man who has been constipated for the past 5 days presents with suprapubic colicky pain. On examination his abdomen is distended and there is marked tenderness in the suprapubic region. Bowel sounds are increased. A plain film supine abdominal film shows dilated loops of large bowel. A barium enema shows an 'apple core narrowing' in the rectosigmoid area. The most likely cause of this man's large bowel obstruction is

    A. Adhesions
    B. Colorectal carcinoma
    C. Volvulus
    D. Faecal impaction
    E. Inflammatory bowel disease

33. Metastatic breast carcinoma

A 50-year-old postmenopausal woman with stage 4 invasive ductal carcinoma of the right breast presents with slight shortness of breath. On clinical examination, you notice that the right lung base is stony dull on percussion coupled with decreased air entry. A chest radiograph confirms pleural effusion of the right lung. A chest drain is inserted and some of the drained pleural aspirate is sent for cytological examination and a computed tomography scan of the chest is performed. The results confirm metastatic spread to the lungs. What is the most likely route of metastases that accounts for the pleural effusion?

- A. Transcoelomic spread *: serosal spread*
- B. Haematogenous spread
- C. Lymphatic spread
- D. Direct extension
- E. None of the above

34. Hormone therapy for breast carcinoma

Which hormone receptor status of breast carcinoma is more likely to respond to hormonal therapy?

- A. Oestrogen receptor negative and progesterone receptor negative
- B. Oestrogen receptor positive and progesterone receptor positive
- C. Oestrogen receptor negative and progesterone receptor positive
- D. Oestrogen receptor positive and progesterone receptor negative
- E. None of the above

35. Endocrine disorders

A 55-year-old man presents with frequency of urine and excessive thirst. He also experiences muscle cramps and has a 5-year history of hypertension that is being managed conservatively. Blood tests show his capillary glucose is 4.1 mmol/L, sodium is 149 mmol/L and potassium is 3.1 mmol/L. The most likely diagnosis is

- A. Hyperparathyroidism
- B. Hypoparathyroidism
- C. Phaeochromocytoma
- D. Conn's syndrome *↑ aldosterone*
- E. Cushing's syndrome

36. Investigation of endocrine disease

A 63-year-old woman presents to the emergency department with episodes of difficulty breathing coupled with flushing and diarrhoea. On taking the history you ascertain that these episodes are precipitated by stress and alcohol. On examination, her blood pressure is 129/83 mmHg and heart rate is 80 beats/min.

Based on this patient's history, select the best distinguishing investigation from the list below.

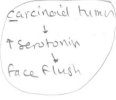

Carcinoid tumur
↓
↑ Serotonin
↓
face flush

A. 24-hour urinary 5-hydroxyindole acetic acid
B. 24-hour urinary vanillylmandelic acid
C. Dexamethasone suppression test
D. Aldosterone and renin levels
E. Short Synacthen test

37. Hunter's canal

During a ward round you are told to list the structures found in the adductor (Hunter's) canal. From the list below, select the statement that best describes the structures found in the adductor (Hunter's) canal. *tunnel around thigh*

V A N
X |
A ∪ N ✓

A. Femoral artery, femoral vein, saphenous nerve and the nerve to the vastus medialis
B. Anterior tibial artery, posterior tibial artery and common peroneal nerve
C. Femoral artery, femoral vein, saphenous nerve and peroneal nerve
D. Femoral vein, anterior tibial artery and saphenous nerve
E. Posterior tibial artery, femoral vein, saphenous nerve

38. Lipodermatosclerosis

Lipodermatosclerosis is commonly associated with which one of the following conditions?

A. Deep vein thrombosis
B. Intermittent claudication
C. Acute leg ischaemia
D. Varicose veins
E. Superficial thrombophlebitis

39. Fontaine's classification

Your senior colleague asks you to see a patient in clinic who has Fontaine's classification stage 3 peripheral vascular disease. Which one of the following options best describes the symptoms associated with stage 3 of Fontaine's classification of peripheral vascular disease?

A. Ischaemic rest pain
B. Ulceration with or without gangrene
C. Asymptomatic
D. Intermittent claudication
E. None of the above

40. Subclavian steal syndrome

You are told that a 40-year-old woman, who has had a 4-month history of left upper limb muscular fatigue, dizziness and vertigo, has been diagnosed with subclavian steal syndrome. The most common cause of subclavian steal syndrome is

    A. Distal occlusion of the left subclavian artery
    B. Proximal occlusion of the left subclavian artery
    C. Distal occlusion of the left brachial artery
    D. Proximal occlusion of the left brachial artery
    E. Proximal occlusion of the left radial artery

41. Upper limb pain

During a ward round one of your patients, who had an elective repair of an abdominal aortic aneurysm 4 days ago, tells you that her left arm is severely painful. On examination, you notice that the proximal forearm is erythematous and swollen, particularly in the region of the left anterior cubital fossa. You are told by a member of staff that it was difficult to insert an intravenous cannula the day before. The patient is apyrexial. What is the most likely diagnosis?

    A. Deep vein thrombosis
    B. Cellulitis
    C. Superficial thrombophlebitis
    D. Tendonitis
    E. Lymphangitis

42. Scrotal swellings (1)

A 30-year-old man presents with a 2-month history of swelling in the left testicle that is associated with an occasional dull ache. On examination, it is possible to get above the swelling, but it is not palpable separate to the scrotal contents. In addition, it transilluminates brightly when a light is shone through it. This is likely to be a

    A. Inguinoscrotal hernia
    B. Spermatocele = epidydymal cyst
    C. Hydrocele
    D. Varicocele
    E. Testicular tumour

43. Urological emergencies

In the initial management of suspected testicular torsion, all of the following are appropriate management steps, except

    A. Intravenous access and fluid resuscitation
    B. Obtain blood for full blood count, urea and electrolytes, clotting, group and save

C. Analgesia
D. Make patient nil by mouth
Ⓔ Ultrasound scan of the scrotum   :delys the tt

44. Complications of urological procedures (1)

As the surgical house officer on call, you are asked to review a 72-year-old man who has undergone transurethral resection of prostate (TURP) earlier in the day, and appears to be very confused. On further questioning, he is disoriented to time and place and reports feeling nauseous. In addition, observations show a blood pressure of 157/95 mmHg and a heart rate of 55 beats/min. A review of his notes indicates that he takes aspirin regularly, but otherwise has no chronic medical problems or past history of confusion. You suspect that this man may have TURP syndrome and request a full set of bloods including urea and electrolytes. Which biochemical marker would you typically expect to be low in this condition?

A. Calcium
Ⓑ Sodium
C. Potassium
D. Chloride
E. Hydrogen

45. Complications of urological procedures (2)

A 36-year-old man presents to the emergency department with a 2-day history of fever, dysuria, frequency and occasional haematuria. He has undergone cystoscopy for investigation of recurrent urinary tract infections 4 days prior to admission. On examination, he is found to be pyrexial with mild tachycardia while rectal examination reveals a swollen, firm and tender prostate gland. Blood tests reveal raised inflammatory markers and a urine dip is positive for nitrites. Antibiotics are commenced and a urological opinion is sought for further management. What inflammatory process is this patient likely to have?

Ⓐ Prostatitis
B. Pyelonephritis
C. Urethritis
D. Epididymitis
E. Cystitis

46. Nephrotic syndrome

A 15-year-old girl known to have minimal change glomerulonephritis (MCGN) presents with a 2-day history of facial swelling and difficulty breathing. On examination, she is able to maintain her airway, but has some shortness of breath and a palpable liver edge. A chest radiograph confirms small bilateral pleural effusions and biochemical markers are suggestive of nephrotic syndrome. All of the following are consistent with this diagnosis, except

- A. Peripheral oedema
- B. Proteinuria
- C. Haematuria
- D. Hypoalbuminaemia
- E. Hyperlipidaemia

47. Median nerve neuropathy

A patient presents with altered sensation over the palmar aspects of the first three fingers of their left hand with associated thenar wasting. You think the patient needs a carpel tunnel release, but wish to confirm your diagnosis. What is your first line investigation?

- A. Anteroposterior and lateral cervical spine films
- B. Magnetic resonance imaging of the cervical spine
- C. Computed tomography of the cervical spine
- D. Nerve conduction studies
- E. Nerve biopsy

48. Upper limb nerve palsy

A patient presents to the outpatient clinic with weakness in their hand. You perform a detailed neurological examination and find the following: generalized wasting sparing the thenar and hypothenar eminence, with normal sensation over the palmar aspect of the fifth finger and the medial aspect of the fourth finger. Sensation to the medial aspect of the palm is spared. The hand is clawed and you elicit a positive Froment's test. The level of the ulnar nerve lesion is therefore

- A. Compression between the heads of flexor carpi ulnaris
- B. Ulnar tunnel
- C. Brachial plexus
- D. Medial epicondyle of the humerus
- E. Wrist

49. Supracondylar fractures

A 7-year-old child is admitted with a supracondylar fracture. His hand is cold and pulseless, however perfusion is restored following fracture reduction. The integrity of which structure is of major concern?

- A. Musculocutaneous nerve
- B. Ulnar artery
- C. Radial artery
- D. Median nerve
- E. Radial nerve

50. Colles' fracture

Which one of the following is not a recognized feature of a Colles' fracture?

- A. Ulnar styloid fracture
- B. Impaction
- C. Volar displacement
- D. Radial tilt
- E. Radial displacement

51. Neck of femur fracture

An otherwise fit 65-year-old patient is admitted following an assault during which he was pushed to the ground and sustained a fractured hip. Your specialist registrar reviews the film and says the fracture is a Garden 2 intracapsular neck of femur fracture. The appropriate management is

- A. Primary total hip replacement
- B. Cannulated screw fixation
- C. Dynamic hip screw fixation
- D. Hemiarthroplasty
- E. Proximal femoral nail

52. Fractures of the proximal femur

A 75-year-old woman is admitted following a fall at home. Her leg is shortened and externally rotated. Radiographs show a fracture line running through both the greater and the lesser trochanters. The appropriate management is

- A. Traction for 8–12 weeks
- B. Cannulated screw fixation
- C. Hemiarthroplasty
- D. Proximal femoral nail
- E. Dynamic hip screw

53. Operative complications

A 93-year-old woman is admitted with an intracapsular fractured neck of femur. The decision was taken to fix the fracture using a cemented hemiarthroplasty. Immediately postoperatively, the patient is short of breath in recovery. Her chest sounds clear. Saturations are 79% on room air, improving to 93% on 6 L of oxygen. The most likely cause is

- A. Pneumonia
- B. Haemorrhage
- C. Pulmonary oedema
- D. Fat emboli
- E. Myocardial infarction

54. Fractures

A 38-year-old man is admitted after falling and sustaining fractures of his tibia and fibula. He is taken to theatre and plate fixation of the fractures is performed. You are called to the ward by the nursing staff, who want you to prescribe morphine patient-controlled analgesia, as the patient's pain has not responded to a current rate of morphine analgesia. You examine the limb; it is in a cast with the forefoot exposed, the skin is warm, but sensation is reduced compared with the non-operative side. You attempt to move the toes, but the patient is in too much discomfort. Your first course of action should be

    A.   Urgent postoperative films
    B.   Increase analgesia
    C.   Remove cast
    D.   Arteriogram/computed tomography angiogram
    E.   Fasciotomy

55. Fracture complications

An 89-year-old woman with multiple medical co-morbidities is admitted after sustaining a fracture of her humerus. The decision is taken not to operate, the arm is placed in a sling and the patient is discharged. The patient re-presents at 3 months after failing to recover normal function in her limb. Radiographs show an absence of callous over the fracture site. The complication is

    A.   Malunion
    B.   Atrophic non-union
    C.   Hypertrophic non-union
    D.   Avascular necrosis
    E.   Delayed union

56. Autoimmune neurological disease

A 27-year-old primary school teacher presents with increasing weakness over the past 3 months. She has been well at the start of each day but feels weaker as the day progresses, with her voice becoming more difficult to understand after several minutes of conversation and an inability to see things clearly at the end of each day. Although the symptoms seem to subside after several hours of sleep they have become worse after a recent bout of flu. On examination, her upper arms are noted to have a reduced bulk and the eyelids appear to droop a few seconds after she is asked to look up or laterally. Her arm reflexes are initially brisk but seem to diminish after repeated testing. An autoimmune disease is suspected as the cause of her symptoms. Against which receptor is she likely to be producing antibodies?

    A. β_2-adrenergic receptor
    B. H_2 histamine receptor
    C.   Presynaptic acetylcholine receptor
    D.   Postsynaptic γ-aminobutyric acid receptor
    E.   Postsynaptic acetylcholine receptor

57. Inherited neurological disease

A 19-year-old girl presents with a recent history of stumbling gait associated with frequent falls and increasing difficulty with her vision, requiring frequent prescription changes. She reports that her grandfather was approximately 40 years old when he died of heart failure, but she and the remainder of her family are otherwise well. Examination reveals bilateral clubbed feet, upward going plantar reflexes, scoliosis and a prominent fourth heart sound. A genetic test is performed, which shows that she is suffering from Friedrich's ataxia. This condition is the result of a defective gene on which chromosome?

    A. Chromosome 4
    B. Chromosome 9
    C. Chromosome 3
    D. Chromosome 10
    E. X chromosome

58. Lumbar puncture

A 41-year-old housewife presents to the emergency department with a severe headache that came on suddenly while driving her son home from a football match. In addition, she reports neck stiffness and some difficulty focusing on objects. She reports that her grandfather died at the age of 50 from chronic renal failure. A subarachnoid haemorrhage is suspected and a head CT scan is requested some 8 hours after the onset of her symptoms, which shows no obvious indication of a haematoma or cerebral mass. A lumbar puncture is performed. Which of the following findings would be diagnostic of a subarachnoid haemorrhage?

    A. Xanthochromia
    B. Bloody appearance in tube 2 of cerebrospinal fluid
    C. Glucose = 1.5 mmol/L
    D. Protein = 5 g/L
    E. Lymphocytosis

59. Neurological infection

A 55-year-old man presents with a 24-hour history of right ear pain, facial weakness and dry tongue. He has previously suffered chickenpox as a child, but otherwise has no significant medical history. On examination, he is unable to close his right eye fully or furrow his brow. Otoscopy is difficult due to pain, but reveals vesicular lesions in the auditory meatus. A clinical diagnosis of type 2 Ramsay–Hunt syndrome is made. The organism causing this condition is a:

    A. Double-stranded RNA virus
    B. Single-stranded RNA virus
    C. Single-stranded DNA virus
    D. Double-stranded DNA virus
    E. Fungus

60. Spinal cord injury

A 17-year-old man presents to the emergency department following a stab injury in the mid-portion of his back 1 hour previously. Following initial assessment and stabilization, a neurological examination is carried out, with signs and symptoms suggestive of Brown–Séquard syndrome. All of the following are classical features of this eponymous syndrome except

A. Ipsilateral motor weakness
B. Ipsilateral extensor plantar reflex (Babinski's sign)
C. Contralateral reduced pain sensation
D. Contralateral loss of proprioception
E. Ipsilateral loss of fine touch sensation

61. Neck lumps (1)

A 72-year-old Asian man presents to his general practitioner with a neck lump noticed when shaving. Of note, he is a smoker of 50 pack years. He denies any symptoms from his ear, nose or throat. He has noticed feeling more tired recently and has lost a few pounds in weight over the last couple of months. He has no previous history of dental abscess or infection. Which one of the following is the most appropriate next management option?

A. Fine needle aspiration cytology
B. Heaf test
C. Referral for ENT assessment
D. Ultrasound scan of the neck
E. Incisional biopsy

62. Neck lumps (2)

A 14-year-old girl presents complaining of a non-painful midline neck swelling. She is otherwise fit and well. On physical examination, the lump moves with swallowing and with tongue protrusion. Clinically, she is euthyroid. Which of the following is the most likely diagnosis?

A. Thyroglossal cyst
B. Dermoid cyst
C. Branchial cyst
D. Cystic hygroma
E. Chemodectoma

63. Thyroid disease

A 40-year-old woman presents with a progressively enlarging midline swelling of her neck over many years. She complains about the cosmetic appearance and states that recently it feels like she is being 'strangled at night' when she lies flat. She does not have dysphagia or dysphonia. Her appetite and weight are unchanged. Her periods are regular. On examination, she has a smoothly enlarged goitre. Which one of the following is the most appropriate management?

- A. Total thyroidectomy
- B. Subtotal thyroidectomy
- C. Radioactive iodine
- D. Oral carbimazole
- E. Oral thyroxine

64. Hoarse voice

A 62-year-old Caucasian man presents to clinic complaining of a recent change in his voice. He has noticed that it is much more hoarse than normal. The symptoms have persisted for more than 4 weeks. He also describes a history of persistent dry cough lasting several months. He is a smoker of 60 cigarettes per day. ENT evaluation reveals an irregular swelling of the left vocal cord which is biopsied. Which one of the following is the best statement regarding laryngeal carcinoma?

- A. Adenoid cystic carcinoma is the most common histological variant
- B. Glottic laryngeal carcinoma is less common than supraglottic carcinoma
- C. Surgical therapy is mandatory
- D. In the absence of cervical nodes, total laryngectomy and radical neck dissection is advocated
- E. None of the above

65. Tongue pathology

A 55-year-old Caucasian woman is referred to the clinic by her dentist. She noticed a painless white spot on her tongue a few months ago, which has failed to heal with topical therapy and is still present 3 weeks later. She smokes 30 cigarettes per day and drinks approximately 30 units of alcohol per week. On examination, she has a small ulcer on the tip of her tongue. Tongue movements are not affected. There is no palpable cervical lymphadenopathy. Which one of the following is the best statement regarding management/diagnosis?

- A. In the absence of tongue fixation, malignancy is unlikely
- B. Any ulcer that has persisted for more than 3 weeks should be biopsied to exclude malignancy
- C. Partial glossectomy is never required
- D. Adenocarcinoma is most common
- E. None of the above

66. Systemic disease and the eye

A 55-year-old Afro-Caribbean man comes to your clinic because of a red right eye. His vision is blurred and he asks you to 'turn down the bright light' as it is causing him pain. The symptoms have been getting progressively worse over the last 3 days. He was diagnosed with sarcoidosis a month ago. He denies fever or night sweats. Respiratory examination reveals bilateral wheeze. Chest radiograph shows hilar lymphadenopathy. Examination of his right eye reveals photophobia and conjunctival erythema. What is the most common eye disorder associated with sarcoidosis?

A. Maculopathy
B. Acute glaucoma
C. Vitreous hemorrhage
D. Anterior uveitis
E. Conjunctivitis

67. The diabetic eye (1)

A 62-year-old African man presents to his general practitioner in the well-man clinic for a routine check-up. His past medical history includes type 2 diabetes mellitus (diagnosed 20 years ago), hypercholesterolaemia and hypertension. He takes metformin 850 mg per day, but does not record his blood sugar regularly. He is additionally taking simvastatin and enalapril. Examination reveals no cardiovascular or respiratory abnormalities and a normal urine dipstick test. Fundoscopy reveals dot retinal haemorrhages, cotton wool spots and neovascularization. His visual acuity is not significantly impaired. Which one of the following best describes this patient's eye disease?

A. Pre-proliferative retinopathy
B. Background retinopathy
C. Diabetic maculopathy
D. Proliferative retinopathy
E. No retinopathy

68. The diabetic eye (2)

Regarding the same patient as in Question 67, which one of the following is the most appropriate management?

A. Increased metformin dose and tight observation of glucose control
B. Vitrectomy
C. Early laser photocoagulation
D. Retinoscopy and deferred laser photocoagulation
E. Retinoscopy and deferred vitrectomy

69. Thyroid eye disease

A 45-year-old Caucasian woman presents to the outpatient clinic complaining of a central neck swelling. She describes being restless and anxious and is always hot. On examination of the neck you detect goitre. She appears also to have clubbing of her nails. Examination of her eyes reveals injected conjunctiva, proptosis, and swelling of the eyelids. Her visual acuity is normal, but there is some restriction of her eye movements. What is the most likely diagnosis?

    A.   Hashimoto's thyroiditis
    B.   Autoimmune thyroiditis
    C.   Graves' disease
    D.   Toxic multinodular goitre
    E.   Toxic adenoma

70. Dry eye

A 68-year-old woman presents to her general practitioner complaining of a constant dry mouth and eyes as well as a gritty sensation in both her eyes. She denies any recent trauma or foreign body injury. Examination reveals a normal visual acuity whilst fluorescein stain excludes abrasion and ulceration. What is the most likely diagnosis?

    A.   Episcleritis
    B.   Scleritis
    C.   Sjögren's syndrome
    D.   Uveitis
    E.   None of the above

71. Neck lumps (3)

A 20-year-old male student attends the surgical outpatient clinic with a pulsatile ovoid swelling just behind the anterior edge of the sternocleidomastoid (SCM) muscle at the level of the hyoid bone. It is elastic in consistency and can be moved from side to side only. This is likely to be a

    A.   Branchial cyst
    B.   Chemodectoma
    C.   Thyroglossal cyst
    D.   Branchial sinus
    E.   Cystic hygroma

72. Neck lumps (4)

A 23-year-old female medical student presents with a 1 cm × 1 cm round swelling in the anterior triangle of the neck. It is smooth and fluctuant with no transillumination or movement on swallowing. The skin is freely mobile over the lump, which is also non-tender to touch. Aspiration of the lump reveals choles-terol crystals. The most likely diagnosis is

A. Sebaceous cyst
B. Dermoid cyst
C. Thyroglossal cyst
D. Cystic hygroma
E. Branchial cyst

73. Neck lumps (5)

A 21-year-old female law student presents with a painless lump, 3 cm × 2 cm in size, in the upper part of the neck. The lump has been growing slowly for the past several months. On examination, it is soft and fluctuant, does not transil-luminate and appears to lie just behind the sternocleidomastoid (SCM) muscle. An aspirate is taken from this lump. The most likely contents are

A. Uric acid crystals
B. Cholesterol crystals
C. Calcium pyrophosphate crystals
D. All of the above
E. None of the above

74. Groin swelling

A slim 60-year-old woman presents to the outpatient clinic with a small (2.5 cm × 1.5 cm), longstanding lump in the right groin, which is only present on standing and walking and usually disappears on lying flat. However, in recent weeks she found that she must reduce it herself when lying down. On examination, the lump is easily reduced with its origin lying below and lateral to the pubic tubercle. Which one of the following structures does not form the femoral canal?

A. Inguinal ligament
B. Lacunar ligament
C. Femoral vein
D. Pectineal ligament
E. Cloquet's node

75. Complications of inguinal hernia repair

A 73-year-old man attends as an outpatient 4 weeks after undergoing a right inguinal hernia repair. He reports good function and the surgical site has healed well. However, he volunteers that since the procedure, he has had a feeling of numbness over the right hemi-scrotum but no such change on the left side. Which one of the following nerves is most likely to be affected?

A. Right ilio-inguinal nerve
B. Left ilio-inguinal nerve

C. Genital branch of genito-femoral nerve
D. Sympathetic nerves
E. Femoral nerve

76. Inguinal hernia surgical anatomy

While assisting in the repair of an inguinal hernia, you are asked to define the boundaries of the Hesselbach's triangle. This anatomical region is defined by

A. Inguinal ligament, inferior epigastric vessels, external oblique muscle
B. Inguinal ligament, inferior epigastric vessels, sartorius muscle
C. Inguinal ligament, inferior epigastric vessels, rectus abdominis muscle
D. Inguinal ligament, adductor longus muscle, sartorius muscle
E. Transversalis fascia, inferior epigastric vessels, rectus abdominis muscle

77. Anatomy of the spermatic cord

Which of the following structures is not found within the spermatic cord?

A. Vas deferens
B. Ilioinguinal nerve
C. Genital branch of the genito-femoral nerve
D. Pampiniform plexus
E. Testicular artery

78. Umbilical swelling

A young couple of Jamaican origin present to the paediatric outpatient clinic with their 3-month-old son, concerned about the presence of a large lump overlying the umbilicus, which appears to enlarge when the child cries. The baby was born at term via an uncomplicated vaginal delivery. On examination, the lump is as described and the child appears otherwise healthy and developed as expected for his age. First-line management of this condition would be

A. Fluid resuscitation
B. Conservative with parental reassurance
C. Antibiotics
D. Digital rectal examination
E. Surgical resection

79. Skin lumps (1)

A 65-year-old woman of Mediterranean origin presents with a longstanding nodule on her left cheek, which has been present for many months but is becoming increasingly unsightly to look at. She is hopeful that it can be treated. On examination, there is a small 0.5 cm × 1 cm round, nodular lesion on the left cheek, the centre of which is collapsed and appears smooth and transparent. The edge of the lesion is rolled and appears 'pearly'. This lesion is likely to be a

A. Basal cell carcinoma
B. Keratoacanthoma
C. Squamous cell carcinoma
D. Solar keratosis
E. Papilloma

80. Skin lumps (2)

A 35-year-old woman, who regularly uses tanning beds, presents with a dark, irregular lesion overlying her left shin. She first noticed it approximately 5 weeks ago. Since then the lesion has become larger and darker. On further examination, it is noted that the lesion is irregular in shape, but approximately 1 cm × 3 cm at its widest and longest points. It is not obviously raised and there appears to be greater pigmentation in the centre of the lesion than at its peripheries. The lesion is likely to be a

A. Nodular melanoma
B. Lentigo maligna melanoma
C. Superficial spreading melanoma
D. Acral melanoma
E. Keratoacanthoma

81. Malignant melanoma

A biopsy of a suspected malignant melanoma shows invasion of the reticular dermis. According to Clark's classification, what level is this lesion?

A. Level I
B. Level II
C. Level III
D. Level IV
E. Level V

82. Skin lesions

A 45-year-old farmer presents with a lump on his wrist that has grown in the last 3 weeks. It has now changed colour and he is worried that it could be something sinister. The lesion is on the radial aspect of the wrist and approximately 2 cm in diameter. It is nodular in shape and firm but with a dark, hard central area. The nodule has a skin-coloured edge and moves freely over the wrist. It is excised and sent for histological analysis. The report confirms that the lesion is benign. This is likely to be what sort of lesion?

A. Ganglion
B. Squamous cell carcinoma

C. Bursa

D. Keratocanthoma

E. Basal cell carcinoma

83. Scrotal swellings (2)

Which one of the following is not a complication of ectopic testis?

A. Increased incidence of torsion

B. Infertility

C. Increased risk of malignancy

D. Delayed development of secondary sexual characteristics

E. Increased incidence of testicular trauma

84. Scrotal swellings (3)

A 6-month-old boy presents with his parents to the paediatric outpatient clinic. The infant's parents have recently become aware that his scrotum appears to be small and underfilled. He was born prematurely at 30 weeks gestation. On examination, the scrotum appears small and hypoplastic, but there is no palpable abnormality within the inguinal regions. An ultrasound scan reports that two ovoid objects lie in the posterior abdominal wall and are consistent with the appearance of bilateral truly undescended testes. The infant's parents are advised that an orchidopexy is indicated to fix the testes in the scrotum. In which age range should this procedure ideally be undertaken to prevent irreparable testicular damage?

A. Within the first year of life

B. 1–2 years of age

C. 2–3 years of age

D. 3–5 years of age

E. After the age of 5 years

85. Testicular pain (1)

A 15-year-old boy presents to the surgical assessment unit (SAU) with a 4-hour history of testicular pain that began after he returned home from a school rugby match. The pain began initially in the lower abdomen, but quickly progressed to involve the testicles, particularly the right. He has vomited twice prior to arrival and remains nauseous. He is unable to recall any recent injury to the groin. On examination the right testicle appears to lie higher in the scrotum than the left. The scrotal skin is warm and the testis extremely tender to touch. This is likely to be:

A. Testicular torsion

B. Torted hydatid of Morgagni

C. Epididymo-orchitis

D. Inguinal hernia

E. Epididymal cyst

86. Scrotal swellings (4)

A 39-year-old man who has previously undergone right-sided orchidopexy as a teenager for an undescended testis presents with a painless swelling in the right hemi-scrotum, which can occasionally cause a dull ache in the groin and heaviness in the testicle. An ultrasound scan of the affected testis reports the appearance as inhomogeneous and cystic. Furthermore, tumour markers confirm the presence of a seminoma. Elevation of which tumour markers is indicative of a seminoma?

A. β-human chorionic gonadotrophin, α-fetoprotein, lactate dehydrogenase

B. β-human chorionic gonadotrophin, α-fetoprotein, CA125

C. β-human chorionic gonadotrophin, placental alkaline phosphatase, lactate dehydrogenase

D. CA19–9, placental alkaline phosphatase, lactate dehydrogenase

E. CA19–9, placental alkaline phosphatase, carcinoembryonic antigen

87. Testicular pain (2)

A 27-year-old office worker presents to his general practitioner with a dull ache in the testes that has been present for the past several weeks and causing a dragging sensation in the scrotum. On examination, the patient reports that the ache is more in the left scrotum than the right. In addition, when the patient stands up, a swelling is present within the left hemi-scrotum that feels like a bag of worms. This is likely to be

A. Haematocele

B. Non-seminomatous germ cell tumour

C. Epididymal cyst

D. Varicocele

E. Epididymo-orchitis

88. Breast lumps

An 18-year-old student presents with a 6-month history of a painless lump in her right breast. She is currently mid cycle and does not report any cyclical change in the lump. On examination a 3 cm × 2 cm lump is found in the inner lower quadrant of the right breast as well as a 1 cm × 0.5 cm lump in the upper outer quadrant of the same breast. Both are smooth on palpation and have sharp edges. They slip easily between the examining fingers of the physician. The primary problem is likely to be a

A. Phylloides tumour

B. Fibroadenoma

C. Breast cyst
D. Fibroadenosis
E. Mammary duct ectasia

89. Treatment of breast lumps

A 25-year-old woman presents to her general practitioner with redness overlying her left nipple and the skin surrounding it. She has been feeling generally unwell for the past several days and has 6 weeks previously given birth to a healthy girl, whom she is breastfeeding. On examination, the redness is confined to the left breast and painful to touch. There is no evidence of the nipple being cracked. The patient's general practitioner suspects that she has developed a lactational breast abscess. The most appropriate action would be to

A. Prescribe an antibacterial agent, e.g. flucloxacillin
B. Advise the patient to stop breastfeeding and review in 2–3 weeks
C. Breast aspiration under local anaesthesia
D. Prescribe an antifungal agent, e.g. ketoconazole
E. Refer to hospital's general surgical team for formal drainage under general anaesthesia

90. Investigation of breast lumps

A 59-year-old woman is undergoing triple assessment for a suspicious lump in the upper outer quadrant of the breast. Which one of the following correctly describes the components of this clinical investigation?

A. Physical examination, lump excision, ultrasonography, computed tomography
B. Physical examination, fine needle aspiration cytology, core biopsy, ultrasonography
C. Physical examination, fine needle aspiration cytology, core biopsy and mammography
D. Physical examination, lump excision, mammography, core biopsy
E. Ultrasonography, fine needle aspiration cytology, mammography

91. Ureteric constrictions

A 54-year-old male presents to the emergency department with intense left loin to groin pain. Following clinical assessment, he is suspected to have a left-sided renal calculus. This is his second presentation. You are able to look at a previous intravenous urogram of the same patient performed 5 years previous to this presentation. This study is normal, however you notice that the ureters have constrictions along their course to the urinary bladder. From the list below, which one of the following is not considered a physiological site of constriction of the ureters?

A. At the pelvic-ureteric junction
B. As the ureter crosses the pelvic brim

C. As the gonadal artery crosses the ureter

D. As the ureter passes anteriorly to the psoas muscle

E. At the vesiculo-ureteric junction

92. Complications of mechanical ventilation

You are in the anaesthetic room observing a 34-year-old lady being prepared for induction of anaesthesia. The consultant asks you to discuss complications associated with mechanical ventilation. From the list below, select the answer which is not a complication of mechanical ventilation.

A. Increased cardiac output

B. Volutrauma

C. Nosocomial pneumonia

D. Barotrauma

E. Parenchymal lung damage

93. Subclavian vein cannulation

A 67-year-old female is taken to theatre for suspected bowel perforation. The on-call anaesthetist is inserting a central venous catheter through the subclavian vein. From the list below which structure is at less risk of damage during this procedure?

A. Subclavian artery

B. Apex of the lung

C. Thoracic aorta

D. Thoracic duct on the left side

E. Phrenic nerve

94. Central venous pressure monitoring

A 45-year-old male who sustained haemorrhagic shock secondary to polytrauma is being fluid resuscitated. A central venous catheter is being inserted. From the list below, choose the answer which correctly describes where the central venous pressure is being measured from.

A. Left ventricle

B. Left atrium

C. Pulmonary veins

D. Aortic arch

E. Right atrium

95. Posterior approach to the hip joint

You are observing an elective right hip replacement. The lead surgeon is accessing the hip joint via the posterior approach. From the list below, choose the correct order (from superficial to deep) and correct structures that are cut through during the posterior approach to the hip.

A. Skin, subcutaneous fat, gluteal fascia, gluteus maximus, short external rotator muscles and the hip joint capsule

B. Skin, gluteus maximus, subcutaneous fat, gluteal fascia, short external rotator muscles and the hip joint capsule

C. Skin, subcutaneous fat, gluteal fascia, short external rotator muscles, gluteus maximus and the hip joint capsule

D. Skin, subcutaneous fat, short external rotator muscles, gluteal fascia, gluteus maximus and the hip joint capsule

E. Skin, gluteal fascia, subcutaneous fat, short external rotator muscles, gluteus maximus and the hip joint capsule

96. Systemic effects of epidural analgesia

A 67-year-old female has been moved to the intensive care unit after undergoing a laparotomy and elective right hemicolectomy for a caecal tumour. The patient is placed on epidural analgesia. From the list below, choose the most likely associated systemic effect of epidural analgesia.

A. Increased functional residual capacity
B. An increased surgical stress response
C. Hypotension
D. Increased cardiac output
E. None of the above

97. Complications of axillary lymph node surgery

A 48-year-old female patient is one day post left axillary lymph node clearance for a left-sided primary breast cancer, which had spread to the left axilla, as confirmed by axillary sentinel lymph node biopsy. She tells you that her left shoulder 'feels funny'. On examination you notice that this patient has winging of the left scapula. From the list below choose the most likely structure which has been injured causing winging of the left scapula.

A. The left long thoracic nerve
B. The left thoracodorsal nerve
C. The right long thoracic nerve
D. The left intercostal brachial nerves
E. None of the above

98. Acid–base disorders

You are asked to see a patient on the ward who has low urine output and blood pressure. She is two days post emergency laparotomy and Hartmann's procedure for faecal peritonitis The patient has a heart rate of 100, blood pressure of 100/60 (mmHg), respiratory rate of 15 and oxygen saturation of 98% on room air. An arterial blood gas performed during your assessment reveals that the patient has a metabolic acidosis. From the list below choose the most likely cause for the patient's acid–base disturbance

A. Acute renal failure
B. Pulmonary oedema
C. Pneumonia
D. Vomiting
E. Hyperaldosteronism

99. Branches of the external carotid artery

As the external carotid artery courses infero-superiorly from the common carotid bifurcation, it gives off the first of seven arterial branches just below the greater cornu of the hyoid bone. From the list below, select the name of the first branch of the external carotid artery.

A. Ascending pharyngeal artery
B. Facial artery
C. Lingual artery
D. Maxillary artery
E. Superior thyroid artery

100. Cardiogenic shock

A 57-year-old male is day 1 post femoral-femoral (left to right) bypass graft insertion for left external iliac stenosis. You are asked to see him because he is complaining of chest pain and difficulty breathing. You alert your seniors and the on-call Intensive Care Registrar who suspects that the patient may be in cardiogenic shock. You are asked to review the patient's chest radiograph. Which one of the following chest radiograph signs is not a characteristic change seen in cardiogenic shock?

A. Hilar shadowing
B. Increased cardiothoracic ratio
C. Right atrial enlargement
D. 'Kerly B' lines
E. Prominent upper lobe pulmonary vessels

ANSWERS

Anticoagulation in surgical patients

1 D Conversion to unfractionated heparin infusion is required

This is a common scenario encountered in any centre where procedural endoscopy is common. Removal of polyps can result in significant bleeding as the lesions are often well vascularized. Patients on warfarin require their INR to be normalized prior to an attempted procedure. In patients receiving warfarin for indications such as atrial fibrillation, warfarin must be stopped 5 days before the procedure. In patients with metal valves, however, the risk of thrombus formation on the valve during this time is too great, and therefore these patients should ideally be admitted and managed on a heparin infusion pump. This allows close, accurate and rapidly reversible anticoagulation which therefore minimizes the time that the patient's anticoagulation is below therapeutic levels in the peri-procedure period.

Low-molecular-weight heparin is not appropriate as it needs to be stopped 48 hours prior to the procedure, during which the patient would not be adequately anticoagulated. The echocardiogram is unnecessary, as is the CT pneumocolon. The patient requires an intervention; finding a further polyp on CT will not affect the need for polypectomy.

Postoperative care in upper gastrointestinal surgery

2 C Restrict oral intake

Following an oesophagectomy, patients commonly become confused, either as a consequence of sepsis or simply due to the huge systemic impact of such major surgery on the body's physiology. Patients removing their own NG tube is a frequent (although not unavoidable) consequence of this and significantly complicates management. The NG tube functions to protect the anastomosis from forceful vomiting and dilatation of the upper gastrointestinal tract. Removal at 4 days is not disastrous but requires careful management; instrumentation of the remnant oesophagus should be avoided and therefore options A and B are inappropriate. A CT scan is unnecessary in the absence of additional indications since NG removal is unlikely to be traumatic, unless an attempt has been made to reinsert.

Sedation does not address the issue highlighted in the case. Also, sedatives may increase the likelihood of ileus and gastrointestinal distension; if sedation is necessary benzodiazepines are probably preferable to antipsychotics such as haloperidol; however, even minor tranquillizers may cause gastrointestinal disturbance. Most important in this case is to limit oral intake and in doing so limit distension and the likelihood of vomiting.

Systemic inflammatory response syndrome

3 D Blood pressure <90 mmHg

Systemic inflammatory response syndrome is a term used to describe the disseminated response to an inflammatory insult such as sepsis, pancreatitis or severe trauma. The criteria for SIRS may be applied in the clinical definitions of certain conditions. For example, a patient may be said to have sepsis if they have the features of SIRS with a likely infective source. A patient is said to have SIRS if two or more of the following are present:

1 Temperature <36°C or >38°C
2 Heart rate >90 beats/min
3 Respiratory rate >20 breaths/min or pCO_2 <4.3 kPa
4 White cell count >12 × 10^9/L or <4 × 10^9/L

Blood pressure is not a consideration. However, if a patient is septic with a systolic BP of less than 90 mmHg, or there is a reduction in their systolic BP of >40 mmHg from their baseline, then they are said to be in septic shock.

Consent

4 C Haemorrhage

Central venous catheters are commonly used in the management of surgical patients as they guide the fluid resuscitation of complex patients and allow the delivery of drugs and concentrated electrolytes which cannot otherwise be given. Therefore, candidates must familiarize themselves with the potential complications of such lines, which occur in approximately 20% of lines inserted.

The question asks specifically for the most common immediate complication; this excludes line-associated sepsis, despite the fact that bacteraemia is by far the most common complication overall. Of those options remaining, the majority of candidates should identify bleeding as the most likely immediate complication.

Note: relative rates of complications differ between line sites. It is commonly held that femoral lines are more often associated with thrombus and infection, subclavian lines are more prone to haemorrhage (due to the risk of arterial damage and the area being incompressible) and internal jugular lines are more prone to pneumothorax. However, in all line types, bleeding is the most common immediate adverse event.

Management of general surgical patients

5 D Attend the emergency department
An important consideration in patient management is that conditions are dynamic and clinical circumstances can easily change.
Management must therefore also be dynamic and change when
appropriate. Reading this scenario, candidates should identify that
the new symptoms described by this unfortunate patient are no longer consistent with his original diagnosis. Rigours suggest abscess
formation or ascending biliary sepsis. Pruritus may indicate obstructive jaundice and it would be appropriate to ask the patient about
jaundice and colour changes in stool and urine. The patient probably
has gallstones, and as such is at risk of obstructive jaundice with or
without ascending cholangitis. A patient with these changes in his
condition warrants reinvestigation and should therefore be readmit-
ted urgently. Option E is incorrect since this patient requires urgent
ERCP with decompression of his biliary tree. Cholecystectomy may
still be deferred for 6 weeks.

Electrolyte replacement strategies (1)

**6 D Maximum concentration of potassium to be given peripherally is
20 mmol/500 mL**
Daily requirements of potassium may be calculated using the formula
1 mmol/kg per 24 hours. This will be increased in certain conditions,
particularly in general surgical patients, in whom electrolyte and
proton loss from the gastrointestinal tract is heavy. Therefore, candidates should be familiar with the safe administration of intravenous
potassium.

The absolute maximum rate and concentration of infusion of potassium through a peripheral cannula is 20 mmol in 500 mL of fluid (normal saline or dextrose) over 2–3 hours. Bolus potassium must never
be given, it acts as a cardioplegic. Faster rates of infusion are possible
in critical care scenarios where up to 40 mmol/100 mL per hour may
be given through a central line. However, this is only advocated in
extreme cases and would therefore be inappropriate in this case.

Electrolyte replacement strategies (2)

7 A May cause hypercalcaemia
Hypophosphataemia may manifest as an arrhythmia, cardiogenic shock,
seizures or even cardiac arrest. Rhabdomyolysis and erythrocyte dysfunction may also occur. Those at risk include the severely debilitated, those on
TPN and those with severe diabetic ketoacidosis. Phosphate replacement
can be problematic as it binds to serum calcium, causing severe hypocalcaemia and precipitating into tissues (metastatic calcification). For these

reasons phosphate should preferentially be given orally. When this is not possible, or the deficit is profound, intravenous phosphate may be given, ideally via a central line, at a rate no more than 30 mmol over 6 hours (usually slower). Because of the potentially fatal, and incipient, consequences of hypophosphataemia these patients should always be treated.

Electrolyte imbalance in special circumstances

8 C Serum magnesium

Candidates should identify that this patient has a low potassium and low phosphate. A patient with a background of poor nutrition who has recently restarted eating should alert one to the possible diagnosis of 'refeeding syndrome'. Those at particular risk are the homeless, alcoholics and those with anorexia nervosa. When the concentration camps of Nazi Germany were liberated, many of the prisoners are thought to have died from this phenomenon on release.

The mechanism is as follows. In the starved state, metabolism is mainly of fat and protein. Insulin levels are minimal due to the lack of dietary carbohydrate. The catabolic state also depletes intracellular stores of potassium and phosphate, with the serum levels usually remaining normal. Once feeding re-commences, insulin levels rise driving potassium and phosphate into cells. The effect is maximal at around day 4. This condition is potentially fatal, primarily from cardiac rhythm disturbance.

Magnesium levels normally closely follow those of potassium and phosphate. Its deficiency predisposes to seizure and arrhythmia. This patient requires close cardiac monitoring and urgent electrolyte replacement.

Fluid replacement

9 E This patient has a metabolic alkalosis

This patient has a metabolic alkalosis. The base excess indicates an increased amount of base (bicarbonate) in the plasma. The rise in CO_2 is due to respiratory compensation; the body aims to retain carbon dioxide to reduce the bicarbonate load. Hartmann's solution contains 29 mmol of bicarbonate and is therefore the likely source of the excess alkali. This patient requires normal saline with potassium replacement; chloride is typically low, and its replacement aids bicarbonate excretion in the renal tubules. Increasing inhaled oxygen concentration might also be of benefit.

Urine output monitoring

10 E The most likely cause is catheter occlusion

The scenario describes a patient with a borderline urine output; a minimum acceptable output may be calculated using the patient's body mass

(= 0.5 mL/kg/h). In all likelihood, this patient is hypovolaemic considering their observations and history. Although options A and C are valid answers, a clinician must complete their assessment of the patient by taking account of the JVP and assessing the lung bases for signs of overload prior to administration of fluid. A better answer is option E: note the sudden cessation of urine output without change in vital parameters. More typical of hypovolaemia would be a gradual tailing of urine output with reciprocal changes in other observations. Sudden cessation such as this is highly suggestive of catheter occlusion; the catheter should be flushed and residual volume recorded. If this remains low and the patient is not in failure, fluid bolus would be the next appropriate course of action.

Paediatric trauma

11 C   Tachycardia
The physiological reserve of children far exceeds that of adults. Therefore, physiological manifestations of haemorrhage occur later, and are more subtle, than in adults. A loss of 30% of circulating volume is required before a child will become tachycardic – this being the earliest indicator of hypovolaemia. At this point the child will typically be peripherally shut down; they will be cold to touch with weak pulses and prolonged capillary refill time. Narrowing of pulse pressure closely follows tachycardia as the child compensates for reduced circulating volume. At this degree of blood loss, a child will go from an irritable state to a state of lethargy, with a diminished pain response which becomes more apparent when inserting a peripheral cannula. Reduced urine output shortly precedes hypotension, as the child's compensatory mechanisms eventually fail. Hypotension in a child indicates that over 45% of circulating volume is lost and that the child is in imminent danger of cardiac arrest.

Paediatric resuscitation

12 A   Intraosseous infusion
Vascular access in paediatric patients is difficult due to the greater amounts of subcutaneous fat and due to the effectiveness of their own peripheral vasoconstriction. The 'shut down' paediatric patient will be difficult for even experienced clinicians to cannulate. Once two attempts have failed, and if the clinical need is adequate, intraosseous infusion may be attempted in any patient, paediatric or adult. The normal position is a fingerbreadth below the tibial tuberosity. Contraindications include fracture proximal to this site or infection/abrasion over the intended site. Intraosseous infusion is preferred as it provides rapid access with fewer complications compared to other techniques. It should be discontinued as soon as peripheral access is achieved.

Alternatives to intraosseous infusion (in order of preference) are femoral line insertion, saphenous cut-down and external jugular cannulation. Central line insertion into the internal jugular or subclavian vein is avoided in children.

Trauma in the elderly patient

13 A Falls

Trauma is the seventh leading cause of death in the elderly population. Falls account for 40% of mortality related to trauma and 60% of all trauma, with the next leading cause of injury being road traffic accidents, followed by burns and assault. There is significant variance in the proportional representation of each mechanism of injury, according to age; falls make up 50% of total traumatic injury in the 65–74 age group, but this increases to over 80% in those over 85. All other modalities of injury reduce in prevalence with increasing age (see the table below for injury-specific incidence by age group).

Mechanism	Number (per cent) 65–75 years	75–84 years	>85 years
Fall	7508 (49.2)	9921 (64.2)	6470 (81.1)
Motor vehicle accident	4648 (30.4)	3349 (21.7)	735 (9.2)
pedestrian	845 (5.5)	713 (4.6)	229 (2.9)
Burns	1928 (12.6)	1242 (8.0)	452 (5.7)
Hit by objects	172 (1.1)	127 (0.8)	49 (0.6)
Assault	168 (1.1)	112 (0.7)	39 (0.5)

Trauma in pregnancy (1)

14 A Blood pressure

Pregnancy induces a variety of physiological changes which prepare the body for the trauma of parturition. These adaptations influence vital signs and normal physiological parameters and therefore the emergency clinician should be familiar with them and able to interpret them accurately in a trauma scenario.

Pregnancy increases the plasma volume disproportionately with a similar increase in numbers of red blood cells. In other words, despite an overall increase in blood volume there is a decrease in haematocrit, so-called 'physiological anaemia of pregnancy'. These changes allow a greater loss of blood volume, approximately 1200–1500 mL, before physiological signs of haemorrhagic shock become apparent. The white cell count increases to levels of 15–25×10^9/L depending on the stage of pregnancy.

Tidal volume increases secondary to actions of progesterone; this lowers the pCO_2 and therefore baseline ABGs in a pregnant woman will typically show hypocapnia. Cardiac output is increased by 1–1.5 L/min due to the increased plasma volume and reduced vascular resistance in the placenta, which receives 20% of blood at full term. There is a consequent increase in heart rate by 10–15 beats/min. Blood pressure initially falls below normal levels in the second trimester, but this resolves by the third term of pregnancy. Therefore hypotension in the third trimester may be due to volume loss, or pressure effects of the gravid uterus compressing the vena cava and reducing venous return to the heart. The so-called 'supine hypotension syndrome' may reduce cardiac output by 30% and therefore pregnant women should be treated lying on their left side, or sat up, if injuries permit.

Trauma in pregnancy (2)

15 E   Explorative laparotomy

Uterine rupture is most common in the third trimester when the uterine wall is at its thinnest and the uterus at its greatest point of expansion and therefore exposure; up to 12 weeks gestation the uterus remains within the bony pelvis, by 20 weeks it reaches the umbilicus, and at 34 weeks the costal margin. Blunt abdominal injury from seat belts is a common cause of uterine rupture and abruptio placentae. Such injuries are more common when the lap belt is worn in isolation, as it compresses the uterus and allows forward flexion of the thorax over the gravid uterus; correct use of shoulder restraints in conjunction with lap belts minimizes risk.

Signs of uterine rupture include those of haemoperitoneum, as well as an abnormal fetal lie and easy palpation of fetal extremities. Features on abdominal radiograph include air under the diaphragm, abnormal fetal lie and extension of fetal extremities outside of the confines of the uterus. In the above case, the certainty of the diagnosis and the compromised state of the mother precludes further delay in definitive treatment; therefore DPL and ultrasound are superfluous and CT should, in any case, be avoided in pregnancy. The choice is therefore between operative techniques, caesarean being inappropriate as it fails to allow sufficient access for a full exploration of the abdomen and exclusion of other compounding injuries. Thus, explorative laparotomy is indicated.

Chronic pancreatitis

16 C   Alcohol

The inherent pathophysiology of chronic pancreatitis is entirely different from acute pancreatitis and the two diseases should be considered different entities. There is continuing chronic inflammation within the gland, which causes the structure to be replaced by fibrous tissue and calcification. Normal function is disrupted, and patients will often develop secondary diabetes, which may be extremely brittle. Patients will often be malnourished not only because of their lifestyle, but also as a consequence of exocrine failure. Obstructive jaundice may also occur.

Incidence is approximately 30/100,000 of the general population; 70% of sufferers have a history of significant alcohol overuse. Other causes are rarer; many cases are idiopathic, some are due to metabolic abnormalities such as hyperlipidaemia and hypercalcaemia, and some are due to congenital or structural abnormalities, such as cystic fibrosis, choledochal cysts and pancreas divisum.

Pancreatic malignancy

17 B Incidence is increasing   *developed*
Pancreatic cancer is a disease of Western living with risk factors including smoking, high-fat diets and exposure to industrial chemicals and dyes. The incidence of pancreatic cancer is increasing; the current incidence is approximately 10/100,000 people. Peak incidence is in the 60–70 year age bracket and there is a male predominance (3:2). The majority of tumours occurs in the head of the gland (85%). Presentation is insidious, and the primary lesion is usually painless and first presentation may be with obstructive jaundice, unintentional weight loss, or back pain/abdominal pain due to infiltration. Other rarer presenting features include acanthosis nigrans and gastric outlet obstruction. Diagnosis is with imaging, although CA19–9 is 90% sensitive, and may be a useful diagnostic adjunct. Unfortunately, over 80% of cases are not resectable at initial presentation, and the prognosis is extremely poor with an average survival of less than 6 months from diagnosis.

Tumour markers

18 C CA19–9
A tumour marker is a substance produced by a tumour which is detectable in the blood or tissues. Such markers may be used in diagnosis or in monitoring response to treatment or detecting recurrence. Types of marker may be divided into hormones (e.g. ACTH, insulin), antigens (e.g. AFP), small peptides (e.g. vanillylmandelic acid, found in the urine of patients with phaeochromocytoma) and enzymes (e.g. PSA). Carcinoembryonic antigen is used to monitor bowel cancer reoccurrence following attempted curative surgery, but may also be raised in smoking, cirrhosis and pancreatitis. α-fetoprotein is raised in 80% of hepatocellular carcinoma and 70% of testicular teratomas. Raised β-hCG is seen in pregnancy, but raised levels in a man suggest a possible

diagnosis of testicular cancer; β-hCG is raised in 70% of teratomas, and 15% of seminomas. CA125 is raised in carcinoma of the ovary, uterus, breast and hepatocellular carcinoma, but may also be raised in peritonitis, cirrhosis and pregnancy. CA19-9 is raised in pancreatic and biliary tract malignancy, but may also be raised in colorectal cancer, biliary stasis and primary sclerosing cholangitis. Tumour markers are therefore non-specific and lack sensitivity, which limits their clinical use.

Peptic ulcer disease

19 D   *Helicobacter pylori*

The most common cause of peptic ulcers is a bacterial infection called *Helicobacter pylori*. It causes 80% of peptic ulcers. *H. pylori* is a spiral-shaped Gram-negative microaerophilic bacterium that infects the stomach and duodenum. It has been postulated that this bacteria is transmitted orally through waste contaminated food and water. *H. pylori* is responsible for causing 95% of duodenal ulcers and 80% of gastric ulcers. It predisposes to peptic ulcers by creating an inflammatory environment within the stomach and duodenal mucosa. The inflammatory process removes the protective lining of gut mucosa, making it more susceptible to acid erosion which eventually leads to peptic ulceration.

duodenal ulcer
duodenal bulb
improves with food

The second most common cause of peptic ulcers is NSAIDs. These drugs are responsible for causing 20% of gastric ulcers and 5% of duodenal ulcers. Cigarette smoking, drinking vast amounts of caffeinated drinks and experiencing high levels of emotional stress are not direct causes of peptic ulcers, but can worsen the clinical symptoms and disease progression of an established peptic ulcer. *H. pylori* infection can be confirmed by a stool antigen test, a urea breath test or tissue biopsy (under endoscopic guidance) of the gastric mucosa. Chronic untreated *H. pylori* infection has been shown to increase the risk of gastric cancer.

Gastric ulcer
in antrum
worsens with food

Management of peptic ulcer disease

20 A   Omeprazole, amoxicillin, clarithromycin

H. pylori-associated duodenal peptic ulcers are best treated using a triple therapy regimen. The NICE guidelines recommend that patients with proven *H. pylori*-associated peptic ulcers should be started on a 7-day triple therapy twice daily dosing of either a PPI with clarithromycin (500 mg) and amoxicillin (1 g) or a PPI with clarithromycin (500 mg) and metronidazole (400 mg). Omeprazole (20 mg) or lansoprazole (30 mg) are generally prescribed but other PPIs (e.g. esomeprazole, pantoprazole) can also be used, but have not been shown to be significantly more effective than omeprazole and lansoprazole which are generally cheaper. Ranitidine (a histamine 2 receptor antagonist) is not as effective in suppressing stomach acid production and hence is not recommended in the treatment regimen of *H. pylori*-associated duodenal ulcers.

Triple therapy has shown to be 85%–90% effective in eradicating *H. pylori* ulcers. Usually after 7 days of treatment, the patient can be placed on a 2-month course of low-dose once daily PPI to further aid healing of the peptic ulcer.

Therefore, from the list, option A (omeprazole, amoxicillin, clarithromycin) is the most appropriate.

Hepatomegaly

21 B **Hepatocellular carcinoma**

Recent weight loss and nodular hepatomegaly coupled with ascites and abdominal discomfort is suggestive that this patient has an underlying malignancy, making the most likely answer hepatocellular carcinoma. Patients can also present with jaundice. Hepatocellular carcinoma is common in countries where chronic hepatitis infection is prevalent and usually occurs against a background of cirrhosis secondary to infective hepatitis, excess alcohol or haemachromatosis. Aflatoxin, a metabolite of the *Aspergillus* species of fungi (mainly *Aspergillus flavus* and *Aspergillus parasiticus*) that grows in nuts, has been shown to be another risk factor for hepatocellular carcinoma.

α-fetoprotein, a tumour marker, is usually raised and imaging (ultrasound, CT, MRI) will confirm the presence of the tumour(s). Treatment involves chemotherapy as well as ablative therapies or surgical liver resection if feasible. Haemochromatosis is an autosomal recessive disorder of increased dietary iron absorption. It is more common in men usually over the age of 40. Systemic iron deposition may lead to cirrhosis, diabetes, heart failure and skin pigmentation resulting in a tanned appearance. Diagnosis can be made with a liver biopsy. Pyogenic liver abscess usually presents with an insidious onset of swinging pyrexia, rigours, a tender palpable liver and jaundice. Diagnosis can be confirmed by blood culturing and imaging. Alcoholic cirrhosis usually presents with jaundice, ascites and a smoothly enlarged liver (in the early stages, fatty liver). In the late stages of cirrhosis, the liver may be impalpable (due to fibrosis) because of chronic inflammation of the liver caused by the alcohol.

Surgery for ulcerative colitis

22 B **Toxic megacolon**

Options A and C should both be regarded as an indication for surgical intervention in ulcerative colitis and therefore cannot be the answer in this case. Previous pelvic surgery can complicate the procedure immensely, but should not prevent lifesaving surgery, although it may change the threshold at which a surgeon may contemplate intervention. Similarly, in cases of young female patients, adequate consideration should be made of the effect on fertility, with an increase in ectopic pregnancy risk and reduction in fertility by 50% due to pelvic adhesions after surgery. Adequate patient counselling is therefore paramount before agreeing on a management strategy, the alternative options being total colectomy with ileo-rectal anastomosis, which carries less risk to fertility, but can result in a symptomatic rectal remnant being left behind.

The only absolute contraindication for this type of surgery is toxic megacolon. In the acute setting, pan-proctocolectomy carries an unacceptably high mortality rate, as well as high leak rate if a pouch anastomosis is attempted. Surgery of this complexity in the acutely unwell patient with an unprepared, inflamed bowel is therefore avoided in favour of a total abdominal colectomy with ileostomy and preservation of the rectum. This removes the diseased bowel, avoids the complex and morbid pelvic dissection, and allows for definitive management once the patient's clinical condition has been stabilized. This may well include a completion proctectomy with ileoanal anastomosis as an elective second operation.

Perianal disease

23 B   Oral and local analgesia and discharge with follow-up
Thrombosed haemorrhoids are painful and uncomfortable, but do not necessitate hospital admission in the acute stages. Appropriate analgesia should be prescribed (avoid opiates as they can cause constipation) along with laxatives and stool softeners. Patients should be advised to use icepacks and elevate the foot of the bed. The majority of haemorrhoids will heal spontaneously with fibrosis, however best practice is to follow up the patient in outpatients, to identify any further haemorrhoids, which may become problematic, and to offer appropriate definitive management.

Fistula *in ano*

24 D   6 o'clock
This question aims to evaluate a candidate's understanding of Goodsall's Rule. This states that the primary (internal) orifice of a fistula can be predicted from the position of its secondary (external) orifice. With the patient lying in the lithotomy position, an imaginary transverse line is drawn from 9 o'clock to 3 o'clock centred on the anal canal. A fistula with its external opening anterior to this line typically has a straight radial tract leading to its internal orifice. Therefore an external orifice positioned at 2 o'clock will have a corresponding

primary orifice also at 2 o'clock. An external orifice posterior to the transverse line will typically follow a curved tract and open internally at the 6 o'clock position, such as in this case.

Pilonidal sinus

25 A   Family history

Pilonidal literally means 'nest of hair' in Latin. They most commonly occur in young adults and there is a male preponderance of 4:1. The aetiology is unclear, but it is thought that implantation of hair occurs in susceptible areas which sets up a foreign body reaction. They are typically asymptomatic until they become infected, when they form abscesses. Risk factors include poor hygiene, obesity and racial origin (Mediterranean, Middle Eastern, Indian subcontinent). Hairdressers are also at risk as they are exposed to large amounts of cut hair, as are those with jobs involving a lot of sitting. There is no genetic link save for preponderance towards body hair.

Right iliac fossa mass (2)

26 D   Psoas abscess

Tuberculosis is re-emerging rapidly in the UK, its prevalence being greatest in large urban areas, especially London. Complications of TB such as psoas abscess are also becoming more common and clinicians must re-familiarize themselves with presentations which were thought to be historical. The at-risk populations are immigrants and the homeless, as well as the immunocompromised.

Psoas abscesses form when pus tracts down the sheath of the psoas muscle, presenting as abdominal pain, fever and an iliac fossa mass. Extension below the inguinal ligament results in a groin swelling. On examination, it is often possible to empty the iliac fossa swelling into the groin swelling, and vice versa. Worldwide, psoas abscesses are most commonly associated with tuberculous abscesses of the lumbar spine, hence the back pain in this case. Psoas abscesses may also be caused by non-mycobacteria; any pyogenic gastrointestinal or urological infection may be causative, although the presentation is typically more acute with sepsis and erythematous, warm swelling of the afflicted area. The examination findings described in the above scenario do not support the diagnosis of hernia.

Management of diarrhoea

27 D   Cholestyramine

Diarrhoea in Crohn's disease may be due to bile acid malabsorption secondary to disease or resection of the terminal ileum. Increased delivery of bile salts into the colon irritates the bowel wall and causes diarrhoea.

Prescribing a bile acid sequester such as cholestyramine can reduce symptoms by 30%–40%.

Antimotility agents such as codeine and loperamide should be avoided in IBD because of the risk of propagating paralytic ileus. A bulking agent in this scenario would not deal with the root cause of the diarrhoea and is unlikely to be effective. As there is no evidence of active inflammation in this patient, methotrexate would be inappropriate.

Surgical anatomy of appendicectomy

28 A Two-thirds of the distance from the umbilicus to the right anterior superior iliac spine

McBurney's point is classically described as 'two-thirds the distance along a line drawn from the umbilicus to the right ASIS'. This point marks the *usual site* of the base of the appendix. The classical incision made over McBurney's point, which is also perpendicular to the imaginary line joining the umbilicus to the right ASIS, is termed a 'grid iron incision'. The 'Lanz incision' is more commonly used now as it has a better cosmetic result and is made horizontally over McBurney's point.

grid iron

lanz

The midpoint between the ASIS and the pubic symphysis marks the landmark of the *mid inguinal point*. The common femoral artery lies beneath this point (±1.5 cm either way at this point due to anatomical variance). The midpoint between the ASIS and the pubic tubercle marks the landmark of the *midpoint of the inguinal ligament*. The deep inguinal ring, which marks the entrance of the inguinal canal, can be found *1.5 cm above the midpoint* of the inguinal ligament. Options D and E are variants of option A and are incorrect.

Mechanical bowel obstruction

29 D Adhesions

Overall, the most common cause of mechanical bowel obstruction (small and large bowel) is adhesions, after which follow hernias, neoplasia and inflammatory conditions such as inflammatory bowel disease (ulcerative and Crohn's colitis) and diverticulitis.

Vascular anatomy of the gallbladder

30 A Cystic artery

The common hepatic artery arises from the coeliac trunk, and along its course gives off the gastroduodenal artery (supplies the pylorus and proximal part of the duodenum). After giving off the gastroduodenal artery, the common hepatic artery becomes the hepatic artery proper which gives off the right gastric artery (supplies the lesser curvature of the stomach). The hepatic artery proper then divides into the left and right hepatic arteries. The right hepatic artery gives off the cystic artery, which supplies the gallbladder. It is worth noting that variations in the origin of the cystic artery exist which will inevitably have consequences on the course of the operative procedure. In 70% of patients the cystic artery arises from the right hepatic artery.

Colorectal surgical resections

31 E Hartmann's procedure

If signs of perforated diverticulitis are present (please see answer to Question 11 in Section 6), the patient is sent to the theatre to have an emergency explorative laparotomy, which will confirm the diagnosis. The abdomen is washed to remove contaminated debris. Hartmann's procedure is commonly performed for perforated diverticulitis or emergency large bowel obstruction. The affected sigmoid colon is resected and the rectal stump is oversewn and left within the pelvis. The proximal end is surfaced and stitched to the skin and usually acts as a temporary left iliac fossa colostomy. The temporary colostomy can be reanastomosed to the rectal stump a few months after surgery; this allows for the inflammation, secondary to bacterial contamination and surgery, to resolve, which improves the rate of success of reanastomosis (if not contraindicated).

High rectal tumours are treated by anterior resection whereby the rectal tumour is removed and the rectal stump is anastomosed with the colon above it. Low rectal tumours are treated with the abdominoperineal resection whereby the rectum and anus are excised and a permanent colostomy is made. See Section 5 for more information regarding colonic resections.

Abdominal distension

32 B Colorectal carcinoma

The apple core lesion seen on the contrast barium enema is highly suggestive of an underlying malignancy, and also the cause of the large bowel obstruction. In the UK, the most common cause of large bowel obstruction is colorectal carcinoma. The colonic luminal diameter decreases as tumour infiltration increases, leading to a narrowing of the bowel lumen, which further results in intraluminal mechanical obstruction of the large bowel.

Metastatic breast carcinoma

33 A Transcoelomic spread

Generally, breast tumours can spread via four main routes:

- Direct extension – To surrounding structures such as muscle and to the chest wall.

- Lymphatic spread – Cancer cells can then block the lymphatic drainage in certain areas of the body causing oedema and changes in the overlying skin.
- Haematogenous spread – Micrometastatic cancer cells can spread via blood vessels and infiltrate bone, lungs, liver and brain.
- Transcoelomic spread – This is a term used to describe invasion of the serosal lining of an organ by malignant cells. The malignant cells trigger an inflammatory response which results in the formation of serous exudates. These exudates then collect in a coelomic cavity, such as the pleural space/cavity.

In this case, the effusion has occurred due to dissemination of malignant cells to the pleura resulting in the formation of malignant pleural seedings. These seedings undergo an inflammatory process which generates serous exudates into the pleural cavity.

Hormone therapy for breast carcinoma

34 B Oestrogen receptor positive and progesterone receptor positive
Studies have shown that tumours that express oestrogen and progesterone receptors show a greater response to hormonal therapy and consequently reduce the growth of tumours that express both of the mentioned receptors. The tumours which express oestrogen alone can respond to hormonal treatment, but to a lesser extent when compared with oestrogen- and progesterone-positive tumours. The tumours which are oestrogen negative tend to express high levels of HER-2 neu transmembrane receptors. These are members of the tyrosine kinase receptors, which have shown to respond to trastuzumab, a monoclonal antibody. Trastuzumab binds to the extracellular portion of the HER-2 neu receptor and thus the cancer cells undergo arrest during the G1 phase of the cell cycle, resulting in decreased cell proliferation.

Endocrine disorders

35 D Conn's syndrome
Polyuria, polydipsia and muscle cramps coupled with high sodium and low potassium suggests that this patient has Conn's syndrome. Conn's syndrome results from an aldosterone-secreting adenoma of the adrenal gland. The excessive amounts of aldosterone leads to increased sodium and water retention and enhances potassium excretion which results in high blood pressure. Hypokalaemia ensues, which is characterized by muscle cramps and polyuria (which occurs secondary to renal tubular damage). This condition can be diagnosed by measuring serum aldosterone and renin levels, which reveal raised aldosterone and renin titres. Managing this patient involves administering an aldosterone antagonist

(e.g. oral spironolactone), and surgical resection of the adenoma once it has been localized with CT.

Cushing's syndrome is the result of raised levels of serum cortisol. Causes include a pituitary adenoma (Cushing's disease), adrenal hyperplasia or neoplasia and ectopic ACTH. The main clinical features of Cushing's syndrome include polyuria, polydipsia, hypertension, increased weight, moon face, central obesity, insulin resistance leading to hyperglycae-mia and diabetes mellitus, thinning of the skin and striae and hirsut-ism. This patient is normoglycaemic and thus Cushing's syndrome can be ruled out.

This patient does not raise or decrease serum calcium levels, which would be seen in hyperparathyroidism and hypoparathyroidism, respectively. Phaeochromocytoma is a neuroendocrine tumour of the adrenal glands originating from the chromaffin cells. Patients present with hypertension, tachycardia and palpitations, anxiety, headaches and weight loss. Diagnosis can be made by measuring catecholamines and metanephrines in blood or urine (24-hour urine collection).

Investigation of endocrine disease

36 A **24-hour urinary 5-hydroxyindole acetic acid**
Paroxysmal flushing, diarrhoea, breathlessness (due to bronchospasm) and abdominal pain, precipitated by stress, alcohol and caffeine, are symptoms highly suggestive of carcinoid syndrome. Carcinoid tumours arise from the enterochromaffin cells of the gastrointestinal tract (mostly small intestine and appendix). Typically, these tumours secrete serotonin (5-HT), which is transported to the liver and broken down into harmless products. When carcinoid secondaries form in the liver, the secreted 5-HT bypasses liver metabolism and is released into the blood stream where the above described symptoms are experienced (also known as carcinoid syndrome). This condition can be diagnosed by measuring 24-hour urinary 5-hydroxyindole acetic acid, a break-down product of serotonin. General management of this condition involves either surgical resection of the primary tumour or, in meta-static disease, with a somatostatin analogue (e.g. octreotide) for symp-tomatic treatment.

The 24-hour urinary vanillymandelic acid test is used in the diagnosis of a phaeochromocytoma. The dexamethasone suppression test is used for diagnosing Cushing's syndrome. Aldosterone and renin levels may be measured for the diagnosis of Conn's syndrome. The short Synacthen test can be used to assess the cortisol-secreting efficiency of the adrenal glands and aid the diagnosis of Addison's disease.

Hunter's canal

37 A Femoral artery, femoral vein, saphenous nerve and the nerve to the vastus medialis

The adductor (Hunter's) canal is usually 15 cm in length and is a narrow fascial tunnel found in the thigh. It is located deep in the middle third of the sartorius muscle and provides an intermuscular passage through which the femoral vessels pass to reach the popliteal fossa, where they become popliteal vessels. The adductor canal begins about 15 cm inferior to the inguinal ligament, where the sartorius muscle crosses over the adductor longus muscle. It ends at the adductor hiatus in the tendon of the adductor magnus muscle. The structures within the adductor canal are the femoral artery, femoral vein, saphenous nerve and the nerve to the vastus medialis. The site at which the femoral artery exits the adductor canal is a common place for the build-up of atherosclerotic plaques. On auscultation of this area, a bruit may be heard. Note that not hearing a bruit does not exclude stenotic vessels.

Lipodermatosclerosis

38 D Varicose veins

Lipodermatosclerosis is characterized by induration, hyperpigmentation and depression of the skin resulting from fibrosis of subcutaneous fat. It is associated with chronic venous insufficiency, occurs just above the ankles, and is commonly seen in patients with varicose veins. The affected area appears erythematous initially and progresses to a purple-brown colour (chronic deposition of haemosiderin coupled with fibrosis of subcutaneous fat), and the overlying skin becomes tight and firm, which may result in pain. Circumferential lipodermatosclerosis may produce the appearance of an inverted champagne bottle. Venous ulcers can develop in areas of lipodermatosclerosis if the chronic venous insufficiency is not corrected.

Fontaine's classification

39 A Ischaemic rest pain

Fontaine's classification is used for clinical categorization according to disease progression of peripheral vascular disease:

- Stage 1 – Asymptomatic patient
- Stage 2 – Patient suffering from intermittent claudication
- Stage 3 – Ischaemic rest pain
- Stage 4 – Ulceration and/or gangrene

Subclavian steal syndrome

40 B Proximal occlusion of the left subclavian artery

Peripheral vascular disease of the upper limbs is less common compared with PVD of the lower limbs. Twice as many patients who have upper limb PVD are women. Subclavian artery occlusion tends to be more common on the left with symptoms of muscular fatigue and pain (similar to what is felt in intermittent claudication of the lower limbs). Occlusion of the proximal subclavian artery can sometimes result in a subclavian steal syndrome whereby blood reaches the affected arm via the ipsilateral carotid artery, the circle of Willis and by retrograde flow down the vertebral artery to the distal subclavian artery. With an increase in upper limb physical activity, there is an increase in the demand for oxygenated blood, and the affected arm 'steals' blood from the posterior arterial cerebral circulation. The resulting symptoms include muscular pain and fatigue in the affected arm, dizziness, vertigo and in some cases, syncope. There are reduced blood pressure measurements in the affected arm and, there may be weak or absent pulses distal to the site of the occlusion. Initial investigations include duplex ultrasound and angiography will usually localize the proximal subclavian occlusion. Percutaneous transluminal angioplasty is usually performed to revascularize the occlusion. If PTA fails, bypass grafting using reversed saphenous vein or synthetic grafts such as PTFE can be used to bypass the occlusion and revascularize the affected arm.

Upper limb pain

41 C Superficial thrombophlebitis

The most likely diagnosis here is superficial thrombophlebitis (inflammation of superficial veins) which is commonly associated with recent trauma (i.e. in this case, multiple attempts of intravenous cannulae insertion), varicose veins, malignancy and thromboangiitis obliterans (a progressive occlusive disease of the blood vessels in the lower extremities associated with cigarette smoking). The patient usually presents with pain and swelling at the site where the superficial vein is inflamed (i.e. site of trauma, varicose veins, etc.). On palpation the vein feels hard and the overlying skin is erythematous and swollen. Management involves removing the underlying cause and treating symptoms with ice packs and NSAIDs. This condition is self-limiting and will usually resolve within 2–3 days. Complications of superficial thrombophlebitis include abscess formation, which will require drainage and antibiotic cover.

Cellulitis is a bacterial infection of the connective tissue underlying the skin. Patients usually present with symptoms similar to superficial thrombophlebitis in addition to fever, nausea and headaches. Common organisms include normal skin flora and Group A streptococcus. If the bacteria penetrate deeper tissues, this can 'lead to necrotizing fasciitis. Lymphangitis is an acute bacterial infection of the lymphatic vessels characterized by painful, red streaks below the skin surface which travel from the site of the infection to the armpits or groin. Associated symptoms include fever, muscle aches and nausea. The most common causative organism is *Streptococcus pyogenes* and in some cases, staphylococci. This is a life-threatening infection and leads to widespread sepsis if prompt treatment is not initiated. Although blood cultures will identify the causative organism, antibiotic therapy should be started immediately if this condition is suspected.

Scrotal swellings (1)

42 C   Hydrocele

Hydrocele is a collection of fluid within the tunica vaginalis. Hydroceles are termed primary, i.e. cause unknown (the predominant type especially in children and those over 40 years of age), or secondary to trauma, infection or neoplasm. Patients present mainly with a swelling in the scrotum or an increase in the size of the testis. On examination, it is possible to get above a hydrocele, but as the swelling is within the testis, it is not palpable as a separate entity. Additionally, is it not possible to reduce the swelling, which would distinguish it from an inguino-scrotal hernia. The fluid within a hydrocele is typically protein-rich and has a clear yellow colour. If large, there is a fluid thrill on palpation and dullness to percussion. Classically, a hydrocele transilluminates brightly when a light is shone through.

Inguino-scrotal hernia occurs as a result of weakness of the deep inguinal ring through which intra-abdominal viscera can pass, exiting through the superficial ring and descending into the scrotum. On examination it is not possible to get above the swelling and a cough impulse will be present. In addition, the swelling is frequently reducible and may be controlled with pressure over the deep ring. The testis and epididymis will also be palpable separate to the hernia and, finally, the structure is opaque to light shone behind it.

Spermatocele is a type of epididymal cyst containing slightly grey, opaque fluid and few spermatozoa. The condition is diagnosed following fluid aspiration and microscopic examination. Physical examination will reveal a swelling in the scrotum above and behind the testis, which is separately palpable. It is usually multilocular and may protrude onto the testicular surface allowing individual loculi to be palpable. Presentation is similar to that of a hydrocele but the ability to palpate the testis separately distinguishes the two conditions.

A varicocele is a bunch of dilated and tortuous veins of the pampiniform plexus (the venous supply of the testis). These are akin to varicose veins of the spermatic cord. They are more common on the left hemiscrotum and may result in a vague, dragging sensation and dull ache in the scrotum/groin. Varicoceles may be primary or secondary to a left-sided renal tumour (testicular artery branches off the left renal artery). The patient with suspected varicocele must be examined standing up as the veins empty on lying flat. The veins are often visible and palpable and classically have the feel of a 'bag of worms'. Management is either conservative with a scrotal support, embolization of the testicular vein under radiological guidance (the preferred method), or surgically by clipping the testicular vein.

Most patients with a testicular tumour will present with a painless lump in the testicle although a small proportion may present with testicular pain. The lump is mostly confined to the scrotum, with the testis and epididymis palpable separately. The lump will also be opaque to light. Definitive diagnosis lies in further tests such as ultrasonography.

Urological emergencies

43 E   Ultrasound scan of the scrotum

Testicular torsion is a surgical emergency most common in males aged 10–25 years. It is commonly preceded by a trivial exertion or trauma, presenting initially as poorly localized pain in the abdomen and loin (the testicle is supplied by the T10 dermatomal level). Severe testicular pain and tenderness follows, usually affecting a single testicle. The pain can be accompanied by severe nausea and vomiting. On examination the testicle can be hot, swollen and extremely tender to touch. Classically the testicle lies horizontally and is high riding. Symptoms progress rapidly over hours and, as the twisting of the testis within the tunica vaginalis compromises the testicular blood supply, leave only a short window in which the testicle is salvageable. A scrotal exploration should be performed as soon as possible in suspected cases of torsion with derotation of the testis and three-point fixation of both the affected and unaffected testicle within the scrotum (orchidopexy).

The first four options for management are appropriate when preparing a patient for most surgical procedures. Given the urgent nature of testicular torsion, requesting an ultrasound scan would cause delay in definitive treatment and could lead to the loss of a potentially viable testis. As a result, in cases of suspected testicular torsion, it is the norm to perform a scrotal examination under general anaesthesia and treat as indicated, i.e. orchidectomy if the testicle is not viable, or orchidopexy.

Complications of urological procedures (1)

44 B   Sodium

Transurethral resection of prostate (TURP) is a commonly performed surgical procedure predominantly to relieve lower urinary tract symptoms that arise due to prostatic enlargement in middle-aged and elderly men. One of the potential major complications of this procedure, affecting some 2% of patients, is TURP syndrome, which occurs during or after the operation as a result of absorption of large volumes of irrigation fluid used in the procedure through the prostatic venous plexus. This process can lead to hyponatraemia, high nitrogen load, dehydration, hypothermia and eventually cerebral oedema. Clinically, patients may become confused, reporting visual disturbances, nausea, vomiting, hypertension, bradycardia and seizures if severe. There is a high mortality associated with this condition and treatment involves supportive measures, fluid restriction, diuretics and an early review by a senior colleague.

Complications of urological procedures (2)

45 A   Prostatitis

Prostatitis is an acute or chronic inflammation of the prostate gland related to bladder outflow obstruction and instrumentation of the urethra and prostate, e.g. with catheterization, cystoscopy, TURP and urethral dilatation. It presents with frequency, urgency, dysuria and occasional haematuria (i.e. symptoms of a UTI) as well as fever, haemospermia and occasionally a tender prostate gland and pain on ejaculation. Organisms causing infection are: *Escherichia coli* (the most common), *Klebsiella*, *Proteus*, *Pseudomonas* and *Serratia*. Treatment is with antibiotics (as per local guidelines) and further investigations such as a transrectal ultrasound may be used to rule out (and if necessary drain) any abscess that has formed as a result of the inflammatory process. Chronic prostatitis occurs more commonly in elderly men with BPH and recurrent UTIs.

Nephrotic syndrome

46 C   Haematuria

Nephrotic syndrome is a clinical entity characterized by proteinuria of >3 g/24 h, hypoalbuminaemia and oedema. It results predominantly from inflammatory conditions that damage renal glomeruli and its filtration process, resulting in proteinuria, hypoalbuminaemia, reduced plasma oncotic pressure and the signs and symptoms associated with the condition.

The condition is the result of either intrinsic or extrinsic kidney disease. Intrinsic kidney disease includes conditions such as minimal change glomerulonephritis (MCGN) and focal segmental glomerulosclerosis (FSGS), while systemic causes include amyloidosis, diabetes mellitus, Henoch–Schönlein purpura and systemic lupus erythematosus. Presenting features of the disease include the following:

- Facial oedema
- Peripheral pitting oedema
- Pleural effusions and ascites
- Xanthelasma and xanthomata (due to hyperlipidaemia)
- Evidence of systemic illness
- Signs of systemic infection
- Acute renal failure/acute kidney injury
- Thromboembolism

Treatment is conservative and medical. Conservative measures include fluid restriction and regulation of dietary sodium, while medical intervention consists of diuretics, steroids to reduce inflammation, antihypertensives, e.g. angiotensin-converting enzyme (ACE) inhibitors, prophylactic anticoagulation in immobile patients and treatment of systemic illness as appropriate.

Median nerve neuropathy

47 D Nerve conduction studies

The only investigation indicated in the first instance when managing carpel tunnel syndrome is a nerve conduction study. This will confirm the site of nerve damage and localize it to the wrist. Only if this investigation identifies more proximal neuropathy should one consider some of the other investigations mentioned above.

Upper limb nerve palsy

48 B Ulnar tunnel

All of the options are common sites of ulnar nerve damage. However, correct interpretation of the neurological findings and knowledge of the functional anatomy of the forearm will allow localization of the lesion. Note that the patient has a clawing deformity of the hand; this occurs in ulnar nerve palsies, which affect the intrinsic muscles of the hands but spare the flexor carpi ulnaris and flexor digitorum profundus. The so-called ulnar paradox refers to lesions of this type; proximal lesions do not spare the long flexors whereas distal injury spares the long flexors, but in doing so allows unopposed action to cause the ulnar clawing, which may be very disabling.

The ulnar nerve lesion is therefore a distal one, branching within the forearm, which therefore excludes options A, C and D. Also, the sensation to the hand is spared. The ulnar nerve branches into various components: the dorsal, palmar and digital branches supply the hypothenar muscles and sensation; and the deep branch supplies the interossei and adductor pollicis and travels through the ulnar tunnel (this is a bony passage between the hook of the Hamate and pisiform bones). Compression at this point can occur following degenerative change (often secondary to a fracture of the carpel bones) or the formation of a ganglion. Suspicions are confirmed by the positive Froment's test (a test of adductor pollicis) and the absence of hypothenar wasting.

Supracondylar fractures

49 D   Median nerve

A fall onto an outstretched hand in childhood may result in a supra-condylar fracture; the fracture pattern is a transverse break just above the level of the epicondyles. The distal fragment is pulled dorsally by the action of the triceps muscle, kinking the brachial artery and inter-rupting the vascular supply to the forearm. Often this is complicated by vessel dissection, and early involvement of a vascular surgeon and urgent open exploration is commonly required. Management requires restoration of flow to prevent ischaemic injury to the muscle compart-ments and permanent disability (Volkmann's ischaemic contracture).

Damage to other structures is common, although not the ulnar or radial arteries; these are distal to the fracture site and therefore cannot be considered valid answers. The musculocutaneous nerve branches from the brachial plexus and travels within the body of the biceps, and is therefore protected from injury. The radial nerve travels posteriorly and therefore does not become bowstringed over the fracture site when the distal segment is displaced by the action of the triceps. This puts it at less risk than the brachial artery, and the closely associated median nerve, which are stretched over the proximal fractured humerus when the distal end is displaced. Therefore, the most commonly damaged structures are the brachial artery and medial nerve, although the ulnar nerve, and less commonly the radial nerve, may also be compromised.

Colles' fracture

50 C   Volar displacement

Colles' fracture is a fracture of the distal radius and is the most com-monly seen fracture pattern in the United Kingdom. The most common mechanism is a fall onto an outstretched hand of an elderly/osteopo-rotic woman. The fracture is diagnosed on the basis of clinical appear-ance ('dinner fork deformity') and radiographic appearance which classically comprises six deformities – dorsal displacement, dorsal tilt, radial displacement, radial tilt, impaction and rotation deformity. Ulnar styloid fracture is a common additional feature. Management is typi-cally with closed reduction under the local haematoma block and cast application. An indication for surgery is displacement of ulnar styloid, which implies serious disruption of the inferior radioulnar joint, or a dorsal tilt of more than 10%, which would severely impair function and predispose to tendon and nerve injury. Operative fixation is by dorsal buttress plating.

Volar displacement is seen in Smith's fracture, which is a similar injury sometimes called a 'reverse Colles'.

Neck of femur fracture

51 B   Cannulated screw fixation

The management of fractures of the femoral neck is a common exam topic, and may easily come up in vivas. The Garden classification is the only fracture classification undergraduates must know. The Garden classification divides intracapsular neck of femur fracture into four groups:

- Garden 1 = Fracture of a single cortex
- Garden 2 = Fracture of both cortices with no displacement
- Garden 3 = Partially displaced
- Garden 4 = Complete displacement

In Garden fractures 1 and 2, the fragments may retain their blood supply and therefore should be managed with cannulated screw fixation in an attempt to save the joint. These patients require regular follow-up for 2 years and if avascular necrosis occurs, these patients should be offered a total hip replacement. Garden fractures 3 and 4 are at much greater risk of avascular necrosis, and therefore hemiarthroplasty is the treatment of choice. The exception is if the patient is very young or has a high level of pre-morbid functionality; in these patients hemiarthroplasty should be avoided and cannulated screws or primary total hip replacements may be considered.

Fractures of the proximal femur

52 E   Dynamic hip screw

Undergraduates often get confused regarding the indications for the different management options in fractures of the proximal femur. Much of this confusion is attributable to incorrect use of the term 'neck of femur fracture' to include extracapsular fractures such as intertrochanteric and subtrochanteric fractures. These fractures are not fractures of the neck of the femur; they do not compromise the vascular supply of the femoral head and therefore they are managed differently. Intertrochanteric fractures are generally fixed using a dynamic hip screw. This device consists of a single screw head which is mobile (i.e. 'dynamic') on a plate attached to the lateral cortex of the femur. The screw is then drilled through the centre of the femoral neck and into the head. This stabilizes the femoral neck, allowing impaction of the fracture surfaces, but not displacement or angle deformity. Subtrochanteric fractures are less common, but typically fixed using a proximal intramedullary nail.

Operative complications

53 D Fat emboli

The scenario describes respiratory failure immediately following surgery. All diagnoses in the list are possible causes with the exception of haemorrhage. Myocardial infarction may cause respiratory failure if complicated by acute left ventricular failure. Intraoperative fluid overload may also complicate immediate postoperative recovery but with both of these one would expect crepitations on listening to the chest, as you would in the presence of pneumonia. The probable cause is therefore a deficit in pulmonary perfusion, which may be due to thromboembolism or fat embolism. Thromboembolic disease is extremely common in hip fracture and surgery complicating up to 50% of cases. However, thromboemboli typically occur 2–3 days postoperatively. Immediately following an operation the cause that must be excluded is fat emboli, which occurs in up to 1% of cases, particularly where cement is used. The distinction is difficult but is important since thromboembolism requires management with anticoagulant therapy, with the obvious propensity for further complications in the postoperative patient.

Fractures

54 C Remove cast

This patient has postoperative compartment syndrome. This is a common complication of operations or fractures in the lower leg or forearm, but may also occur elsewhere. The most obvious clinical sign is pain, which is out of all proportion with what one would expect. Paraesthesia and the sensation of tightness are additional symptoms patients will complain of. The most sensitive feature on examination is pain on passive flexion of the affected compartment. If this is encountered on the ward, first remove all bandages and casts to try to relieve the pressure. Increasing analgesia is important, but secondary to saving the limb. Neither postoperative films nor an arteriogram will be helpful, and both will delay important definitive management. Once the cast is removed involve a senior surgeon, who will decide on whether a fasciotomy is indicated.

Fracture complications

55 B Atrophic non-union

Various problems with fracture union can occur and candidates should be able to identify the main features of each to distinguish between them on radiographs. Avascular necrosis occurs when a fracture interrupts the blood supply to a part of a bone. This only occurs in a small number of sites because the bones typically receive a good supply from various sources and are therefore protected from this phenomenon. The 'at risk' sites are the femoral neck and head, scaphoid and talus. Radiographically the appearance is of sclerosis with distortion of shape and structure. Malunion is when a fracture heals in an abnormal position. Delayed union is when a fracture heals normally but takes a prolonged period of time. Non-union is when the fracture surfaces fail to unite; there are two types, hypertrophic and atrophic. In hypertrophic non-union there is an abundance of callus but no union; this may be due to excess movement across the fracture site or due to interposed tissues. Atrophic non-union occurs when the body makes no effort to heal and no callus forms. The bony ends often appear osteopenic, and this is more common in the elderly, the malnourished or generally debilitated.

Autoimmune neurological disease

56 E Postsynaptic acetylcholine receptor

This is a two-stage question which requires a clinical diagnosis to be made, followed by knowledge about the disease, for the question to be answered.

The description is of myasthenia gravis, a rare autoimmune disease in which antibodies develop against the postsynaptic acetylcholine receptor, resulting in reduced receptor numbers at the neuromuscular junction. Young adults are most susceptible, presenting with increasing muscle fatigability that initially is worse with exertion and relieved by rest but can progress to a permanent weakness. Muscles of the eye (presenting with ptosis and diplopia), face, neck, trunk and distal limbs can be affected. Twenty per cent of individuals will have an associated tumour of the thymus (which is involved in T-lymphocyte production). Incidence is also increased in patients with other autoimmune conditions such as hyperthyroidism, RA and SLE. Treatment takes a variety of forms:

- Symptomatic control is obtained by using anticholinesterase agents such as pyridostigmine, edrophonium (also a diagnostic agent) and neostigmine, which increases the amount of available acetylcholine, but can be associated with cholinergic toxicity.

- Immunosuppression with prednisolone or azathioprine can be beneficial in some individuals.
- Thymectomy in the presence of a thymoma can produce disease remission in around 33% of patients and symptom reduction in another 40%.
- Plasmapheresis is used in emergency cases for short-term symptomatic relief.

The β_2-adrenergic receptor is found in many body cells and its agonists include adrenaline and noradrenaline (together with many pharmacological agents). Its effects include smooth muscle relaxation and dilatation of small blood vessels. The H_2 histamine receptor is located on gastric parietal (oxyntic) cells. Binding of histamine to this receptor results in the production of gastric acid and intrinsic factor. The presynaptic acetylcholine receptor may be affected in the myasthenic syndrome, a condition associated with bronchial small cell carcinoma (together known as Eaton–Lambert syndrome). Here, the muscle strength and reflexes are improved by repeated contractions, unlike true myasthenia gravis. γ-amino butyric acid (GABA) is the chief inhibitory neurotransmitter in the human body and acts on the GABA receptor, of which three varieties (A, B, C) are known.

Inherited neurological disease

57 B Chromosome 9

Friedrich's ataxia is a hereditary ataxia inherited in an autosomal recessive fashion due to a gene defect on chromosome 9 coding the protein frataxin. This results in the loss of dorsal root ganglia cells and degeneration of peripheral sensory fibres, the lateral corticospinal tracts and dorsal columns. It usually presents in early adulthood with progressive difficulty walking due to muscle wasting, a broad based (ataxic) gait, reduced visual acuity, nystagmus, dysarthria, loss of fine touch and proprioception (due to effects on the dorsal columns), loss of deep tendon reflexes and an extensor plantar response (Babinski's reflex). Associated systemic features include diabetes, scoliosis, pes cavus (club foot) and hypertrophic cardiomyopathy. Treatment is symptomatic only and most patients die in their mid-thirties.

Genetic defects on chromosome 4 are associated with Huntington's chorea, an autosomal dominant disease resulting in an expansion of the CAG trinucleotide repeat. The condition usually presents with depression, cognitive impairment, poor memory and jerky, involuntary, dance-like movements. The accumulation of trinucleotide repeats increases with successive generations causing symptoms and death to occur at a younger age in children as compared to their parents. Von Hippel-Lindau disease is an autosomal dominant neurocutaneous syndrome associated with mutation in the *raf-1* oncogene on chromosome 3. The disease results in the formation of haemangioblastomas in the cerebellum. The spinal canal and retina, which can cause hydrocephalus, ataxia, cord compression and subretinal haemorrhage (leading to blindness), respectively. The condition is also associated with systemic pathology such as renal cell carcinoma and phaeochromocytoma. Death is often the result of these many varied systemic pathologies.

Lumbar puncture

58 A   Xanthochromia

The CSF is a clear, watery fluid that surrounds the spinal cord and brain, cushioning the latter from contact with the skull and reducing its weight. It is produced by the choroids plexus in the lateral, third and fourth ventricles and circulates there, in the central canal and in the subarachnoid space. It is absorbed by the arachnoid villi that project into the superior sagittal sinus. The CSF normally has a clear appearance, a white cell count of <5 cells/mm^3 (predominantly mononuclear cells), a glucose of 2.8–4.2 mmol/L (about half to two-thirds of the blood glucose level) and a protein count of 0.15–0.45 g/L.

Subarachnoid haemorrhage (SAH) is the accumulation of blood in the subarachnoid space. It is the result of either trauma or a spontaneous process. Most spontaneous bleeds are the result of rupture of intracranial berry aneurysms (~75%), which occur at the bifurcations of the circle of Willis in association with polycystic kidney disease/connective tissue disorders; a further minority result from arterio-venous malformation, vasculitis, clotting disorders and an extending carotid dissection. In approximately 20% of cases, the cause is unknown. Subarachnoid haemorrhage most commonly presents with a sudden onset (thunderclap) headache, often described as the worst headache ever experienced by the patient, signs of meningism (i.e. neck stiffness and photophobia), focal neurological deficit and a depressed consciousness level. The presence of a greater number of these signs carries a higher mortality.

The investigation of choice is a head CT scan, which will detect approximately 98% of bleeds. If there is no haematoma, mass lesion or hydrocephalus, a lumbar puncture is performed 12 hours after the onset of symptoms. This will usually demonstrate equal numbers of blood cells (and a similar appearance) in tubes 1 and 3 on CSF collection. However, this may also occur in a traumatic tap, although the CSF should normally be clear. A bloody tap is spun down and the supernatant decanted to test for xanthochromia (yellow colour), which is the result of the breakdown of the haemoglobin within red blood cells, and diagnostic of SAH. Treatment can be medical and/or surgical depending on the severity of the bleed. An urgent neurosurgical opinion is needed if there is reduced consciousness or focal neurology to consider haematoma evacuation. Further surgical intervention is considered to reduce the risk of re-bleeding, which occurs in around 30% of patients and can be more severe and life-threatening than the initial bleed. Surgical methods include clipping of identifiable aneurysms or insertion of coils into their lumen to promote thrombosis.

Neurological infection

59 D   Double-stranded DNA virus

Ramsay–Hunt syndrome is the eponymous name given to herpes zoster (or shingles) of the geniculate or facial ganglion. Infection is the result of the varicella zoster virus (VZV), a double-stranded (ds) DNA virus, responsible for chickenpox (varicella) and shingles. Following a bout of childhood chickenpox, the virus lies dormant in the dorsal root ganglion of the spinal cord, trigeminal or geniculate ganglion. Reactivation of the virus can lead to shingles, Ramsay–Hunt syndrome or herpes zoster ophthalmicus (trigeminal herpes zoster). Classically, Ramsay–Hunt syndrome presents with a vesicular rash in the external auditory meatus (or over the pinna), sudden facial paralysis in a lower motor neurone distribution which can be preceded by severe pain, loss of taste sensation in the anterior two-thirds of the tongue and dry mouth and eyes. The symptoms are the result of loss of sensory, motor and parasympathetic functions of the facial nerve. The vestibulocochlear nerve lies close to the geniculate ganglion, such that the zoster virus may also affect its function, resulting in deafness and tinnitus. Treatment is with systemic steroids, e.g. prednisolone, and antiviral agents, e.g. aciclovir, if symptoms are severe. Most patients make a complete recovery if treatment is started promptly.

Spinal cord injury

60 D   Contralateral loss of proprioception

A Brown–Séquard syndrome is a clinical presentation resulting from lateral hemisection of the spinal cord particularly in the cervical and thoracic regions. Hemisection has many causes including: spinal cord trauma, tumour, disc herniation, cervical spondylosis, meningitis, syphilis and multiple sclerosis. Classically, cord hemisection affects the three major neural systems, that is:

- Upper motor neurone pathway of the corticospinal tract
  - Ipsilateral motor weakness and spastic paralysis below the level of the lesion
  - Brisk reflexes
  - Clonus
  - Extensor plantar reflex (Babinski's sign)

- Dorsal columns
  - Loss of ipsilateral fine touch, vibration and proprioception (lesion in fasciculus gracilis/cuneatus) below the level of the lesion
- Spinothalamic tract
  - Loss of contralateral pain and temperature sensation one to two segments below the lesion

Although the classical presentation is described here, this is a rare finding. Instead a mixed presentation with asymmetrical distribution of signs and symptoms is more common in clinical practice. The long-term prognosis is dependent on the ability to rapidly treat the causative factor but overall recovery is poor.

Neck lumps (1)

61 C Referral for ENT assessment

This patient should be referred for full ENT assessment. This would include inspection, radiology and biopsy of any primary sites in the head and neck. If the primary sites are clear, then an ultrasound along with fine needle aspiration cytology may assist the diagnosis. Otherwise the lesion must be biopsied by excision, as incisional biopsy carries the risk of seeding malignant cells. If malignancy is confirmed in the absence of an obvious primary site, a radical neck dissection is usually recommended to remove all the lymph node bearing tissue in the anterior and posterior triangles of the neck between the prevertebral tissues and platysma. The Heaf test will help to establish the tuberculosis status but should be conducted following a comprehensive clinical assessment.

Neck lumps (2)

62 A Thyroglossal cyst

Thyroglossal cysts are remnants of the thyroglossal duct, and can arise anywhere from the tongue (foramen caecum) to the thyroid gland itself. Most are asymptomatic, but secondary infection may cause pain. The most common site is under the hyoid and the cyst will move on swallowing and on tongue protrusion. Dermoid cysts do occur in the midline but tend not to move on swallowing or tongue protrusion. Branchial cysts and cystic hygromas are causes of lateral neck swelling in children. Chemodectomas are extremely rare benign tumours arising laterally in the carotid bulb in the region of the carotid bifurcation.

Thyroid disease

63 B Subtotal thyroidectomy

This patient has goitre and is euthyroid clinically. Patients with goitres may require subtotal thyroidectomy if they are causing compressive symptoms. Total thyroidectomy is reserved for the management of thyroid carcinoma. Carbimazole and radioactive iodine is prescribed to treat hyperthyroidism.

Hoarse voice

64 E None of the above

None of the above. Squamous cell carcinoma is the most common histological variant. Adenoid cystic carcinoma, sarcoma and lymphoma are rare. Sixty per cent occur in the glottis and present with dysphonia. Radiotherapy is advocated for virtually all glottic tumours. T1 lesions have over a 95% cure rate with this modality. Total laryngectomy and radical neck dissection is reserved for recurrent and metastatic disease.

Tongue pathology

65 B Any ulcer that has persisted for more than 3 weeks should be biopsied to exclude malignancy

Any ulcer on the tongue that persists should be biopsied to exclude malignancy. The most common variant is squamous carcinoma. Tongue fixation and mandibular infiltration are late features. Partial glossectomy may be required for larger lesions. Small lesions may be treated with surgery or radiotherapy.

Systemic disease and the eye

66 D Anterior uveitis

Sarcoidosis is associated with a number of ocular problems. Acute uveitis is the most common. This may progress to chronic uveitis and cataract formation, glaucoma and bands of calcium deposition in the cornea (band keratopathy). Lacrimal gland infiltration may lead to chronic dry eyes with the need for artificial tear replacement. Optic nerve infiltration is also a recognized complication.

The diabetic eye (1)

67 D Proliferative retinopathy

This patient has proliferative retinopathy indexed by neo-vascularization. Background retinopathy is characterized by microaneurysms, dot haemorrhages and hard yellow exudates. These changes do not have much of an effect on vision when they occur in the peripheral retina. However, when they occur in the vicinity of the macula ('diabetic maculopathy') vision can be severely affected. Pre-proliferative retinopathy is characterized by tiny abnormal blood vessels and retinal haemorrhages. Visual acuity may be preserved until a large haemorrhage occurs, so specialist referral is required.

The diabetic eye (2)

68 C Early laser photocoagulation

The patient has proliferative retinopathy which should be managed with referral for early laser photocoagulation. Deferred laser photocoagulation is an acceptable management strategy in patients with non-proliferative diabetic retinopathy. Tight regulation of glucose control may help prevent progression of retinopathy but further treatment is indicated. Vitrectomy is the surgical removal of the vitreous. It is used to treat the complications of diabetic retinopathy such as vitreous haemorrhage and retinal detachment.

Thyroid eye disease

69 C Graves' disease

Graves' disease is an autoimmune condition causing goitre, hyperthyroidism and eye disease. The ocular features include swelling of eyelids, chemosis, proptosis ophthalmoplegia and optic neuropathy. Hashimoto's and autoimmune thyroiditis are causes of hypothyroidism. Toxic multinodular goitre and toxic adenoma are not associated with thyroid eye disease.

Dry eye

70 C Sjögren's syndrome

Sjögren's syndrome is an autoimmune disorder affecting exocrine glands secreting saliva and tears. It is associated with rheumatoid arthritis. The Schirmer test measures the wetness of tear production and confirms the diagnosis. Treatment includes artificial tear drops and mucolytic agents.

Neck lumps (3)

71 B Chemodectoma

The description is classical of a chemodectoma, a rare tumour of the chemoreceptor tissue in the carotid body. It is elastic in consistency, pulsatile and can be moved from side to side but not up and down. It is usually found behind the anterior border of the SCM at the level of the hyoid bone.

A thyroglossal cyst is a remnant of the thyroglossal duct. It occurs as a smooth, midline swelling 2–3 cm in diameter at or below the level of the hyoid bone. It commonly presents between the ages of 15 and 30 years. It moves up on swallowing and on protrusion of the tongue. A branchial sinus is a tract leading from a focus of infection to the surface of the skin.

It is formed from the second branchial cleft (as are branchial cysts) and is seen as a small dimple at the junction of the middle and lower third of the anterior edge of the SCM and can discharge a thick, clear mucus. Cystic hygroma is a congenital collection of lymphatic sacs (also known as lymph cyst or lymphocele). It usually presents within the first few years of life as a large lump behind the clavicle that transilluminates brightly.

Neck lumps (4)

72 E   Branchial cyst
All of the listed swellings are found in the anterior triangle of the neck, except cystic hygroma, which is a lymphatic cyst usually found in the posterior triangle behind the clavicle (most commonly in young babies) that transilluminates brightly. Thyroglossal cysts, although consistent with the above description, tend to occur in the midline, with movement on swallowing or tongue protrusion. Sebaceous cysts occur in hair bearing areas of the skin and classically (although not always) contain a central punctum through which a cheesy keratinous substance can be exuded. Dermoid cysts are large swellings in the midline of the neck and are rare beyond adolescence. Branchial cysts are squamous epithelium remnants of the second pharyngeal cleft, usually found in the anterior triangle of the neck behind the upper third of the SCM muscle. The cysts are usually fluctuant and opaque due to the presence of desquamated epithelial cells and definitively diagnosed by aspiration of cholesterol crystals.

Neck lumps (5)

73 B   Cholesterol crystals
This question requires knowledge about two things: (i) the description is that of a branchial cyst, which is commonly associated with the presence of cholesterol crystals and (ii) uric acid and calcium pyrophosphate crystal aspirates are associated usually with gout and pseudogout respectively.

Groin swelling

74 E   Cloquet's node
The description is of a femoral hernia. An inguinal hernia will reduce to lie above and medial to the pubic tubercle (the origin of the superficial ring). All of the listed structures form the femoral canal, except Cloquet's node. This is a lymph node transmitted within the femoral canal together with a plug of fat.

Complications of inguinal hernia repair

75 A   Right ilio-inguinal nerve
The inguinal canal is an oblique, inferomedially directed passage between the deep (internal) and superficial (external) inguinal rings through the

inferior part of the anterior abdominal wall. The canal lies superior and parallel to the medial half of the inguinal canal. Its contents are

- Spermatic cord in men
- Round ligament in women
- The ilio-inguinal nerve
- Blood vessels
- Lymphatic vessels

The ilio-inguinal nerve arises from the first lumbar nerve and over- lies the spermatic cord/round ligament during its passage through the inguinal canal. On exiting the superficial inguinal ring it is distrib- uted to the skin of the upper and medial part of the thigh and to the following:

- Males – Skin over the root of the penis and upper scrotum
- Woman – Skin covering mons pubis and labium majus

The ilio-inguinal nerve supplies the ipsilateral hemi-scrotum and can become entrapped during the repair of the hernial defect at the time of surgery, resulting in long-term numbness ± pain over the hemi- scrotum. Other complications of hernia repair include wound infection, haematoma formation, mesh infection and ischaemic orchitis.

Inguinal hernia surgical anatomy

76 C **Inguinal ligament, inferior epigastric vessels, rectus abdominis muscle**

Inguinal hernias are the most commonly occurring hernias. They are divided into direct (25%) and indirect (75%). Indirect hernias occur when a viscus (usually bowel) protrudes through the deep ring and tra- verses the inguinal canal and may eventually exit through the superfi- cial ring into the scrotum. Direct inguinal hernias occur as a result of abdominal wall weakness and protrusion of viscus directly through the posterior wall of the inguinal canal, medial to the deep (internal) ring. Clinically, the two may be indistinguishable and can only be defined at the time of repair with reference to Hesselbach's triangle. The borders of this anatomical landmark are:

- Medial: Rectus abdominis muscle
- Superior/lateral: Inferior epigastric vessels
- Inferior: Inguinal ligament

The defect in an indirect hernia is in the internal ring, which is lateral to the inferior epigastric vessels, whereas the defect in direct hernias is through Hesselbach's triangle, which is medial to the inferior epigastric vessels.

Anatomy of the spermatic cord

77 B   Ilioinguinal nerve

The inguinal canal transmits the spermatic cord in males from the abdomen to the testes, while in females it is replaced by the round (uterine) ligament that travels from the uterus to the labium majorum. While all the structures are within the inguinal canal, the ilio-inguinal nerve is transmitted on top of the spermatic cord, whereas the remaining structures are found within the cord. The spermatic cord is covered in three fascial layers derived from the anterior abdominal wall, and contains the following structures:

- Vas deferens
- Testicular artery
- Testicular veins (pampiniform plexus)
- Testicular lymph vessels
- Autonomic nerves
- Remains of the processus vaginalis (tunica vaginalis)
- Cremasteric artery
- Artery of the vas deferens
- Genital branch of the genito-femoral nerve (supplies cremasteric muscle, which allows retraction of the testicle)

Umbilical swelling

78 B   Conservative with parental reassurance

The description is of a congenital umbilical hernia, which is especially common in black and Afro-Caribbean children (as well as those with Down's syndrome and congenital hypothyroidism). *In utero*, the developing gut grows more rapidly than the coelomic capacity, resulting in temporary herniation of the gut into the wide base of the umbilical cord. The abdominal cavity then continues to grow and by week 12 of development the herniated abdominal contents return to the abdominal cavity. The umbilical ring then constricts with a small defect for the umbilical vessels that nourish the developing fetus. After birth, the vessels thrombose and fibrous tissue plugs the defect. The failure of this process results in a congenital umbilical hernia.

The hernia can commonly enlarge when a child cries but rarely strangulates due to the presence of a wide base. They require no specific treatment and the defect usually closes by the age of 4. However, surgical repair can be considered should the hernia persist after the age of 3.

Skin lumps (1)

79 A   Basal cell carcinoma

Basal cell carcinoma (rodent ulcer) is a slow growing malignant tumour of the skin, predominantly affecting the central portion of the face and is directly related to sun exposure. It begins as a raised nodule with venules crossing its central portion, which can collapse and ulcerate and invade locally to form large lesions (the rodent ulcer). The classical presentation is with a rolled pearly edge. Treatment is dependent on the site and the size of the ulcer but most commonly consists of surgical excision, curettage and radiotherapy, if large.

Keratoacanthoma (molluscum sebaceum) is a lesion occurring in middle-aged individuals, most commonly in hair-bearing areas. It is related to sun exposure and consists of a lesion that grows over many months as a domed swelling with a central plug of keratin. The keratin plug can fall off, leaving a bleeding floor. If managed conservatively, it usually regresses over many months to leave a small scar. Excision allows a definitive diagnosis between keratoacanthoma and malignancy. Squamous cell carcinoma occurs commonly on exposed areas of the body such as the head, neck, hands and trunk, which are repeatedly exposed to sunlight. It consists of an ulcer that has an everted edge (unlike the rolled edge of BCC) and is dark brown in colour. Squamous cell carcinoma commonly begins as a small nodule on the skin, becoming necrotic in its centre as it enlarges and forms an ulcer. Solar (senile) keratoses are scaly lesions occurring mainly in elderly individuals who have had chronic sun exposure. Malignant change can occur in 25% of lesions, necessitating excision. Papilloma are small epidermal tumours relating to human papilloma virus (HPV) infection. They are benign lesions that occur as sessile or pedunculated structures.

Skin lumps (2)

80 C Superficial spreading melanoma

Melanoma is a malignant tumour of the pigment producing cells of the body (melanocytes). Spread can be to lymph nodes, liver and other parts of the body. Incidence is increased in individuals with fairer skin tones and increased exposure to UV radiation. This presentation is of a superficial spreading melanoma, which makes up 70% of melanomas. It spreads superficially in the epidermis initially and becomes invasive after many months or years. The lesion margin and surface tend to be irregular and pigmented. It can be surrounded by an area of inflammation and generally carries a poor prognosis.

Lentigo maligna melanoma is a slow growing, irregularly pigmented macule that can be present for many years and usually occurs in exposed areas in elderly individuals. Nodular melanoma consists of a dark nodule, commonly occurring in middle-aged men. It has a poor prognosis because of invasive growth from the start of its development. Acral melanoma occurs on the palms and soles and in the nail bed of affected individuals. Prognosis depends on the lesion thickness (i.e. depth) as measured from the granular layer to the deepest layer

of invasion, using Clark's and/or Breslow classification. Overall 5-year
survival is 75% in women and 60% in men.

Malignant melanoma

81 D   Level IV

Clark's classification is one of two classification systems (the other
being Breslow's depth) used to determine the prognosis of malignant
melanoma. The level is determined by lesion depth measured in mil-
limetres from the granular layer, i.e. base of epidermis to the deepest
layer of invasion:

- Level I   – Within epidermis
- Level II – Few melanoma cells within the dermal papillae
- Level III – Many melanoma cells in the papillary dermis
- Level IV – Invasion of the reticular dermis
- Level V   – Invasion of the subcutaneous tissue

Skin lesions

82 D   Keratocanthoma

A keratoacanthoma is a self-limiting overgrowth of hair follicle cells
producing a central plug of keratin with subsequent spontaneous regression. Keratoacanthomas grow rapidly over 2–4 weeks and then regress
spontaneously over approximately 6 months. Keratoacanthomas can be
found in any area containing sebaceous glands and are usually solitary, consisting of a skin-coloured conical lump that develops a necrotic
centre. The lump is confined to the skin and freely mobile over the
subcutaneous tissue. The central core eventually separates causing the
lesion to collapse and leave an indrawn scar. They are usually excised
to differentiate from a squamous cell carcinoma. The descriptions of the
other lesions are discussed in earlier answers.

Scrotal swellings (2)

83 D   Delayed development of secondary sexual characteristics

The testes develop intra-abdominally in the posterior abdominal wall
from nephric tissue. They are guided by the gubernaculum into the scrotum, usually entering this structure at between 28 and 34 weeks gestation. Ectopic testis refers to the deviation of a descending testicle from its
normal line of descent into an abnormal position. As a result, the testicle
may lie at the base of the penis, in the superficial inguinal pouch, within
the perineum or in the femoral triangle of the thigh. Individuals may
present with an absent testis or pain, if the ectopic testis (a smooth, sensitive, ovoid swelling) is on a site that is likely to be rubbed or pressed in
the course of normal daily activity.

When a testis follows the correct anatomical path of descent but does not reach its final position in the scrotum, it is referred to as a truly undescended testis. Undescended testes are more commonly found in premature babies, 30% of whom may have undescended testes. In term infants, the incidence decreases to 3%, while in children of 1 year of age, this is further reduced to 1%. Spontaneous descent after that age is very rare. The line of testicular descent crosses the external inguinal ring and neck of the scrotum, where 80% of undescended testes are typically found and can be palpable on examination. Presence in either of these areas is an indication for orchidopexy, whereby the testis is fixed in the scrotum between the dartos muscle and skin, by the age of 18 months, to prevent testicular damage. After age 2 years, the testis can become damaged and incapable of spermatogenesis. Truly undescended and ectopic testes are potentially complicated by:

- Infertility – A near inevitability in individuals with bilateral undescended (and common in those with unilateral undescended) testes
- Torsion
- Trauma
- Inguinal hernia
- Malignant disease

Although failure of descent/ectopic testes are associated with abnormal spermatogenesis and infertility, hormone-producing cells of the testes function normally, resulting in puberty and the development of secondary sexual characteristics.

Scrotal swellings (3)

84 B   1–2 years of age
When a testis follows the correct anatomical path of descent but does not reach its final position in the scrotum, it is referred to as a truly undescended testis.

Patients usually present in early childhood with an absence of one or both testes from the scrotum and an underdeveloped, flat scrotum is a common clinical finding. The testicle itself may be small and accompanied by a patent processus vaginalis, presenting as a congenital hernia. Occasionally, patients can present as adults with infertility and are found to have undescended testicles.

The line of testicular descent crosses the external inguinal ring and neck of the scrotum, where 80% of undescended testes are typically found and can be palpable on examination. Presence in either of these areas is an indication for orchidopexy, whereby the testis is fixed in the scrotum between the dartos muscle and skin, by the age of 18 months, to prevent testicular damage. After age 2 years, the testis can become damaged and incapable of spermatogenesis. Impalpable testes can be investigated using ultrasound scanning, CT and laparoscopy to determine whether a testicle is present or absent and also determine its exact location. See also the answer to Question 83.

Testicular pain (1)

85 A Testicular torsion

The tunica vaginalis normally covers the anterior and lateral testis and part of the epididymis, thereby fixing it in the scrotum and preventing twist. Normal variations in the extent that the tunica vaginalis covers the body of the testis means that the testicle is liable to twist on its attachment. Testicular torsion is most common in males aged 10–25 years. It is a surgical emergency, preceded by a trivial exertion or trauma, presenting initially as poorly localized pain in the abdomen and loin (the testicle is supplied by the T10 dermatomal level). Severe testicular pain and tenderness follows, usually affecting a single testicle. The pain can be accompanied by severe nausea and vomiting. On examination, the testicle can be hot, swollen, extremely tender to touch and is classically high riding with a horizontal lie. Symptoms progress rapidly over hours and, as the twisting of the testis within the tunica vaginalis compromises the testicular blood supply, leave only a short window in which the testicle is salvageable. A scrotal exploration should be performed as soon as possible in suspected cases of torsion with derotation of the testis and three point fixation of both the affected and unaffected testicle within the scrotum.

Torted hydatid of Morgagni (also known as torsion of the testicular appendage) is the commonest lesion presenting in a similar manner to testicular torsion (however, it does not result in compromise of the testicular blood supply). The appendix testis (or hydatid of Morgagni) is a vestigial remnant of the Müllerian duct, present on the upper pole of the testis in 90% of men and attached to the tunica vaginalis. The testicular appendage can become torted, causing acute one-sided testicular pain and requiring surgical excision to achieve relief. A third of patients present with a palpable 'blue dot' discoloration on the scrotum, which is diagnostic of the condition.

Epididymo-orchitis is an inflammation of the testis and epididymis secondary to infection, e.g. mumps in the young and bacterial infections such as *Escherichia coli*, *Chlamydia* and gonorrhoea in adults and the elderly. Patients can present with acute onset testicular pain, fever, malaise, urethral discharge and symptoms of UTI. The testis itself can be tender, red and warm to touch. The epididymis will be swollen and is palpable separate to the testis. Treatment is supportive with bed rest, antibiotic cover, and analgesia. Pain can also be relieved by elevation of the testis, which is not possible in cases of torsion.

An epididymal cyst is a fluid-filled swelling arising from the collecting tubules of the epididymis. Patients tend to be middle-aged and present with a normally painless swelling (although occasionally painful in younger adults) in the scrotum that has grown larger over many years. The cyst occurs supero-posteriorly to the testis and can be palpated separately, while the spermatic cord can be felt superior to the swelling. The cyst may be loculated and fluctuant to palpation and is irreducible. The presentation of inguinal hernia is discussed elsewhere in this section.

Scrotal swellings (4)

86 C   β-human chorionic gonadotrophin, placental alkaline phosphatase, lactate dehydrogenase

Testicular tumours are broadly divided into seminomas (carcinoma of the seminiferous tubules accounting for 42% of testicular tumours) and non-seminomatous germ cell tumours (these account for 58% of testicular tumours), of which teratomas are the most common. Teratomas present in patients aged 15–35 and can be solid or cystic, arising from primitive totipotent cells. AFP, β-hCG and LDH are elevated in 70% of patients affected by this cancer. Seminomas tend to affect an older population, in the age range of 20–40. They arise from germinal cells in the testes and are usually solid and slow growing. These tumours are associated with an elevation primarily of placental alkaline phosphatase but approximately 15% of patients will have a raised β-hCG level.

Testicular tumours occur more commonly in individuals with undescended testicles, infertile parents and in the presence of a contralateral testicular malignancy. Patients typically present with a painless testicular mass that is irregular, firm, fixed and does not ransilluminate. These tumours are staged according to the Royal Marsden Classification:

- Stage 1 – Tumour confined to testis
- Stage 2 – Abdominal nodal spread
- Stage 3 – Nodal disease outside the abdomen
- Stage 4 – Extralymphatic spread

Five-year survival for metastatic disease is 75% and 45% for seminomas and teratomas, respectively. CA125 is associated with ovarian carcinomas and upper gastrointestinal carcinomas. CA19–9 is most commonly elevated in cases of pancreatic carcinoma. Carcinoembryonic antigen (CEA) is raised primarily in individuals with colorectal carcinoma and also those with gastric, pancreatic, lung and breast carcinoma.

Testicular pain (2)

87 D   Varicocele

A varicocele is a bunch of dilated and tortuous veins of the pampini-form plexus (the venous supply of the testis). These are akin to varicose veins of the spermatic cord. They are more common on the left hemi-scrotum, resulting in a vague, dragging sensation and dull ache in the scrotum/groin. Varicoceles may be primary or secondary to a left-sided renal tumour (testicular artery branches off the left renal artery). The patient with suspected varicocele must be examined standing up as the veins empty on lying flat. The veins are often visible and palpable and classically have the feel of a 'bag of worms'. Varicoceles are managed either conservatively with a scrotal support, via embolization of the testicular vein under radiological guidance (the preferred method) or surgically by clipping the testicular vein.

A haematocele is a collection of blood in the tunica vaginalis, with bleeding usually secondary to trauma or underlying malignant disease. In the acute phase, patients will present with a large scrotal sac and a firm, painless swelling which the examiner can reach above (as a hydrocele). The testis will not be felt separately. When the blood clots, a small, hard mass is formed that can be mistaken for a malignant mass. Patients with a testicular tumour typically present with a painless tes-ticular mass that is irregular, firm, fixed and does not transilluminate. For discussion of epididymal cysts and epididymo-orchitis, see the answer to Question 85.

Breast lumps

88 B   Fibroadenoma

Fibroadenoma is a benign breast neoplasm primarily affecting young women aged 15–35. It results from a dominant fibromatous element in breast tissue with a cut surface revealing lobules of whorled, white fibrous tissue that bulge out of their capsule. Two histological vari-ants are documented: pericanalicular in which fibrous tissue dominates and intracanalicular where glandular tissue is more prominent. The two types are clinically indistinguishable. Presentation is as a painless, slow-growing and well-defined lump of rubbery consistency. The lumps can be hypermobile and are also known as 'breast mice'. Reassurance is usually sufficient as most lesions regress spontaneously. However, lesions >4 cm in size or occurring in older women should be excised to exclude malignancy.

Phylloides (Brodie's) tumour is a variant of fibroadenoma found in older women. These slow-growing tumours can grow extremely large but remain as a smooth swelling. They are usually excised to exclude malignancy and for cosmesis. They can also result in skin necrosis in advanced cases. Breast cysts are fluid-filled cavities in the breast without a demonstrable endothelial lining or capsule. Their presentation is similar to that of fibroadenoma, but they occur more commonly in women in their forties to early fifties as a result of a changing hormonal environment in preparation of the menopause. Women may present with a history of a sudden large swelling that may or may not be associated with pain and tenderness. Solitary cysts are smooth, spherical and of a variable consistency from soft/cystic to hard. Large cysts can be visible through the skin. An immediate aspiration of a cyst will reveal a yellow to dark green coloured fluid, which will confirm the clinical diagnosis and relieve patient symptoms.

Fibroadenosis is a condition that occurs as part of the normal spectrum of breast changes associated with the menstrual cycle. It occurs in young women, usually between the ages of 15–35 years, and is associated with lumpiness, especially in the upper outer quadrant of the breast, with or without cyclical pain. Physical examination can reveal single or multiple tender lumps. Investigation is with triple assessment: clinical examination, fine needle aspiration cytology and mammography (or ultrasound scan if the patient is younger than 35 years). If the assessment is normal, the patient can be reassured as to the benign nature of the condition. Medical treatment may include anti-inflammatory agents, contraceptive pill and evening primrose oil.

Mammary duct ectasia is dilatation of the mammary ducts, which become filled with macrophages and chronic inflammatory debris. Patients can present with lumpiness in the breast and chronic inflammation, which results in nipple retraction and an eventual slit-like appearance of the nipple that can be confused with DCIS (ductal carcinoma *in situ*). Acute inflammation can cause abscess formation which discharges at the areolar margin and eventually forms a sinus, acting as a focus for further inflammatory attacks.

Treatment of breast lumps

89 A   Prescribe an antibacterial agent, e.g. flucloxacillin
Lactational breast abscess formation is most commonly the result of infection with *Staphylococcus aureus* (a cluster forming Gram-positive organism) during breastfeeding. The organism can enter the breast through a cracked nipple, resulting in increasingly severe pain, malaise, fever and lost sleep. Examination will reveal a tender, warm, red segment and occasionally a cracked nipple. Fluctuation occurs only when the abscess is advanced and can cause skin necrosis.

The case described is that of acute mastitis, which is initially treated with anti-staphylococcal antibiotics such as flucloxacillin. Breastfeeding does not need to be stopped unless there is obvious damage to the nipple, in which case the mother would be advised to express milk from healthy segments on the opposite breast. Continuing pain and loss of sleep, despite treatment with antibiotics, would be an indication of abscess formation that can be aspirated using a wide-bore needle under local anaesthesia. Skin changes such as thinning and areas of necrosis requires drainage of the abscess under general anaesthesia with loculi broken down to prevent recurrence.

Investigation of breast lumps

90 C Physical examination, fine needle aspiration cytology, core biopsy and mammography
Triple assessment is the mainstay of investigation of breast lumps. It comprises the following:

- Physical examination
- Imaging – Ultrasound (women below 35) or mammography (women over 35)
- Pathology – Fine needle aspiration cytology and/or core biopsy

This patient is over the age of 35 and therefore physical examination followed by mammography and fine needle aspiration and core biopsy would have been conducted as part of the triple assessment. Ultrasonography is preferred as an investigation tool in women younger than 35 years as the breast tissue is usually too dense for small lesions to be seen on mammography. In addition, ultrasound is useful for evaluating palpable lumps.

Ureteric constrictions

91 D As the ureter passes anteriorly to the psoas muscle
During the course of the ureters from the kidneys to the urinary bladder, there are four main sites at which the ureters constrict or are narrowed. Physiologically, this usually does not pose a problem but renal calculi (>4 mm in size) can become lodged at these constrictions causing pain, hydronephrosis and subsequent acute kidney injury on the affected side.

The four main sites where the ureters are constricted are (1) the pelvic-ureteric junction, (2) as the ureter crosses the pelvic brim, (3) as the gonadal artery crosses the ureter and (4) as the ureter enters the bladder obliquely at the vesiculo-ureteric junction.

There is no constriction of the ureters as they pass anterior to the psoas muscle and therefore Answer D is the correct option here.

Complications of mechanical ventilation

92 A   Increased cardiac output

The complications of ventilation include parenchymal lung damage, hospital acquired (nosocomial) pneumonia, volutrauma (damage to the lungs caused by overdistention secondary to high mechanical tidal volumes) and barotrauma (physical damage to the lung/mediastinal tissues caused by differences in pressure during ventilation, which can cause pneumothorax, pneumomediastinum, pneumopericardium, surgical emphysema and acute lung injury).

Positive alveolar pressure caused by mechanical ventilation increases lung volume and intrathoracic pressure which causes compression of the heart by the inflated lungs. Venous return is reduced due to increased intramural pressure of the heart cavity. This ultimately decreases cardiac output and hence Answer A is the correct option here.

Subclavian vein cannulation

93 C   Thoracic aorta

The thoracic aorta is usually not at risk of damage during subclavian vein cannulation due to the fact that it is positioned within the posterior aspect of the mediastinum. However, the subclavian artery, apex of the lung, phrenic nerve and thoracic duct (on the left side) lie in close proximity, or on route, to the subclavian vein and hence are at higher risk of damage during subclavian vein cannulation.

Central venous pressure monitoring

94 E   Right atrium

Central venous pressure is the pressure, measured in either mmHg or cmH_2O, in the right atrium. It is also referred to as right atrial filling pressure. The normal value of CVP ranges from 0 to 10 mmHg or 0 to 8 cmH_2O. It is worthwhile noting that the absolute value of CVP is not as helpful as measuring the change in CVP in response to a fluid challenge. It is also worth noting that CVP is not accurate in critically ill patients, especially those who suffer from cardiac and pulmonary diseases, and in these patients readings must be interpreted cautiously.

Posterior approach to the hip joint

95 A   Skin, subcutaneous fat, gluteal fascia, gluteus maximus, short external rotator muscles and the hip joint capsule

Systemic effects of epidural analgesia

96 C Hypotension

Epidural analgesia carries many systemic effects of which the main ones include decreased surgical stress response, reduced cardiac output, hypotension and reduction in functional residual capacity. Reduction in postoperative deep venous thrombosis rates also occurs, mainly owing to the use of intravenous fluids to maintain arterial pressure.

Complications of axillary lymph node surgery

97 A The left long thoracic nerve

The long thoracic nerve (of Bell) supplies the serratus anterior muscle which is responsible for pulling the scapula anteriorly to the posterior upper chest wall. Injury to this nerve leads to posterior protrusion of the scapula and deformity of the upper extremity. Damage to this nerve causes ipsilateral deformity of the shoulder. The intercostal brachial nerves may be sacrificed/injured during axillary lymph node clearance and this leads to ipsilateral numbness to the medial aspect of the arm. The thoracodorsal nerve innervates the latissimus dorsi muscle.

Acid–base disorders

98 A Acute renal failure

From the patient's clinical history and initial assessment, a pulmonary problem is least likely of all the possible answers. Furthermore, pulmonary oedema will tend to cause a respiratory alkalosis whereas pneumonia will lead to a respiratory acidosis. Vomiting and hyperldosteronism lead to loss of hydrogen ions and hence result in a metabolic alkalosis. Therefore, the most likely option is Answer A. This is very likely due to hypovolaemia and this patient requires fluid balance assessment. Please refer to Chapter 1 for more information on fluid balance management.

Branches of the external carotid artery

99 E Superior thyroid artery

The external carotid artery has seven main arterial branches. From first to last branch these are

- Superior thyroid artery
- Ascending pharyngeal artery
- Lingual artery
- Facial artery
- Occipital artery
- Posterior auricular artery
- Maxillary artery

- Superficial temporal artery.

The mnemonic 'Some Anatomists Like Freaking Out Poor Medical Students', among others, is useful in helping to remember the divisions of the external carotid artery.

Cardiogenic shock

100 C Right atrial enlargement

On a postero-anterior chest radiograph the following changes can be seen in patients with cardiogenic shock: (1) an increase in cardiothoracic ratio (this is due to a dilated left ventricle secondary to volume overload); (2) 'Kerly B' lines which are small line shadows seen above the costophrenic angle representing interstitial oedema; (3) interstitial shadowing of the lung fields secondary to pulmonary oedema; (4) hilar 'bat's wing' shadowing which is further evidence of oedema; and (5) prominent upper lobe pulmonary vasculature indicating venous congestion and left atrial enlargement owing to enlargement of the left atrial appendage.

Index

Abdomen, organs of, 4, 12
Abdominal aortic aneurysm (AAA), 207
  management of, 161–162, 171–172
  repair, 57, 65–66, 207–208, 218–219
  ultrasound scanning, 218
Abdominal CT scan, postoperative pyrexia,
  27, 36–37
Abdominal distension, 21, 31, 362, 397
Abdominal emergency, perforated duodenal
  ulcer, 106, 118
Abdominal exercise, gastro-oesophageal reflux
  disease, 108, 121
Abdominal pain
  computed tomography scan, 166, 179
  constipation and, 163, 174
  diagnosis of, 178–179
  diarrhoea and, 164, 175
  explorative laparotomy, 165–166, 177
  management of, 159, 168
  mesenteric atherosclerosis, 135–136,
    145–146
  and vomiting, 160, 169–170
Abdominal surgery, vitamin B_1 deficiency,
  105, 116–117
Abdominal wall anatomy, 338, 346–347
  falciform ligament, 106, 119
  rectus abdominis, 138, 150
ABPI, see Ankle-brachial pressure index
Absence seizures, 296
Achalasia, dysphagia, 104, 114
Acid-base balance, 23, 32
Acid-base disorders, 382–383, 428
Acute cholecystitis, Murphy's sign, 161, 171
Acute closed angle glaucoma, 319, 326
Acute hypocalcaemia, cardiac monitoring,
  61, 70
Acute limb ischaemia, 206, 214, 215, 217
Acute limb pain, 264, 277
Acute lower limb pain
  diagnosis of, 215–216
  management of, 206, 216–217
Acutely hot joint, 265, 278–279
Acute mesenteric ischaemia, 210–211, 225
  rectal bleeding, 161, 170–171
Acute otitis externa, 304, 311
Acute otitis media, 311–312
Acute pancreatitis, 163, 174
  complications of, 111, 128–129
  epigastric pain, 160–161, 170
  gallstones, 166–167, 179
  serum amylase, 104, 114

Acute renal failure, 383, 428
Acute respiratory distress syndrome,
  60–61, 70
  pancreatitis, 111, 128
Acute upper limb pain, 206–207
Acute urinary retention
  bladder outflow obstruction, 164–165, 176
  urinary catheterisation, 165, 176–177
Acute visual disturbance, 321–322, 329
Addison transpyloric plane, 5, 13
Adductor pollicis, 261, 271
Adenohypophysis, hormones
  released by, 298
Adenolymphoma, 345
Adhesions, 362, 396
Adhesive capsulitis, 273
β_2-Adrenergic receptor, 410
Adult polycystic kidney disease, 246
Age-related macular degeneration, 322, 329
Airway adjunct selection, 78, 88
Airway compromise, 77–78, 87
Airway protection, 78, 88
Alcohol, 358, 390–391
Alcoholic cirrhosis, 393
Alcoholism, 261, 271
Alkaline chemicals, 321, 328
Alkalinization process, 242
Amaurosis fugax, 209
  causes of, 222
  investigation of, 222–223
American Society of Anaesthesiologists (ASA)
  grading, 58, 67
γ-Amino butyric acid (GABA), 410
Amoxicillin, 359, 392–393
Amputation, 206
  indications for, 216
  types of, 216–217
Anaesthesia, 338, 346
  stages of, 56, 64
Anal fissure, propranolol, 138, 149
Analgesia, 360
Anal squamous carcinoma, 136–137, 147
Anaplastic carcinoma of thyroid, 336,
  342–343
Anaplastic thyroid carcinoma, 342
Anastomotic leakage, postoperative pyrexia,
  22–23, 32
ANCA, see Antineutrophil cytoplasmic
  antibody
Aneurysm, 218
Angiography, 213

Ankle-brachial pressure index (ABPI), 214
    measuring, 204, 205, 212
Anterior cruciate ligament injury, 259, 268
Anterior uveitis, 373, 414
Antibacterial agent, 380
Antibiotic ear drops, 304, 311
Antibiotic prophylaxis, 162, 172
Anticoagulant effects of aspirin, 217
Anticoagulation in surgical patients, 354, 384
Antineutrophil cytoplasmic antibody (ANCA),
    341
Anti-thyroglobulin antibody, 341
Anti-thyroid-stimulating hormone receptor
    antibody, 334, 340–341
Aortic aneurysm, 207, 218
Aortic dissection, 63, 73
    investigation of, 210
Aortic rupture, chest trauma, 80, 91
Apical lung tumour, 319, 327
Appendicectomy, surgical anatomy of,
    361, 396
Appendicitis, Murphy's sign, 138, 150–151
Appendix mass, percutaneous drainage, 136,
    146–147
Arterial ulcers, 215
Arthritis
    and hand, 261, 272
    septic, 265
Aspirin, anticoagulant effects of, 217
Astrocytoma, 301
Asymptomatic varicose veins, 219
Atelectasis, splenectomy, 126
Atherosclerosis, 212
    mesenteric, 135–136, 145–146
Atrophic kidney, 232, 244
Atrophic non-union complication, 369, 409
Autoimmune neurological disease, 369,
    409–410
Autosomal dominant gene chromosome 16,
    233, 246–247
Avascular necrosis, 409
Axillary lymph node
    clearance, 3–4, 11
    surgery, complications of, 382, 428

Basal cell carcinoma, 377, 418–419
Basal skull fracture, 285, 295–296
Benign paroxysmal positional vertigo (BPPV),
    314
Benign prostatic hypertrophy, 255
Biliary cirrhosis, cholangiocarcinoma, 109,
    124–125
Birefringent crystals, 243
Bladder cancer, TNM classification of, 251
Bladder carcinoma, treatment of, 251–252
Bladder malignancy, 235, 250–252
Bladder outflow obstruction, acute urinary
    retention, 164–165, 176
Bleeding
    per-rectal, 133, 141

upper gastrointestinal bleeding, 119
    variceal, 106, 117–118
β-Blockers, 210, 224–225
Blood loss, estimation of, 79, 89
Blood pressure, 358, 385, 389
Blood supply to rectum, 8, 17
Blood transfusion, 21, 30
    complications of, 42, 49–50
    preoperative, 24, 34
Bohr effect, 69
Bone
    disorders of, 263, 275
    Paget's disease of, 275–276
Bone disease, 264, 276
Bone pathology, 263, 274–275
Bony infarct, 264, 277
Bowel habit, change in, 134, 142–143
Bowel obstruction
    constipation and abdominal pain, 163, 174
    hernia, 139–140, 153
    paralytic ileus, 164, 175–176
    sigmoid volvulus, 167, 180
Brain injury, extradural haematoma, 82, 95–96
Branchial cyst, 375, 416
Breast abscess, 184, 192
Breast cancer, management of, 189, 198
Breast carcinoma
    breast lumps, 185, 193
    hormone therapy for, 363, 398
    invasive, 187, 195–196
Breast cysts
    breast pain, 185, 193
    management of, 187, 196
Breast enlargement, phyllodes tumour, 186, 194
Breast infection
    breast abscess, 184, 192
    flucloxacillin, 187–188, 196–197
Breast lumps, 379–380, 424–425
    assessment, 187, 195–196
    breast carcinoma, 185, 193
    fibroadenoma, 184, 192
    investigation of, 425–426
    treatment of, 380
Breast pain
    breast cyst, 185, 193
    cyclical mastalgia, 186, 195
    fat necrosis, 184, 192
Breast pathology
    core biopsy, 191, 201
    mammography, 188–189, 197
    ultrasound, 185–186, 194, 199
Breast surgery, complications of, 190, 200
Breathing
    difficulty in, 56, 64–65
    shortness of, 57–58, 66
Breathlessness
    management of, 45, 53
    postoperative, 21, 30
Brodie's tumour, *see* Phyllodes tumour
Brown-Séquard syndrome, 412

Burn injury, management of, 84–85, 100
Burns management, 84, 98
    intubation, 84, 98–99
Burn victim, management of, 84, 99
Bypass grafting, 12–13

Calcium, 335
Calcium oxalate, 230, 241
Campylobacter-like organisms (CLO) test, 359
Cannulated screw fixation, 368, 407
Carcinoembryonic antigen (CEA), 423
Carcinoid syndrome, 399
Carcinoid tumours, 140, 155
Carcinoma
    of bladder, 250
    of parotid gland, 345
    of penis, 236, 253–254
Cardiac monitoring, acute hypocalcaemia, 61, 70
Cardiac output, 381
Cardiac tamponade, muffled heart sounds,
        60, 69–70
Cardiogenic shock, 383, 429
Cardiomyopathy, inflammatory bowel disease,
        135, 145
Carotid artery disease, 222
Carotid artery territory, 209, 222
Carotid bruit, 322, 329–330
Carotid duplex, 322, 329
Carotid endarterectomy, 209, 223
    postoperative complications of, 210, 223
Carpal tunnel, 261, 271
    decompression, 8, 16
    syndrome, 262, 271–273
Catheter occlusion, 357
CA19-9, tumour markers, 359, 391–392
Cauda equina syndrome, 266, 279–280
Cavernous sinus thrombosis, 305, 312
Cellulitis, 401
Central line sepsis, 44–45, 53
Central venous cannula, uses of, 56, 64
Central venous catheters, 385
Central venous pressure monitoring, 381, 427
Cerebral blood supply, 282, 290–291
Cerebrospinal fluid, 283, 291
Cervical spine trauma, 83–84, 98
Chemodectoma, 374, 415
Chest drain insertion, 5, 11
    complications of, 80, 91–92
Chest trauma
    aortic rupture, 80, 91
    pericardiocentesis, 79–80, 90
Chlamydia, 323, 330–331
Chloramphenicol, 320, 327–328
Cholangiocarcinoma, primary biliary cirrhosis,
        109, 124–125
Cholangitis, right upper quadrant pain,
        162–163, 173
Cholelithiasis, 108
    complications of, 122–123
    smoking, 122

Cholesterol crystals, 375, 416
Cholestyramine, 361, 395–396
Chordee, 247
Chronic granulomatous inflammation, 222
Chronic otitis externa, 311
Chronic pancreatitis, 358, 390–391
Chronic pyelonephritis, 244
Clarithromycin, 359, 392–393
Clavicle, 336, 343
Cloquet's node, 343, 375, 416
Coeliac trunk, 6, 14–15
Colles' fracture, 368, 406–407
Colonic carcinoma
    gadolinium-enhanced liver magnetic
        resonance imaging, 133, 141–142
    management of, 139, 152
Colonic resections, extended right
        hemicolectomy, 134, 142
Colorectal carcinoma, 362, 397
Colorectal surgical resections, 362, 397
Computed tomography (CT) scan, 210, 224
    abdominal pain, 166, 179
    diverticular abscess, 167, 181
    head injury, 58–59, 67
Conductive deafness, right-sided, 306, 313
Confusion, 28, 38
    postoperative, 24, 34
    postoperative acute, 57, 65
Conjunctivitis, 318, 325
Conn's syndrome, 363, 398–399
Consent, patient, 355, 385
Constipation
    and abdominal pain, 163, 174
    neoplasia, 134–135, 143–144
Contralateral loss of proprioception, 371,
        412–413
Conus syndrome, 280
Core biopsy, 237
    breast pathology, 191, 201
Coronary heart disease, 205
Corticosteroids, severe head injury, 83, 96–97
Cranial anatomy, 282, 289
Craniopharyngioma, 301
Cremaster muscle, 347
CREST syndrome, erythematous malar rash,
        104–105, 115
Critical limb ischaemia, 205, 214
Crystalline arthropathy, 265, 278
Cyclical mastalgia, breast pain, 186, 195
Cysteine stones, 241
Cystic artery, 362, 396–397

Dacron artificial graft, 219
D-dimers, 221
Deep vein thrombosis, 208, 220–221
Denys-Drash syndrome, 248
Desmopressin, endocrine disease,
        190, 200
Dextrose/saline, fluid therapy, 47
Diabetes, 262, 273

Diabetic eye, 373, 415
Diabetic foot ulceration, 204, 212
Diaphragm, 3, 10
    left crus of, 105, 115
Diarrhoea, 52
    and abdominal pain, 164, 175
    management of, 361, 395–396
Diethylene triamine pentaacetic acid (DTPA)
    scan, 242
Dimercaptosuccinic acid (DMSA) scan, 242
Disc prolapse, 284, 293–294
Discrimination, 262, 273
Disseminated intravascular coagulation, 60,
    68–69
Diverticular abscess, computed tomography
    scan, 167, 181
Diverticular disease, 135, 145
Diverticulitis, left iliac fossa pain,
    162, 172
Dizziness, 307, 314
Doppler ultrasound, 214
Double-stranded DNA virus, 370, 412
Dry eye, 374
Ductal carcinoma, 199
    in situ, 189, 198
Dukes' stage A, 139, 152
Duodenal ulcers, Zollinger-Ellison
    syndrome, 107, 120
Duodenum, 6, 15
Duplex ultrasound scanning, 209, 213
    amaurosis fugax, 222–223
Dupuytren's contracture, 260, 270
DVT, risk factors for, 221
Dynamic hip screw, 368, 407–408
Dysphagia, 104
    achalasia, 114
    upper gastrointestinal endoscopy, 113

Ear disease
    diagnosis of, 306, 307, 313
    management of, 305, 311–312
    pathogens involved in, 304, 311
Ear infections, causative pathogens in,
    306, 312–313
Ear pain, 305, 312
    management of, 304, 311
Ecchondromas, 274
Ehlers-Danlos syndrome, 224
Elective abdominal aortic aneurysm repair,
    207–208, 218–219
Electrolyte imbalance in special circumstances,
    356, 387
Electrolyte replacement strategies, 355,
    356, 386
Emboli, 217
Emergency department, 355, 386
Emergency preoperative management,
    25–26, 35
Emphysema, 260, 269
Enchondroma, 274, 275

Endocrine disease
    desmopressin, 190, 200
    investigation of, 363–364, 399
    management of, 190–191
Endocrine disorders, 363, 398–399
Endometrium, 287, 300
Endoscopic retrograde
    cholangiopancreatography, 20–21, 30
    complicated gallstones, 109, 123–124
Endoscopy, oesophageal cancer, 103, 112
Endotracheal tube insertion, 80, 90–91
Endovascular aneurysm repair (EVAR), 219
Enteral feeding, complications of, 46, 54
Enteral nutrition, complications of, 43–44, 52
Epidural analgesia, systemic effects of, 382,
    428
Epigastric pain, diagnosis of, 160–161, 170
Epilepsy, 285–286, 296–297
Epileptics, 297
Epispadias, 247
Epistaxis, 308–309, 314, 315
Erythema nodosum, 260, 269–270
Erythematous malar rash, 104–105, 115
Erythrocyte sedimentation rate (ESR),
    287, 300
Escharotomy, 84–85, 100
Escherichia coli, urological infection, 232,
    243–244
ESR, *see* Erythrocyte sedimentation rate
EVAR, *see* Endovascular aneurysm repair
Ewing's sarcoma, 275
Exercise programmes, 213
Exostosis, 263, 275
Explorative laparotomy, 81, 92–93, 358, 390
    abdominal pain, 165–166, 177
    splenic trauma, 93–94
Extended right hemicolectomy, colonic
    resections, 134, 142
External carotid artery, 383, 428–429
External laryngeal nerve, 3, 11
External oblique muscle, 8, 17
Extradural haematoma, brain injury, 82,
    95–96
Eye
    infection, 323, 330–331
    nerve palsy and, 319, 327
    pain, diagnosis of, 318, 325
    systemic disease and, 373

Facial swelling, 337, 344–345
Facial trauma, 308, 314
Falciform ligament, abdominal wall anatomy,
    106, 119
Falls mechanism, trauma, 358, 389
FAST, *see* Focused assessment with
    sonography for trauma scan
Fat emboli, 368, 408
Fat necrosis of breast, 184, 187,
    192, 196
Femoral canal, 348

Femur fracture, neck of, 368
α-Fetoprotein, 393
Fibrinolysis, 221
Fibroadenoma, 379, 424–425
    breast lumps, 184, 192
    management of, 188, 197
Fibroadenosis, 425
Fibromatoses, 270
Fibrotic stricture, gastric outflow obstruction,
    107–108, 120–121
Fistula *in ano,* 360, 394–395
    treatment of, 137–138, 149
Flail chest, 80, 90–91
Flexible cystoscopy, 242
Flexible sigmoidoscopy, per-rectal bleeding,
    133, 141
Flucloxacillin, 380
    breast infection, 187–188, 196–197
Fluid management
    balance, 41, 48–49
    and nutrition management, 40–41, 48
    in trauma patient, 40, 47
Fluid replacement, 356, 387
Fluid resuscitation, in critically ill,
    41–42, 49
Fluid therapy, 40
    cross-matched blood, 47
    postoperative, 41, 47–48
Focused assessment with sonography for
    trauma (FAST) scan, 81–82, 94
Follicular carcinoma, 342
Fontaine's classification, 364, 400
Foramen ovale, 282, 290
Foramen spinosum, 7, 15
Foramina of skull base, 282, 290
Foreign bodies, 320, 327–328
Fournier's gangrene, 233, 245
Fractures
    complications, 369, 409
    of head of radius, 267
    lower limb, 7–8, 16
    patterns, 260, 270
    of proximal femur, 368
    remove cast, 408
Friedrich's ataxia, 410
Furosemide, 339, 347–348

Gadolinium-enhanced liver magnetic
    resonance imaging, 133, 141–142
Gallbladder, 103, 112
    vascular anatomy of, 362
Gallstones
    acute pancreatitis, 166–167, 179
    complication of, 109, 123–124
    disease, 108, 121–122
Ganglion, 262, 272, 338, 346
Gastric cancer, 103, 112
Gastric outflow obstruction, fibrotic stricture,
    107–108, 120–121
Gastrin pancreas, 110–111, 127

Gastroduodenal artery, upper gastrointestinal
    bleeding, 119
Gastrointestinal haemorrhage, 105–106, 117
    lower, 139, 152–153
Gastro-oesophageal obstruction, vomiting and
    left upper quadrant pain, 165, 177
Gastro-oesophageal reflux disease, abdominal
    exercise, 108, 121
Gastro-oesophageal sphincter, left crus of
    diaphragm, 105, 115
Gene mutation, 236, 254
General surgical patients, management of,
    355, 386
Genitofemoral nerve, genital branch of, 2, 9
Germ cell tumours, 252
Giant cell, 300
Giant cell arteritis, 222
Giant cell tumours, 275
Gigantism, 298
Glandular fever, 340
Glasgow Coma Scale, 283, 284
    score, evaluation of, 82, 94–95
Glaucoma, 324, 331
Glucose-fermenting Gram-negative coccus,
    232, 244–245
Glucose tolerance test, 287, 298–300
Glycaemic control
    optimisation of, 212
    perioperative, 26, 36
Gold standard test, 300
Gout, 243, 276
Grafting, bypass, 12–13
Gram negative bacteria, 61, 71
Grand mal seizures, 296
Graves' disease, 340, 341, 374, 415, 416
Groin swelling, 339, 349, 375
Growth hormone, 298–299
Gynaecomastia, 338, 347–348

Haematemesis, 159, 168
Haematocele, 424
Haematuria, 235, 250, 367, 404–405
Haemochromatosis, 393
Haemolytic transfusion reaction, 24, 34
Haemophilus influenzae, 304, 311
Haemorrhage, 355, 385
Hartmann's procedure, 362, 397
Hartmann's solution, 42–43, 50–51
Headache, 323, 330
Head injury, 284–285, 294–295
    CT scan, 58–59, 67
    uncal herniation, 83, 97
Hearing
    decline in, 306, 313
    difficulty, 307, 313
Helicobacter pylori, 359, 392
Heparin infusion, 207, 217, 354, 384
Hepatic duct, upper gastrointestinal surgery,
    110, 125
Hepatocellular carcinoma, 359, 393

Hepatomegaly, 359, 393
Hereditary colon carcinoma, 139, 151–152
Hernia
  anatomy of, 338, 346–347
  bowel obstruction, 139–140, 153
  inguinal, 339, 348
Hip joint, posterior approach to, 381, 427
Hoarse voice, 372, 414
Horner's syndrome, 319, 327
Hospital-acquired infection, 133, 141
β-Human chorionic gonadotrophin, 379, 423
Human papilloma virus, 236, 253
Hunter's canal, 364, 400
Hutchinson's sign/rule, 325
Hydrocele, 365, 402–403
5-Hydroxyindole acetic acid, 364, 399
Hypercalcaemia, 356, 386
Hyperlipidaemia, 205
Hypernatraemia, 233, 245–246
Hypertension, 210, 223
Hyperuricaemia, 243
Hypervolaemia, postoperative acute
  confusion, 57, 65
Hypocalcaemia, 42, 49–50
Hypokalaemia, 248–249, 398
  small P-waves, 59, 68
Hyponatraemia, 43, 51
Hypophosphataemia, 386
Hypospadias, 234, 247
Hyposplenism bite cells, 110, 125
Hypotension, 382, 428
Hypothermia
  thyroid storm, 59, 68
  warmed peritoneal lavage, 84–85, 100

Ilioinguinal nerve, 376, 418
  right, 375
Infection stones, 242
Infectious mononucleosis, 334, 340
Inferior mesenteric artery, 5, 13–14
Inferior oblique muscle, 321, 328–329
Inflammatory bowel disease
  cardiomyopathy, 135, 145
  change in bowel habit, 134, 142–143
  lead piping, 140, 156
  6-mercaptopurine, 136, 146
Informed surgical consent, 23–24, 33
Inguinal canal, 2, 9, 349
Inguinal hernia, 339, 348
  management of, 163, 173
  repair, complications of, 375, 416–417
  surgical anatomy, 376
Inguinal ligament, 339, 348–349
Inguino-scrotal hernia, 402
Inherited neurological disease, 370, 410–411
Inherited urological disease, 233
Initial assessment, 77–78, 87
Injection sclerotherapy, 219
Intermittent claudication, 204–205, 213–214
Intermuscular lipomata, 274

Internal iliac artery, 236, 254
Internal pudendal artery, 8, 17
Intervertebral disc, 293
Intra-abdominal injury, diagnosis of,
  80–81, 92
Intracranial haemorrhage, pregnancy, 83, 96
Intracranial tumour, 287–288, 300–302
Intramural urethra, 240
Intramuscular haematoma, 274
Intra-ocular pressure (IOP), 326
Intraoperative complication, 63, 73
Intraosseous infusion, 357, 388–389
Intravenous access, in trauma patient, 40, 47
Intravenous antibiotics, 305
  high-dose, 319, 326–327
Intravenous urography (IVU), 242
Intubation, burns management, 84, 98–99
Intussusception, management of, 166, 178
Iritis, 318, 325
Ischaemia, 213
Ischaemic rest pain, 364, 400
IVU, *see* Intravenous urography

Jacksonian seizure, 286, 296–297
Jaundice, obstructive, 109, 123
Juvenile nasal angiofibroma, 309, 315

Keratoacanthoma, 378, 419, 420
Kidney
  anatomy of, 238
  covering layers of, 229
  vascular supply of, 239–240
Kidney ureter bladder (KUB) radiograph,
  urinary calculi, 231, 241–242
Kiesselbach's plexus, 315
KUB radiograph, *see* Kidney ureter bladder
  radiograph

Lacerations to eyelids, 320, 327
Lactate dehydrogenase, 379, 423
Lactic acidosis, 62, 72
Lactose-fermenting gram-negative rods, 244
Laminar flow ventilation, 22, 31
Laparoscopic cholecystectomy, presurgical
  optimization for, 27–28, 37
Laparotomy
  explorative, 81, 92–94
  midline, 2, 9–10
Large bowel obstruction
  constipation and abdominal pain, 163, 174
  sigmoid volvulus, 167, 180
Laryngeal mask airway, 78, 88
Laser photocoagulation, 373, 415
Laser trabeculoplasty, 324, 331
Latissimus dorsi, 239
Lead piping, inflammatory bowel disease,
  140, 156
Left bundle branch block, 234, 248–249
Left crus of diaphragm, gastro-oesophageal
  sphincter, 105, 115

Left iliac fossa pain
  diagnosis of, 162, 172
  management of, 173
Left phrenic nerve, 3, 10
Left subclavian artery, proximal occlusion
  of, 365
Left upper limb, movement and sensation
  of, 217
Left upper quadrant pain, vomiting and,
  165, 177
Leg ulcers, 205–206, 214–215
Lesch-Nyhan syndrome, 278
Lipodermatosclerosis, 364, 400
Liver, 229, 238
  laceration, 5–6, 14
LMWH, *see* Low-molecular-weight heparin
LOAF muscles, 271
Local anaesthetic, 62–63, 72–73
Looser's zones, 276
Lower gastrointestinal haemorrhage,
  oesophagogastroduodenoscopy, 139,
  152–153
Lower gastrointestinal infection,
  pseudomembranous colitis, 167, 180
Lower limb
  fracture, 7–8, 16
  pain, 204, 212–213
  vascular anatomy of, 4–5, 12–13
Lower urinary tract symptoms (LUTS), 255
Low-molecular-weight heparin (LMWH), 208,
  220, 384
Lumbar disc herniation, 266, 280
Lumbar puncture, 283, 292, 370, 411–412
Lumps, 337–338, 346
LUTS, *see* Lower urinary tract symptoms
Lymphangitis, 402
Lymph nodes, 340
Lymphoedema, 210, 225

Magnetic resonance
  cholangiopancreatography, pancreatitis,
  111, 127–128
Male urethra, 230, 240–241
Malignant bladder cancers, 250
Malignant bone tumours, 275
Malignant melanoma, 377, 420
Malignant otitis externa, 306, 312
Malignant ulcers, 215
Mammary duct ectasia, 188
  nipple discharge, 185, 193
Mammography, breast pathology,
  188–189, 197
Mandibular nerve, 4, 11
Manubriosternal junction, 8, 17
Marfan's disease, 224
Marginal artery of Drummond, 5, 13–14
MCGN, *see* Minimal change glomerulonephritis
Mechanical bowel obstruction, 362, 396
Mechanical ventilation, complications of,
  381, 427

Meckel's diverticulum, pancreatitis, 140,
  154–155
Median nerve, 406
  neuropathy, 367, 405
Mediastinum, 6, 14
Medullary carcinoma, 342
Medulloblastoma, 302
Melanoma, 377, 419–420
Membranous urethra, 240–241
Meningeal artery, middle, 285, 289, 294
Meningioma, 288, 301
Meningitis, 286, 297–298
6-Mercaptopurine, inflammatory bowel
  disease, 136, 146
Mesenteric artery, superior and inferior, 5,
  13–14
Mesenteric atherosclerosis, abdominal pain,
  135–136, 145–146
Metabolic alkalosis, 357, 387
Metacarpal bone, 261, 270
Metastatic breast carcinoma, 363, 397–398
Midline laparotomy, 2, 9–10
Mikulicz's syndrome, 345
Minimal change glomerulonephritis
  (MCGN), 366
Molluscum sebaceum, *see* Keratoacanthoma
Muffled heart sounds, 60, 69–70
Multiple endocrine neoplasia syndrome II,
  139, 151–152
Murphy's sign
  acute cholecystitis, 161, 171
  appendicitis, 138, 150–151
Muscle hernia, 263, 274
Muscle lumps, 263, 274
Musculoskeletal pathology, 259, 260,
  268–269
Myasthenia gravis, 409
Mycobacteria, 231, 242–243
Mycobacterium tuberculosis, 286, 297–298
Myoglobin, 246
Myoglobinuria, 246
Myringotomy, 312

Nasal obstruction, 308, 314–315
Nasojejunal feeding, 43, 51–52
Neck
  anatomy, 336, 343
  of femur fracture, 368, 407
  lumps, 334, 335, 340–342, 371, 374–375,
  413, 415–416
  swellings, 336, 343
Necrotizing fasciitis, 216
Neisseria gonorrhoeae, 244
Neisseria meningitides, 61, 71
Neoplasia, constipation, 134–135, 143–144
Nephroblastoma, *see* Wilm's tumour
Nephrotic syndrome, 366–367, 404–405
Nerve conduction studies, 367, 405
Nerve palsy, 328
  and eye, 319, 327

Neurohypophysis, hormones released by, 298
Neurological infection, 370, 412
Neuropathic ulcers, 215
Neurovascular visual disturbance, 322,
    329–330
Nipple discharge, mammary duct ectasia,
    185, 193
Nutrition, 61, 71
Nutrition management
    commence total parenteral nutrition, 44, 52
    fluid and, 40–41, 48
    nasojejunal feeding, 43, 51–52
    percutaneous gastrostomy tube, 45, 54

Obstruction, 140, 154
Obstructive jaundice, 109, 123
Occlusive disease, 217
Ocular trauma, 320–321, 328–329
Oesophageal cancer, endoscopy, 103, 112
Oesophagitis, 109
    high dose PPI and repeat endoscopy, 124
    proton pump inhibitor, 105, 116
Oesophagogastroduodenoscopy, lower
    gastrointestinal haemorrhage, 139,
    152–153
Oesophagus, surgical anatomy of, 103,
    113
Oestrogen receptor, 363, 398
Oligodendrogliomas, 301
Omeprazole, 359, 392–393
Operative complications, 368, 408
Ophthalmic emergencies, 319, 326
Oral antibiotics, 305, 311–312
Oral aspirin, 322, 329
Orbital 'blow out' fracture, 321, 328
Oropharyngeal airway, 78, 88
Orthopaedic disease, 259, 267
Orthopaedic examination, 259
Osteoarthritis, 259, 268
Osteoclastoma, see Giant cell tumours
Osteomalacia, 264, 276
Osteomyelitis, 263, 274–276
Osteoporosis, 276
    management of, 264, 276–277
Osteosarcomas, 275
Otitis media, complications of, 305, 312
Oxygen dissociation curve, 60, 69
Oxytocin, 286, 298

Paediatric ophthalmology, 319, 326
Paediatric patients, vascular access in, **388**
Paediatric resuscitation, 357, 388–389
Paediatric trauma, 357, 388
Paediatric urology, 233, 234, **247–248**
Paget's disease
    of bone, 263, 275–276
    rash, 186, 194–195
Pain, postoperative pyrexia and, 27, 37
Pancreas, gastrin, 110–111, 127
Pancreatic malignancy, 358, 391

Pancreatic pseudocyst, 111, 128–129
Pancreatitis, 48, 111
    acute respiratory distress syndrome, 128
    burns management, 84, 98
    magnetic resonance
        cholangiopancreatography, 127–128
    Meckel's diverticulum, 140, 154–155
Papillary carcinoma, 342
Para-aortic lymph nodes, 235, 253
Paralysis, 205, 214
Paralytic ileus, bowel obstruction, 164,
    175–176
Paraphimosis, 247
Paresthesia, 205, 214
Parotid carcinoma, 310, 316
Parotid gland, 4, 11
    carcinoma of, 345
    pathology, 337
Parotid swelling, 310, 316
Patient-controlled opiate analgesia (PCA),
    20, 29
PCA, see Patient-controlled opiate analgesia
Pectineal ligament, 2, 9
Pectoralis minor, 262, 273
Pelvi-ureteric junction (PUJ), 239
Penile urethra, 241
Penis, carcinoma of, 253–254
Peptic ulcer disease, management of,
    359, 392
Percutaneous drainage, appendix mass, 136,
    146–147
Percutaneous gastrostomy tube, 45, 54
Perforated duodenal ulcer, abdominal
    emergency, 106, 118
Perform positional test, 307, 314
Perianal anatomy, 137, 147–148
Perianal disease, 360, 394
    diagnosis of, 136–137, 147
Perianal pathology, supralevator abscess,
    137, 148–149
Pericardiocentesis, chest trauma, 79–80, 90
Pericranium, 282, 289
Perineal urethra, 247
Perioperative glycaemic control, 26, 36
Perioperative steroid therapy, 21–22, 31
Peripheral access, 79, 89–90
Peripheral perfusion, 78, 87–88
Per-rectal bleeding, flexible sigmoidoscopy,
    133, 141
Peyronie's disease, 236, 254
Pfeiffer's disease, 340
Phimosis, 247
Photocoagulation, laser, 373
Phrenic nerve, left, 3, 10
Phyllodes tumour, 424
    breast enlargement, 186, 194
Pilonidal abscesses, 346
Pilonidal sinus, 360, 395
Pituitary disease, 286, 298–300
Placental alkaline phosphatase, 379, 423

Plain film radiograph, abdominal pain, 160, 169
Plantar ulcer, 204
Platelets, 60, 68–69
Pleomorphic adenoma, 337, 344–345
Polycystic kidney disease, 246
Popliteal aneurysms, 207, 218
Portosystemic anastomoses, 7, 15
Posterior cerebral artery, 282, 290–291
Posterior interosseous nerve, 8, 16
Posterolateral herniation, 293
Postoperative acute confusion, 57, 65
Postoperative analgesia, 20, 29
Postoperative breathlessness, 21, 30
Postoperative confusion, 24, 34
Postoperative fluid therapy, 40, 41, 47, 48
Postoperative pyrexia, 32
    abdominal CT scan, 27, 36–37
    anastomotic leakage, 22–23
    central line sepsis, 44–45, 53
    and pain, 37
    systemic inflammatory response syndrome, 25, 34–35
    systemic response to surgical trauma, 22
Postoperative wound dehiscence, 23, 32–33
Postsurgical patient, colloid replacement in, 42, 50
Postsynaptic acetylcholine receptor, 369, 409–410
Pregnancy
    intracranial haemorrhage, 83, 96
    trauma in, 358, 389–390
Preoperative assessment, 234, 248–249
Preoperative blood transfusion, 24, 34
Preoperative coagulation assessment, 25, 35
Preoperative starvation, 59, 67–68
Pre-prostatic urethra, 240
Presbycusis, 307, 313
Presurgical assessment, 28, 37–38
Primary angle closure glaucoma, *see* Acute closed angle glaucoma
Primary biliary cirrhosis, cholangiocarcinoma, 109, 124–125
Primary lymphoedema, 225
Primary survey, 77, 87
Progesterone receptor, 363, 398
Proliferative retinopathy, 373, 414–415
Prolonged ileus, 52
Prophylaxis, antibiotic, 162, 172
Propranolol, anal fissure, 138, 149
Prostate cancer, 237, 256
Prostate gland, anatomy of, 236, 254
Prostatic disease, 236–237, 255–256
Prostatic urethra, 240
Prostatitis, 245, 366, 404
Prothrombotic effect, 220
Proton pump inhibitor, oesophagitis, 105, 109, 116
Proximal femur, fractures of, 368, 407–408

Proximal leg vein ultrasound scan, 221
Proximal occlusion of left subclavian artery, 365, 401
Pseudofractures, 264
Pseudomembranous colitis, lower gastrointestinal infection, 167, 180
Pseudomonas aeruginosa, 306, 312–313
Psoas abscess, 361, 395
Psoas muscle, 229, 238, 239, 381
Ptosis, 327
PUJ, *see* Pelvi-ureteric junction
Pulmonary contusion, 77, 87
Pulmonary embolism, 62, 72
Purine metabolism, 278
    disorder of, 243
PVD
    diagnostic investigation for, 213
    effect of, 212–213
Pyelography, 242
Pyelonephritis, 244
Pyloric stenosis, 62, 72
Pyrexia, postoperative, *see* Postoperative pyrexia

Quadratus lumborum, 239

RA, *see* Rheumatoid arthritis
Radiculopathy, 265, 279
Ramsay-Hunt syndrome, 412
Rash, Paget's disease, 186, 194–195
Raynaud's syndrome, 210, 224–225
Rectal bleeding, diagnosis of, 161, 170–171
Rectum
    blood supply to, 8, 17
    colonic carcinoma, 139, 152
Rectus abdominis, abdominal wall anatomy, 138, 150
Recurrent laryngeal nerve, 3, 10–11
Red eye, 318, 325–326
Reiter's syndrome, 330
Renal cell carcinoma, 234, 249–250
Renal colic, 241
    abdominal pain, 166, 178–179
Renal stone disease, 230, 231
    calcium oxalate, 241
    mycobacteria, 242–243
    uric acid, 243
Renal tract
    anatomy of, 239
    stones, 241
Reproductive system, anatomy of, 230, 240
Respiratory alkalosis, 57–58, 66
Respiratory failure, 62, 72
Resuscitation of injured patient, 77, 86–87
Retinal detachment, 321, 329
Rhabdomyolysis, 233, 245–246
Rheumatoid arthritis (RA), 260, 269
    systemic manifestations of, 269–270

Rheumatoid disease, signs of, 272
Right atrium, 381, 427
Right iliac fossa mass, 361, 395
    ulcerative colitis, 138, 151
Right upper quadrant pain, 20–21, 30
    cholangitis, 162–163, 173
    ultrasound, 164, 176
RNA viruses, 337, 345

SAH, *see* Subarachnoid haemorrhage
Salivary gland swellings, 336–337, 344
Sarcoidosis, 414
Scalp, formation of, 289
Scarpa's fascia, 5, 11
Scleroderma, erythematous malar rash,
    104–105, 115
Sclerosants, 219
Scrotal exploration, 8, 17
Scrotal swellings, 365, 378, 379, 402–403,
    420–421, 423
Scrotum, ultrasound scan of, 366
Secondary sexual characteristics, 378,
    420–422
Seminoma, 235, 253
Sengstaken-Blakemore tube, 106, 117–118
Sensorineural deafness, left-sided, 307, 313
Sepsis, 62, 71–72
Septic arthritis, 265, 277–279
Serum amylase, acute pancreatitis, 104, 114
Serum magnesium, 356, 387
Serum potassium, causes of low, 248
Severe head injury, management of, 83, 96–97
Severe limb ischaemia, 205, 214
SFJ, 222
Shock, 78–79, 89
Shoulder
    anatomy of, 262, 273
    pathology, 262–263, 273–274
Sialogram, 337, 344
Sigmoidoscopy
    with flatus tube insertion, 135, 144
    flexible, 133, 141
Sigmoid volvulus, large bowel obstruction,
    167, 180
Silver nitrate cautery, 309, 315
Sjögren's syndrome, 345, 374, 415
Skin lesions, 377, 420
Skin lumps, 376–377, 418–420
Skull foramina, 7, 15
Smoking, cholelithiasis, 108, 122
Sodium, 366, 404
Soft tissue pathology, 261–262, 272
Sore throat, 307–309, 314, 315
Spermatic cord, 2, 9
    anatomy of, 376, 418
Spermatocele, 402
Sphenoid bone, lesser wing of, 282, 289
Spinal cord compression, 266, 279–280
Spinal cord injury, 265, 279, 371, 412–413
Spinal stenosis/claudication, 216

Spinal tap, *see* Lumbar puncture
Spine, anatomy of, 283, 292
Splenectomy
    atelectasis, 126
    tetanus, 110
Splenic trauma, explorative laparotomy,
    81, 93–94
Squamous cell carcinomas, 250
Squaring of thumb, 261, 272
Staghorn calculi, 242
Staphylococcus, 320, 328
Staphylococcus aureus, 265, 277–278
Starvation, preoperative, 59, 67–68
Status epilepticus, 297
Sternocleidomastoid, 7, 16
Steroids, high-dose, 323, 330
Steroid therapy, perioperative, 21–22, 31
Stomas, 134, 143
Stones, 241
Strangulated groin swelling, 339, 349
Subarachnoid haemorrhage (SAH), 411
Subarachnoid space, 283, 291
Subclavian steal syndrome, 365, 401
Subclavian vein cannulation, 381, 427
Subcutaneous nodules, 260, 268–269
Subdural haemorrhage, 285, 294–295
Subtotal thyroidectomy, 372, 414
Superficial thrombophlebitis, 365, 401–402
Superior gluteal, 259, 267
Superior mesenteric artery, 5, 13–14
Superior thyroid artery, 3, 10, 383, 428–429
Supracondylar fractures, 367, 406
Supralevator abscess, perianal pathology, 137,
    148–149
Supraspinatus, 262, 274
Supraspinous ligament, 283, 292
Surgical environment, health and safety in,
    22, 31
Surgical trauma, systemic response to, 22
Symptomatic carotid artery stenosis, 209,
    223
Syphilis, 260, 270
Systemic disease, 67
    and eye, 373, 414
Systemic inflammatory response syndrome,
    25, 34–35, 354, 385

Tachycardia, 357, 388
Temporal arteritis, 300
Temporal lobe epilepsy, 296
Tension pneumothorax, 58, 66
Testicular malignancy, 235, 252–253
Testicular pain, 159–160, 168–169, 378, 379,
    422–424
Testicular torsion, 378
Tetanus, splenectomy, 110, 126
Thoracic aorta, 6, 14–15, 381, 427
Thoracic nerve, 382, 428
Thyroglossal cyst, 334, 340, 371, 413, 415
Thyroid carcinoma, 335, 342

Thyroid disease, 335, 342–343, 371–372, 414
Thyroid eye disease, 374, 415
Thyroid gland, 3
  recurrent laryngeal nerve, 10–11
  superior thyroid artery, 10
Thyroid storm, 59, 68
Thyroid surgery, complications of,
  334–335, 341
Thyrotoxic crisis, *see* Thyroid storm
Thyrotoxicosis, 341
Tongue pathology, 372, 414
Total parenteral nutrition, 52–53
  central venous cannula, 56, 64
  commence, 44, 52
Toxic megacolon, 164, 175, 360, 393–394
Tracheostomy, insertion of, 7, 16
Transcoelomic spread, 363, 397–398
Transition zone, 237, 255–256
Transurethral resection of prostate
  (TURP), 404
Transversus abdominis, 239, 338, 346–347
Trauma, 283–284, 293
  in elderly patient, 358, 389
  and management, 77, 86
  patient, intravenous access in, 40, 47
Traumatic ulcers, 215
Trendelenburg's tourniquet test, 209, 222
Trigeminal neuralgia, 290
Triple phosphate stones, 241
Troisier's sign, 336, 343
Tumours
  carcinoid, 140, 155
  markers, 359, 391–392
  phyllodes, 186, 194
Tunica vaginalis, 230, 240
TURP, *see* Transurethral resection of prostate
Tympanic membrane, 306, 313

Ulceration, causes of, 212
Ulcerative colitis
  right iliac fossa mass, 138, 151
  surgery for, 360, 393–394
Ulnar paradox, 405
Ulnar tunnel, 367, 405–406
Ultrasound
  breast pathology, 188–189, 197, 199
  KUB, 242
  right upper quadrant pain, 164, 176
Ultrasound scan
  abdominal aortic aneurysm, 207, 218
  chest drain insertion, 80, 91–92
  of scrotum, 366, 403
Umbilical swelling, 376, 418
Upper gastrointestinal bleeding,
  gastroduodenal artery, 119
Upper gastrointestinal endoscopy, dysphagia,
  104, 113
Upper gastrointestinal haemorrhage, 107,
  119–120
Upper gastrointestinal surgery

hepatic duct, 110, 125
  postoperative care in, 354, 384–385
Upper limb nerve palsy, 367, 405–406
Upper limb pain, 365, 401–402
Urea-splitting organisms, 242
Ureteric constrictions, 380, 426
Ureters, 4, 12, 239
Urethral discharge, 232
Uric acid, 231, 243, 278
  stones, 241
Urinary calculi, investigation of, 230–231,
  241–242
Urinary catheterization, 77, 86–87
  acute urinary retention, 165, 176–177
Urinary retention
  bladder outflow obstruction, 164–165, 176
  urinary catheterisation, 165, 176–177
Urinary tract defence mechanisms, 243
Urinary tract infections (UTIs), 240
Urinary tract sepsis, delirium secondary to,
  24, 34
Urine alkalization, 246
Urine dipstick test, 231, 244
Urine output, 20, 29–30
  monitoring, 357, 387–388
Urological disease, 232, 245
  inherited, 233, 246–247
Urological emergencies, 365, 403
Urological infection, 231–232
  atrophic kidney, 244
  Escherichia coli, 243–244
Urological procedures, complications of,
  366, 404

Variceal bleeding, Sengstaken-Blakemore tube,
  106, 117–118
Varicella zoster corneal ulcer, 318, 325–326
Varicocele, 379, 403, 424
Varicose veins, 208, 209, 222, 364, 400
  surgery, 219–220
Vascular access in paediatric patients, 388
Vascular anatomy of gallbladder, 362,
  396–397
Vascular claudication, 213
Vascular supply of kidney, 239–240
Vasculitis, 287
Vas deferens, 240
Vasectomy, 240
Venous disease, 225
Venous embolism prophylaxis, 208
Venous hypertension, 214
Venous stasis, 220
Venous thromboembolism prophylaxis, 24,
  33–34
Venous ulcers, 206, 214–215
Ventilation, assessing, 78, 87–88
Vertebral artery, 291
Vesico-ureteric junction (VUJ), 239
Virchow's node, 343
Visual field deficit, investigation of, 323, 330

Vitamin A, 61, 71
Vitamin B_1 deficiency, abdominal surgery, 105,
    116–117
Volar displacement, 368, 406–407
Volvulus
    sigmoid, 167, 180
    sigmoidoscopy with flatus tube insertion,
        135, 144
Vomiting
    abdominal pain and, 160, 169–170
    and left upper quadrant pain, 165, 177
VUJ, *see* Vesico-ureteric junction

WAGR syndrome, 248
Warfarin, 220

Warmed peritoneal lavage, hypothermia,
    84–85, 100
Warthin's duct, 336, 344
Warthin's tumour, 345
Whipple's procedure, 125
Wilm's tumour, 234, 248
Wound dehiscence, postoperative, 23, 32–33

Xanthine oxidase, 278
    deficiency, 265, 278
Xanthine stones, 241
Xanthochromia, 370, 411–412

Zollinger-Ellison syndrome, 107, 120